Qualitative Research Methods in Mental Health

Maria Borcsa · Carla Willig
Editors

Qualitative Research Methods in Mental Health

Innovative and Collaborative Approaches

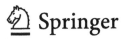 Springer

Editors
Maria Borcsa ⓘ
Institute of Social Medicine
Rehabilitation Sciences and Healthcare Research
University of Applied Sciences Nordhausen
Nordhausen, Germany

Carla Willig ⓘ
Department of Psychology
City, University of London
London, UK

ISBN 978-3-030-65330-9   ISBN 978-3-030-65331-6 (eBook)
https://doi.org/10.1007/978-3-030-65331-6

This Springer imprint is published by the registered company Springer Nature Switzerland AG
The registered company address is: Gewerbestrasse 11, 6330 Cham, Switzerland

Foreword

This book is very timely and much needed, and in this foreword, I will explain why I think so.

Mental health has finally come out of the shadows. There is an increasing understanding globally that mental health and well-being are not anymore in the margins of policies and human development. Mental health, as a new priority, appears now to be often the focus of policies relating to health, social welfare, education and other areas of societal life. Recently, there have been many high-level global, regional, and national decisions about the central role of mental health and well-being in shaping the future of societies. It is strange that the world had to wait so long to come to its conclusion about this importance, and now, we have the opportunity to reflect on what may have been behind such a long delay. In addition, the time has come to invest more in the promotion of mental health of individuals and societies, and to develop effective ways of prevention, support, care and recovery in the field of mental health.

There seems to be a broad consensus regarding this part of the new discourse about mental health as an emerging priority. This is, actually, an easier part of the discourse. However, when we move to the next issue, which is about how to invest and how not to invest in mental health, the global community, including experts, appears to be far from consensus. There is disagreement about how resources should be used, which interventions are effective, what kind of balance should we have between biomedical, psychological and social interventions, and whether coercion is justified in mental health care. The list of questions without clear answers, but to which there could be agreement, is very long.

I had the unique opportunity during the last 6 years to be in the center of this fascinating global discourse, with a huge variety of opinions, with passionate experts and entire organizations formulating and presenting their versions of truth, with quite dramatic interaction of science, practices, policies as well as power struggles. In 2014, I was appointed by the UN Human Rights Council as a UN Special rapporteur on the right to physical and mental health. This means that I became a mandate holder, and the rule of the game is that the Special rapporteur should keep informing the UN, the member states and other stakeholders about how the right to physical and mental health should be realized–and how it should not. Because mental health was already emerging as a new priority, because of the legacy of undermining the importance of mental health during previous decades, and because my own professional background is in mental health (I am a child and adolescent psychiatrist), I decided to make mental health a priority of my rapporteurship. Therefore, I started to explore the global situation and to work on my reports to the UN.

I have learned a lot from my previous work including insights produced from my critical analysis of the situation in the field of mental health in Central and Eastern Europe. In this region, the field of mental health has been and remains–for different historical reasons–affected by a legacy of stigma, discrimination, institutionalization and social exclusion. In addition, I have been observing for many years how ideology was influencing practices, but also outcomes of research. At that time when I was studying medicine and started to work as a young psychiatrist and researcher, mental health was used by the Soviet Union as one of the "battlefields" of the Cold War. It was of utmost importance for Soviet ideology to prove that mental health problems can be prevalent in the west, but not in the Soviet Union which, according to that ideology, have been eradicated by the political system. The researchers had to prove that in the country which was supposed to be on the way to building communism, social and psychological risk factors in the society do not exist anymore. Hence, mental disorders or mental health problems could emerge only in individuals who have biologically determined mental disorders. This is how schizophrenia and other diagnostic categories started to be misused, which lead finally even to the political abuse of psychiatry in that part of the world. This was one of the lessons I learned– that a lot of statistics and biased research can perfectly hide the real problems.

However, since 2014 my mandate was global, so I could not focus on just one region any longer. I needed to capture global challenges and opportunities.

I was traveling to many countries, meeting representatives of governments, mental health professionals, users and ex-users of mental health services. I was attending numerous meetings and visiting a large number of mental health facilities. Based on consultations, site visits and collected information I prepared several reports to the UN. This was my duty—the Special rapporteur prepares and presents thematic reports to the UN Human Rights Council (HRC) and to the General Assembly.

One of these reports—the report which I presented to the UN HRC in June 2017, sparked so many responses, and these responses were characterized by such a broad spectrum of views–ranging from extremely positive to extremely negative–that it could be interesting for someone to explore these responses as something very unique and meaningful "food for thought".

How it could happen that one group of experts, well known in the world of mental health research and mental health policy, decides that the main messages of the report of the UN Special rapporteur are correct and should be taken up by governments, while the other group of experts, who are also prominent researchers and advisers for politicians, conclude that this report should be disqualified and that its main messages are wrong and misleading?

The huge polarization, which was revealed through responses to the report, is a reflection of long-standing tensions with regard to the status quo in global mental health and to the way, the global community should proceed.

While many organizations and experts supported the main messages of the report, one group of experts and organizations that did not agree with those messages, was mainly representing the professional group of psychiatry.

This was not a surprise. My assessment of the current situation in global mentalhealth was very clear about this status quo being unacceptable. I questioned the central statement of the movement for globalmental health, which was about the "heavy burden of mental disorders" and the main goal of investments that need to be increased, which is to address the treatment gap. One of my conclusions was that the main problem is not the burden of mental disorders, but the burden of obstacles for the realization of the right to mental health. Three main obstacles that I have identified were reflecting the dominance of the neurobiological model during the last four decades in mental health care and psychiatry. One obstacle was the obvious overuse of the biomedical model and biomedical interventions (mainly treatment with psychotropic medications) dominating mental health care practices. Another obstacle was huge power asymmetries—especially between service providers and services users in mental health care, but also between psychiatrists and other mental healthcare workers. The third obstacle was biased use of knowledge and evidence in mental health care, resulting in informing everyone that, for example, depression is about chemical imbalances in the brain.

Is this all about denouncing or demonizing the medical model in the field of mental health? No, I think that the medical model and psychotropic medications do have their role in providing care and support to people with mental health needs. The problem I was raising was about overuse and misuse of some interventions, and about a human rights-based approach being undermined by the dominant idea that first of all mental disorders should be fixed by doctors, voluntarily or by force, and only then dignity and human rights can be exercised.

The dominance of the biomedical model and biomedical interventions is based, as we know, on research. Here we approach the main theme of the foreword— why qualitative research is so much needed. The reason is that one more important imbalance was created by the excessive reliance and overuse of quantitative research. As it appears now, findings of that research have been strongly influenced by the pharmaceutical industry, and have failed to keep to its promises. We know, and I have elaborated on this issue in other reports (such as my report on corruption and right to health), that large numbers of findings of research that were informing the stakeholders have been biased. Medications may have their role in the management of mental health conditions. However, evidence about their effectiveness has been biased, and for many years, patients, doctors and politicians have been receiving misleading information about what could be the most effective way to manage mental health conditions.

To restore the balance in research and in informing the general public, politicians and medical doctors, good qualitative research is very much needed. It is becoming evident nowadays, that mental health is strongly about the context. It is about relationships, diversities, power issues, effects of discrimination, inequalities and violence. It is about the emotional and psychosocial environment in which we live. This environment can and should be healthy, rich in supportive and respectful relationships.

Unfortunately, quite often this environment can also be toxic and contaminated with hatred, mistrust, violence, xeno-, homo- and all other kinds of phobia. Largely, mental health depends on these contextual and social factors, which can be investigated with social sciences and qualitative methods. Behind the phenomenon that nowadays is called depression–considered one of the most prevalent health conditions-power imbalances might be more important factors, than so-called chemical imbalances which are still presented in medical textbooks as targets for the management of depression.

Sadly, during recent decades, the context of the societal fabric was largely ignored, and we should understand that this was because of focusing excessively on the brain and on the dominance of the reductionist idea that neurosciences will eventually provide a cure for mental health conditions. The attempt to present mental health care as a classical field of medicine, with a desperate search for a "cure of mental diseases" has failed. Behind this failure stood mainly the fact that research on societal and contextual issues was undermined and was considered not as important as research on brain.

There is still a long way to go for this systemic error to be corrected. Despite increasing evidence that essential changes in mental health policies and services are needed, the lion's share of mental health budgets in most countries of the world continues to be allocated to cover expenses of psychotropic medications, psychiatric hospitals and long-term care institutions. The expert opinions of persons with lived experience (users and ex-users of mental health services), and non-medical mental health professionals are often ignored or undermined. According to existing "unwritten rules" shaped by decades of the status quo, psychiatrists are the experts as they are medical doctors and this is why they know more and better. Interestingly, among psychiatrists there is an increasing variety of views as well. However, as a consequence of decades of dominance of the biomedical-neurobiological model, the power in decision making belongs to those professionals who hold the view that psychiatry is a field of biomedicine and that it should continue to be so.

This is not a black-and-white matter. However, we should agree that the time has come for another paradigmatic shift in globalmental health. This is how the field of mental health is developing; we know from history that mental health care and psychiatry has been marked by shifts of paradigm. On the one hand, each such shift was bringing some improvement to the lives and human rights of people who had mental health conditions and mental health needs. On the other hand, the pendulum was often moving to the other extreme, and after some time a critical mass of evidence was in place that something has gone wrong (again), and that change is needed (again). There has been a continuous search of optimal balance within the bio-psycho-social model, to avoid moving too far either to "mindless brain" or to "brainless mind". So now, in the 20s of the twenty-first century, we have quite a lot of evidence to identify harmful imbalances and asymmetries in the global mentalhealth scene and to move to vitally important changes. These changes need to be guided by evidence, which includes outcomes of social sciences and qualitative research, and by fully embracing a human rights based approach which has been undermined so far by the status quo in global mentalhealth.

To conclude this foreword, let me share some suggestions which might inspire researchers to contribute even more than before, with a combination of qualitative and quantitative research, to the development of effective and human rights-based mental health care and support services.

Analysis of power issues and the heavy reliance on involuntary (forced) measures in mental health care could shed more light on how to abandon this legacy of paternalism, coercion and disempowerment of users of mental health services. Analysis of issues related to relationships, diversities, indivisibility of human rights, therapeutic alliance and trust could provide creative solutions to how the mental health of society and individuals, including those with mental health challenges, could be effectively promoted.

While the tradition of investing in quantitative research, focusing on assessment of global burden of mental disorders, is still quite strong, in order to establish a better balance more qualitative research is needed to critically address the categorical approach of diagnosing mental health conditions and the excessive focus on targeting individuals and their brains with biomedical interventions. Protective factors and how to invest in resilience should be explored, so that we do not excessively rely on highlighting risk factors.

Given that there is quite a lot of evidence regarding the crisis of biological psychiatry and the neurobiological paradigm, the importance of modern social psychiatry is increasing. Here, research is needed to pave the way for effective practices that could be free from coercion and respectful of the human rights of persons with mental health needs, including persons with psychosocial, intellectual and cognitive disabilities.

Suicide should be investigated as a form of (self-directed) violence and as a public health issue, and more research in this direction could be helpful to balance reductionist biomedical explanation of depression and suicide. The impact of adverse childhood experiences on physical and mental health should become a central theme of modern health research all over the world.

With regard to stigma, there is still quite a strong myth that persons with mental health conditions and psychosocial disabilities are dangerous to "normal society". We need more concerted efforts, with research and advocacy, to address this kind of "common sense error" based on a legacy of stigma and discrimination. I would suggest the hypothesis, that it is first of all the so called "normal society" that may be dangerous to groups in vulnerable situations, but also to itself, with all these prejudices, fears and myths that work as self-fulfilling prophecies and are reinforced by outdated mental health systems.

One of the important meetings I had was a meeting in 2019 with leaders of German psychiatry. This meeting took place in Berlin, in Luisenstrasse, famous for many important events and discoveries in the history of medicine. Among monuments to famous researchers, not that far from each other, I had the pleasure to symbolically meet and pay tribute to two people who contributed with their discoveries and insights to two equally important sides of medicine and health care. They were Robert Koch and Rudolf Virchow. Robert Koch discovered specific causative agents for several infectious diseases and thus contributed to the successes of biomedicine. Rudolf

Virchow reminded, and continues to remind us, never to forget that medicine is a social science. It is very important to nurture the fragile balance within these two significant parts of science and practice—so that the global community is effective and successful in protecting physical and mental health of everyone.

August 2020

Dainius Pūras
Former UN Special Rapporteur on the right to health (2014–2020)
Professor, Clinic of Psychiatry, Vilnius University
Vilnius, Lithuania

Contents

Editors and Contributors

Angela Abela is a Professor and founding Head of the Department of Family Studies at the University of Malta where she teaches and supervises clinical psychology, and family therapy trainees. She is also a registered clinical psychologist, family therapist and a systemic supervisor. Angela has acted as a consultant for Parliament and the Maltese government on family affairs and is lead author of the Strategic Policy on Positive Parenting for Malta. She now sits on the Task Force mandated with its implementation. Angela has served as an expert for the Council of Europe in the area of children and families for many years. She has published widely and her research projects include studies on marital satisfaction, couple conflict and family violence, families living in poverty, families where one of the members faces mental illness, lone parent families, parenting, and children in out-of-home care. In 2014, she was lead editor for *Contemporary Issues in Family Studies: Global Perspectives on Partnerships, Parenting and Support in a Changing World* by Wiley-Blackwell and in 2020 for *Couple Relationships in a Global Context: Understanding Love and Intimacy Across Cultures* by Springer. She co authored *Intervening After Violence, Therapy for Couples and Families* with Springer (2017). She is an international advisory editor of *Contemporary Family Therapy, Children Australia* and other journals. In 2021 she is lead chair for the qualitative research conference on mental health (QRMH8).

Rebecca Aloneftis is as a Counselling Psychologist at Hertfordshire Partnership University NHS Foundation Trust (HPFT) in Adult Community Mental Health Services, currently in a specialist Early Intervention in Psychosis Service. Her research interests are predominantly focused on psychosis and qualitative methodology. She has published on the role of embodiment in third wave mindfulness-based cognitive therapies, and on negotiating the voice hearing identity. She is currently researching the use of mobile app technology for Treatment Resistant Obsessive Compulsive Disorders and Body Dysmorphic Disorder (BDD) at HPFT in collaboration with the University of Cambridge.

Felice Bisogni is a clinical psychologists, specialist in psychoanalytic psychoterapy, Ph.D. in Social Psychology and founder member of GAP, an association based in Rome (Italy) that provides action-research services for the organizational development and the staff training on behalf of organizations of the National Health System, schools and third sector organizations.

Maria Borcsa, Ph.D., is Professor of Clinical Psychology at the University of Applied Sciences in Nordhausen (UASN), Germany, licensed psychological psychotherapist (CBT), family therapist, trainer and supervisor and founding member of the Institute of Social Medicine, Rehabilitation Sciences and Healthcare Research at UASN.

She is the editor (with M. Ochs and J. Schweitzer) of '*Systemic Research in Individual, Couple, and Family Therapy and Counseling*' (2020, Springer Int.), (with P. Rober) of '*Research Perspectives in Couple Therapy. Discursive Qualitative Methods*' (2016, Springer Int.) and (with P. Stratton) of '*Origins and Originality in Family Therapy and Systemic Practice*' (2016, Springer Int.). She is member of the Editorial Board of the journals *Testing, Psychometrics, Methodology in Applied Psychology* and *Contemporary Family Therapy*, advisory editor of *Family Process*, international associate editor of the *Journal of Family Therapy*, associate editor of *Encyclopedia of Couple and Family Therapy*, and founding editor of the *EFTA Family Therapy Book Series* (Springer Int.).

She has published research papers, books and book chapters in the domain of family therapy and systemic practice also in German, French, Spanish, Italian and Greek. She has been board member of the European Family Therapy Association (EFTA) (2007–2016) and President of EFTA from 2013 to 2016.

She was awarded for her 'Excellence in the Research Field of Family Therapy and Systemic Practice' from the European Family Therapy Association in 2019.

Fiorella Bucci Psy.D, is a clinical psychologist and psychotherapist, lecturer at the School of Specialisation in Psychoanalytic Psychotherapy of SPS (Rome, Italy). Her doctoral research at Ghent University focuses on Emotional Textual Analysis, the roots of this method in psychoanalytic theory and its usage as a tool for psychosocial research and intervention. The culture of mental health care in Italy and Japan has been a main subject of her past research and publications.

Julianna Challenor is Director of Studies (Research) and Co-Director for the Doctorate in Counselling Psychology and Psychotherapy by Professional Studies at Metanoia Institute in London. She teaches, researches and publishes in the fields of counselling psychology, qualitative research methods, psychotherapy and mental health. She is particularly interested in working with critical and social constructionist research approaches together with pluralistic or integrative methods, as well as psychoanalytically informed case study approaches. She is a member of the conference organising committee for Qualitative Research in Mental Health (QRMH). She has published in journals such as *European Journal of Psychotherapy and Counselling, Journal of Health Psychology, Health* (UK) and *Psychodynamic Practice*.

She is a chartered psychologist with the British Psychological Society and HCPC registered Counselling Psychologist in the UK, and has over 12 years' experience practising in NHS, educational and private clinical settings.

Helena Curran is a Trainee Counselling Psychologist nearing the end of her doctorate at City, University of London, UK. She has a research interest in women's health, the body and the intersection of physical and psychological health, and has worked clinically in various NHS, charity and private settings. She contributed as an Honorary Research Assistant to the Tavistock Adult Depression Study. She has a Masters in the History of Design from the Royal College of Art and the V&A Museum, and was awarded the Thames and Hudson Prize for her work exploring the psychological intention and effect of objects designed with a connection to pain in either a healing or harming capacity—namely surgery and corporal punishment in the seventeenth century.

Nobuhle "Dedani" Dlodlo is a Counselling Psychologist, registered in the UK with the Health and Care Professionals Council. She holds a Masters in Psychology from University of East London, and focused her postgraduate Masters research on creativity and recovery in postmodern society. She also holds a Counselling Psychology Doctoral qualification awarded by City, University of London. Her doctoral thesis explored the role of psychologists in employability enhancement and vocational rehabilitation efforts that target individuals at risk of social exclusion. Dedani is particularly interested in research focusing on the intersection of mental health challenges, social integration and creative arts. As a psychological professional, Dedani has worked in the NHS and with statutory services to offer psychological support to children, families and adults experiencing mild to severe psychological difficulties. She is currently working with Children Looked After by London Borough Sutton Local Authority. Dedani has a personal interest in social justice, writing and storytelling. She has collaborated with ZimHealth (Zimbabwe Network for Health in Europe) to promote awareness about mental health in Zimbabwe, her home country, and has shared a stage with artists like Oliver Mtukudzi to perform spoken word pieces about mental health in Zimbabwe.

Francesca Dolcetti clinical psychologist and psychotherapist; lecturer at the School of Specialization in Psychoanalytic Psychotherapy of SPS (Rome, Italy), where she teaches Emotional Textual Analysis models and techniques. CEO of the Studio RisorseObiettiviStrumenti that provides services for supporting transformation of organisational cultural models in contexts such as health and educational services, and in the field of social economy.

Eugenie Georgaca is Associate Professor in Clinical Psychology at the School of Psychology of the Aristotle University of Thessaloniki, Greece. She teaches, researches and publishes in the fields of clinical psychology, psychotherapy and mental health, especially community mental health and critical perspectives on psychopathology. She is interested in using discursive, dialogical and biographical narrative ideas to examine the construction, experience and management of mental distress, as well as of psychotherapy process. She has published in international journals, including *Journal of Constructivist Psychology, Feminism & Psychology, Journal of Mental Health, Mental Health & Prevention, Psychosis, Qualitative Research in Psychology*. She has served as associate editor of the *International Journal of Dialogical Science* and is a member of the editorial board of international journals. She is co-chair of the 1st Conference of the Association of European Qualitative Researchers in Psychology (EQuiP), to be held in Thessaloniki in 2021, and has co-chaired the 5th and 6th Qualitative Research in Mental Health (QRMH) conferences in 2014 and 2016. She has served as coordinator of the Clinical Psychology Section of the Hellenic Psychological Society and is currently serving on the Society Board as Treasurer.

Dewi Hannon, M.Sc., graduated in 2018 from Ghent University, Belgium, in clinical psychology, where she also contributed to the Single Case Archive as a student assistant. Afterwards, she worked as scientific researcher at the department of Experimental Clinical and Health Psychology, where she was involved in various European projects such as MentALLY and ACCOMPLISSH. She is currently working as a clinical psychologist at a mental health care center in Ostend.

Dr. Kirsi Heimonen is an artist-scholar in the field of artistic research. In the research project Engraved in the Body. Finnish people's memories from mental hospital, she focuses on the corporeal method, and attunes to the affective atmospheres that the memories entail producing articles and works of art. Her other research interests include slowness, the silence of corporeality and the connection between experience and language. She is currently acting as a Senior Researcher at the Center for Artistic Research (CfAR) at the University of the Arts Helsinki, Finland.

Saara Jäntti, Ph.D., is a Senior Researcher in the Department of Language and Communication Studies at the University of Jyväskylä, Finland. She is the PI of the Engraved in the Body. Finnish people's memories from mental hospital research project. She has a background in English and literary studies. Her current research interests include psychiatric cultures, representations and narratives of mental ill-health and, especially, the culturally and historically shifting notions of mental distress and their relation to spatialities and materialities of belonging. Her other previous and on-going research projects explore these through arts-based methods, especially applied drama.

Bernadetta Janusz, Ph.D., is Assistant Professor at the Jagiellonian University, Medical College, Family Therapy and Psychosomatics Department, Kraków, Poland, clinical psychologist, ethnologist, licensed psychotherapist in systemic and psychodynamic approach, psychotherapy trainer. She is a co-editor of the scientific journal "Psychoterapia" (since 2018), member of the Editorial Board of the "Frontiers of Psychology: Psychology for Clinical Settings". Her research interests focus on grieving, psychotherapy research, personality disorders, and on the anthropological concept of rituals. She is interested in applying qualitative methodologies to clinical settings (Conversation Analysis, Linguistic Approach to Grounded Theory).

Saskia Jünger is a professor for health research methods at the Department of Community Health (DoCH), University of Applied Health Sciences, Bochum (Germany). She is a health scientist with expertise as a research associate and a psychologist in the field of psychosomatics, palliative care, and general practice. During her Ph.D. in health research at Lancaster University (UK), she has examined the role of consensus building and scientific knowledge production in healthcare. Her particular interests comprise questions related to mental health, and a sociology of knowledge approach to health and disease.

Penelope Kinney NZROT, Ph.D., is the Head, Occupational Therapy, College of Health, Otago Polytechnic, Dunedin, New Zealand. Penelope's Ph.D. explored how clients psychologically adapt to living in the community after spending significant time within forensic psychiatric hospitals. She utilised walking interviews as a data collection method in this research. Her other research interests include the transition process, forensic mental health and ethical research.

Juri Krivzov, M.Sc., M.Res., is Ph.D. candidate at the Department of Psychoanalysis and Clinical Consulting at Ghent University, Belgium. He graduated from Radboud University and Leiden University in clinical psychology and worked afterwards at a specialized psychosomatic unit in Fliedner Hospital in Ratingen, Germany. Currently, he works on the Single Case Archive project and pursues his Ph.D. on interpersonal functioning and therapeutic relationships in patients with Medically Unexplained Symptoms.

Sari Kuuva, Ph.D., is a scholar in art history and cognitive science in the Department of Music, Art and Culture Studies at the University of Jyväskylä, Finland. Her earlier investigations have focused particularly on the cultural aspects of emotions. Kuuva has also been interested in the relationship between emotions, pictures and corporeal knowledge. In the research project Finnish people's memories from mental hospital Kuuva has investigated corporeal knowledge in photographs of mental hospitals and the emotional experiences of the children of mental hospital personnel. Key emotions in her analysis have been nostalgia, melancholia, fear, feelings of security, topophobia, topophilia and empathy.

Mariya Lorke is a research associate at the Cologne Center for Ethics, Rights, Economics, and Social Sciences of Health (ceres), University of Cologne. She is an ethnologist and social anthropologist with experiences in field work, qualitative research, education and training. Currently she works on a dissertation in the field of health sciences examining the concepts of health at risk and health literacy from an ethnological perspective.

Karoliina Maanmieli holds a Ph.D. in creative writing. She is also a poetry therapy instructor and practical psychiatric nurse and is working in the Department of Music, Art and Culture Studies at the University of Jyväskylä, Finland. For the past three years she has engaged with the mental hospital memories in Finnish people's memories from mental hospital and now coordinates an Erasmus + -project "HEROINES: Empowerment of Women with Mental Illness Living in Rural Areas through Writing Therapy". She has twelve years of experience as a poetry therapy instructor and trainer. Her Ph.D. thesis (2015) dealt with poetry therapy as a rehabilitation tool for psychoses.

Giulia Marchetti is a specialist in psychoanalytic psychotherapy and a clinical psychologist. She has worked as a psychologist in several organizational contexts in the fields of healthcare, education, business (goods and services production) and public administration. Since 2017, she collaborates with the Association GAP in research and reporting activities using the ETA methodology.

Reitske Meganck, Ph.D., is associate professor at the Department of Psychoanalysis and Clinical Consulting at Ghent University, Belgium. She completed her Ph.D. on validity of alexithymia measures in 2009. She is one of the originators of the Single Case Archive and the Ghent Psychotherapy Study—an RCT with emphasis on mixed methods studies. Next to her research activities, she is also a supervisor, a postdoctoral psychotherapy trainer, and a psychotherapist in private practice, working from Freudian-Lacanian perspective.

Rosa Maria Paniccia is Associate Professor at Sapienza University of Rome and member of the scientific and teaching board of the School of Specialisation in Psychoanalytic Psychotherapy of SPS (Rome, Italy). Editor of Rivista di Psicologia Clinica. Author of more than 100 publications. Her scientific work currently focuses on how the prevelance of a medicalized and diagnostic culture in many sectors of social life is broadening phenomena of marginalization of low-power groups.

Stefano Pirrotta is a clinical psychologists, specialist in psychoanalytic psychoterapy and founder member of GAP, an association based in Rome (Italy) that provides action-research services for the organizational development and the staff training on behalf of organizations of the National Health System, schools and third sector organizations.

Anu Rissanen is a Ph.D.-student in the Department of History and Ethnology at the University of Jyväskylä, Finland and member of the Finnish people's memories from mental hospital research group. Her research interests include the history of medicine and psychiatry, particularly in the twentieth century, and she takes special interest in researching and challenging the notions of normality, abnormality, otherness and inequality in relation to broad social issues such as citizenship and institutions and at the level of everyday life.

Katia Romelli, Ph.D., MSc Psychotherapy, Trained in Lacanian psychoanalysis. Department of Maternal & Infant Health, ASST Valle Olona Hospital, Busto Arsizio (Italy), AGAPE Social Cooperative, Treviglio (Italy). She investigates the discursive construction of subjectivity in the mental health domain. Critical psychology perspective, with peculiar references to Critical Discourse Analysis and Lacanian Discourse Analysis, drives her research.

Janice Sargent holds a first class (honours) degree in Psychology and obtained an MPsy in Counselling Psychology with distinction from the University of Malta. She works as a practitioner in counselling psychology at Richmond Foundation, a mental health NGO in Malta. Previously having worked as a mental health recovery officer within the same foundation, she became interested in the impact of the mental health system and the society's view of mental illness on the well-being of those diagnosed with mental illness. Currently, she is taking part in the planning of a psychosis anti-stigma campaign. She also runs a support group for individuals diagnosed with psychosis and is also interested in conducting qualitative research in this area.

Sebastian Schröer-Werner, Ph.D., is Professor of Social Work with focus on methods of Empirical Social Research and as of April 2020 President of the Protestant University Berlin, Germany. He is a licensed Dipl. Social Worker / Certified Social Pedagogue (FH). Since 2018 he has been one of the speakers of a section on promoting doctorates in the German Association of Social Work (DGSA). As former visiting professor at the University of Applied Sciences Nordhausen (UASN), Germany, he was a founding member of the Institute of Social Medicine, Rehabilitation Sciences and Healthcare Research. Scientific interests: social change and resilience, post-traditional communities, grounded theory.

Carolin Schwegler is a postdoctoral researcher in applied linguistics at the Institute for German Studies at the University of Koblenz-Landau (Koblenz) and a research fellow at ceres, University of Cologne. Her research interests are conversation and discourse analysis, language in (predictive) medicine and in the field of sustainability. For her doctoral thesis in German linguistics at the University of Heidelberg and McGill University Montreal, she received a scholarship from the German Federal Environmental Foundation (DBU) and the German Academic Exchange Service (DAAD).

Carla Willig, Ph.D., is Professor of Psychology at City, University of London, UK. She is also a Chartered Health Psychologist and a registered Counselling Psychologist in private practice. She is an associate editor of the *Journal of Health Psychology*, a member of the editorial board of *Qualitative Research in Psychology*, and a member of the International Advisory Board of the *Journal of Psychological Therapies.*

A major theme in her work to date has been a concern with research methodology. She has published empirical and theoretical papers and book chapters concerned with epistemological and methodological questions. She is the editor of *'Applied Discourse Analysis. Social and Psychological Interventions'* (1999) published by

Open University Press and the author of the best-selling textbook *'Introducing Qualitative Research in Psychology. Adventures in Theory and Method'* (2001, 2008, 2013, Open University Press), a fourth edition of which is due to be published in 2021 (McGraw Hill/ Open University Press). She is the editor (with Wendy Stainton-Rogers) of the *'The SAGE Handbook of Qualitative Research in Psychology'*, first published in 2008, with a second edition in 2017, and the author of *'Qualitative Interpretation and Analysis in Psychology'* (2012, McGraw Hill/ Open University Press) which is concerned with the theoretical, practical and ethical challenges associated with the use of interpretation in qualitative research.

She was awarded the British Psychological Society's Qualitative Methods in Psychology Section's 'Lifetime Achievement and Contribution to Qualitative Methods' researcher prize in 2019.

Chapter 1
Introduction: Qualitative Research in Mental Health—Innovation and Collaboration

Maria Borcsa, Carla Willig, and Sebastian Schröer-Werner

Abstract This introductory chapter explicates the conceptual background of the volume. It describes the tradition of the Qualitative Research in Mental Health (QRMH) conferences and illuminates the transdisciplinary field of mental health as well as the current discourse of mental health as global challenge. Innovative elements of the book chapters are pointed out and related to main features of qualitative research in general and in mental health research specifically, like power issues and ethical considerations, the meaningfulness of process research and naturalistic settings, how to accumulate knowledge by doing metasynthesis and how research can become an intervention. Finally, the chapter gives an outline of the book's structure.

Keywords QRMH conferences · Global mental health · Qualitative research · Metasynthesis · Naturalistic setting · Transdisciplinarity · Power · Ethics

> *Good mental health is related to mental and psychological well-being. WHO's work to improve the mental health of individuals and society at large includes the promotion of mental well-being, the prevention of mental disorders, the protection of human rights and the care of people affected by mental disorders.* (WHO, October 2019)

Introduction

There is broad agreement in contemporary scientific discourse that the topic and focus of any research project determines the methodology used. If amounts, frequencies,

M. Borcsa (✉)
Institute of Social Medicine, Rehabilitation Sciences and Healthcare
Research, University of Applied Sciences Nordhausen, Nordhausen, Germany
e-mail: borcsa@hs-nordhausen.de

C. Willig
Department of Psychology, City, University of London, London, UK
e-mail: C.Willig@city.ac.uk

S. Schröer-Werner
Protestant University, Berlin, Germany
e-mail: schroeer@eh-berlin.de

© Springer Nature Switzerland AG 2021
M. Borcsa and C. Willig (eds.), *Qualitative Research Methods in Mental Health*,
https://doi.org/10.1007/978-3-030-65331-6_1

1

and statistical relationships are of interest, quantitative methods are the methods of choice. However, if research focuses on structures of meaning, patterns of action, and associated processes, then the only option is to choose qualitative methods. In this context, traditional quality criteria of research derived from natural sciences like objectivity, validity, and reliability play a subordinate role. For qualitative research, instead, it is essential to define criteria linked to the respective research questions (see Flick, 2014; Strauss & Corbin, 1998; Strübing, Hirschauer, Ayaß, Krähnke, & Scheffer, 2018). Polemic discussions between scientists about what is "true" science should be a footnote of history (Kromrey, 2005). Nevertheless, it seems still important to emphasize the advantages and potentials of qualitative approaches in the field of social and health sciences (see e.g., Loewenthal & Avdi, 2018).

Classical approaches of qualitative research are often related to language and text, for example by conducting and analyzing interviews. In recent years, we witness two so-called turns: (1) a corporeal/body turn and (2) a visual turn. First, more attention is paid to the body as one particular field of research, as a theory category (e.g., within the context of conceptions of identity), as well as a tool to acquire knowledge about an area of research (Giardina & Donnelly, 2018; Gugutzer, 2006). Second, the importance and relevance of visual data is supported by an increasing significance of media in everyday life (Banks, 2001; Pauwels, 2000); Mey and Dietrich (2016), for example, transferred considerations and procedures of grounded theory onto visual data. In this book, Saara Jäntti, Kirsi Heimonen, Sari Kuuva, Karoliina Maanmieli, and Anu Rissanen present their research on Finnish people's memories from mental hospitals; one of their foci is the body, in which experiences are metaphorically "engraved" (see Chap. 10). Another project, introduced by Penelope Kinney (Chap. 4), describes the method of "walking interviews". Here as well, the body can be seen as a central tool of data collection and source of knowledge at the same time. Following the second development, Julianna Challenor, Eugenie Georgaca, Rebecca Aloneftis, Helena Curran, and Nobuhle Dlodlo (Chap. 6) present, besides other studies, a visual discourse analysis of childbirth images posted by postnatal women on Instagram. The example of giving birth as one primary affective lived experience shows that some realities "cannot or ought not to be reduced to discourse" (p. 107 in this book).

Nevertheless, in many other chapters of this book, the importance of word-based analysis is highlighted, reminding us that much meaning is communicated by language in social life, and this includes the construction of meaning around mental health.

The Tradition of Qualitative Research in Mental Health (QRMH) Conferences

Hosted by the Protestant University Berlin, Germany, the seventh Qualitative Research on Mental Health conference (QRMH7) took place in September 2018.

These biennial conferences[1] have grown from a modest beginning some fourteen years ago, being organized by a network of researchers. The 1st and 2nd Qualitative Research on Mental Health conferences were held 2006 and 2008 in Tampere, Finland, the 3rd and 4th followed 2010 and 2012 in Nottingham, UK, and the 5th and 6th in 2014 and 2016 in Chania, Greece. Successive events have attracted steadily growing international interest, both by novices as well as by experienced researchers. Contributors have come from a diversity of backgrounds: health and social care professionals, social scientists and health policy makers, mental health service users, and others, creating a space for lively and enriching discussions.

The QRMH conferences have developed in response to the wide acknowledgment that a fuller understanding of mental health difficulties, their origins, and their treatment entails a comprehensive range of epistemologies and research methodologies. As mentioned, qualitative methods offer essential insight into highly relevant mental health related topics, such as relationship issues, power, social exclusion, and other social phenomena, which quantitative approaches are typically not able to deliver. Therefore, they are an important complement to biomedical models and research methodologies, which can be considered as mainstream in mental health research these days. We agree with del Rio Carral and Tseliou (2019, p. 332) that "collective efforts are needed internationally to increase the participation of qualitative researchers" in a wide range of research areas, one of special importance being mental health themes. This awareness has been the motivation to engage in editing this book.

The Transdisciplinary Field of Mental Health

In this book, and in line with the tradition of the QRMH conferences, mental health is referred to as a field of phenomena that requires multiperspectivity and a transdisciplinary stance to grasp the diversity of aspects contained in this concept. Moreover, even if health legislations (still) follow national policies, a field has been established within public health which tries to transcend national perspectives, "one that aimed to improve treatments, increase access to services, and reduce human rights abuses of people experiencing mental disorders" (Cohen, Patel, & Minas, 2014, p. 3). This global mental health approach grounds in the consensus, that neither pure biological, nor pure cultural processes are able to fully explain mental health conditions. We follow the above-mentioned premises, seeing mental health in a socio-ecological framework (Petersen, Barry, Lund, & Bhana, 2014), resulting from *intrapersonal* (genetic make-up, physical health, cognitions, emotions, skills, and behavior), *proximal* (interpersonal and immediate factors related to family, peer, school, and community), and *distal factors* (culture and policies, e.g., economic and environmental policies—representing national and the global level in terms of macrostructural factors).

---

[1]Due to the COVID-19 pandemic, QRMH8 was postponed to 2021.

According to Rutz (2001, cited in Coskun, 2017, p. 17), "the type of mental health services offered and how mentally ill people are treated and integrated into society is one of the most sensitive indicators of the level of democracy, pluralism, and tolerance in a society." Starting from clients or patients and their concrete interaction with professionals, we have to incorporate mental health services in their intersectionality into our considerations (Wahlström, 2017). Moreover, we have to be aware of the influence of societal discourses regarding mental health and illness on individuals and social systems. These different phenomenological levels require a diversity of research approaches as "the context of where research is carried out, by whom, for what reason(s), from what position, with what aims, and in what manner are some of the, many, factors that affect its quality and usefulness" (Loewenthal & Avdi, 2017, p. 2).

Cultural and social practices co-construct how people understand mental health, be it as "service user," "service provider," or "decision-maker" (Coskun, 2017). Subsequently, research in this field has to be considered as cultural and social practice, too (Loewenthal & Avdi, 2017; Wahlström, 2017), providing the researcher(s) with responsibility and a certain amount of power. Self-reflexivity, which is essential in qualitative research, goes hand in hand with an emancipatory attitude, trying to enrich the social discourses on mental health with wisdom "from within" and "bottom-up," instead of "top-down," in its double sense: theory-driven as well as hierarchical.

Besides clarifications from a methodological standpoint, this task requires adequate methods with regard to the respective levels of analysis. That is why, among others, psychological, sociological, historical and linguistic disciplines, with their respective qualitative research approaches and specificities are needed to embrace the empirical complexity. Most often, this multiperspectivity cannot be achieved by one researcher alone, but needs collaboration. Chaps. 6–10 in Part II of this book illustrate how fruitful it can be to cooperate in studying one phenomenon, in its best case transcending disciplinary boundaries.

Mental Health as a Global Challenge

"*Globally, it is estimated, that only 7% of health budgets are allocated to address mental health difficulties. Most investment is focused on long-term institutional care and psychiatric hospitals, resulting in a near total policy failure to promote mental health holistically for all. (…) Public policies continue to neglect the importance of the preconditions of poor mental health, such as violence, disempowerment, social exclusion and isolation and the breakdown of communities, systemic socioeconomic disadvantage and harmful conditions at work and in schools.(…) For any mental health system to be compliant with the right to health, the biomedical and psychosocial models and interventions must be appropriately balanced, avoiding the arbitrary assumption that biomedical interventions are more effective.*" (United Nations, Human Rights Council; Report of the Special Rapporteur Dainius Puras, March 2017, p. 3ff)

The right to mental health as a universal right is a regulating idea according to Kant, as humankind might never reach this aim. As with all regulating ideas of humanity, the challenge is not to surrender in front of the task, but to the contrary, to show perseverance in approaching this goal. In this context, Di Nicola (2019) refers to a "slow psychiatry"; from his point of view, a redefined social psychiatry is needed, which is phenomenological (instead of technocratic), is emic (experience-near), creates thick descriptions, is heuristic (instead of developing algorithms), accumulates knowledge (instead of emphasizing the pragmatic impact), focuses on comprehension (instead on mastery), and which is methodologically pluralistic. His position is clear: "The vaunted biopsychosocial (BPS) approach, offering an integration of three domains, became a convenient cover for psychopharmacology and neuroscience research to appear inclusive, yet in practice, as DSM-IV chairman Allen Frances later observed, BPS became "bio-bio-bio"." (ibid., p. 9). Also Janice Sargent and Angela Abela (Chap. 2) point out that "psychiatric diagnosis do not explain aetiology, prognosis and treatment but merely classify them" (p. 19 in this book). By asking research questions like "Where do psychiatrists locate themselves on the continuum between the biology-only perception of schizophrenia and its recovery and the biopsychosocial perspective of the disorder and its recovery?" and "how are such perceptions in turn manifested in their clinical practice?" (p. 20), we can trace psychiatrists' habitus and their influence on their professional work, as done in Sargent and Abela's research on the island of Malta. As shown in their study, "despite all participants holding a medical view of schizophrenia, those who focused more on the disease and its medical treatment as opposed to viewing the person as a whole and incorporate diverse interventions, appeared to develop a more pessimistic view of recovery in schizophrenia" (p. 28). Obviously, as mental health treatment is always provided through interaction (even if it is merely medication), a more pessimistic view is in danger of creating negative effects on the therapeutic relationship and consequently, on the patient himself/herself. However, we also need to widen the perspective: "The mental health system in which psychiatrists operate seems to greatly influence their decisions when it comes to treating individuals diagnosed with schizophrenia. Although the mental health act (2012) states that treatment should primarily take place in the community, the participants [of the study; i.e. psychiatrists] claimed that community support is lacking, (….) and the mental health system in Malta is still hospital-based" (p. 29). This is confirmed by the number of beds in psychiatric hospitals.[2] At the same time, multidisciplinary teams and a structure of community treatment are lacking. Taken these factors together, we see that even if some of the psychiatrists wished to adopt a different, less trauma-inducing and more recovery-oriented treatment, they might fail due to the deficiency of resources. Here, there is no other option than to change the system of intervention from medical to political.

---

[2]Malta having 185 per 100,000 inhabitants while the European average lays by 72 (ibid.).

Giving Voice—The Inside and Outside

What it means to be a "service user" shows itself in different ways, depending on whether it relates to one's own experience, an experience we witness or an experience accessed second or third-hand—researchers are mostly in the latter position. As Carla Willig states, "suffering is not a passive state but a project in which the person is actively engaged" (p. 98 in this book). How can we approach this suffering in an ethically appropriate way? In her chapter, Penelope Kinney presents a participant-focused data collection method, which is compatible with different epistemological backgrounds; here, in the center of attention is not the researcher with his/her (scientific) worldview, but the subject of inquiry. Kinney learned as an occupational therapist within forensic psychiatric services, that "living with major mental illness often affects a person's ability to hold spontaneous conversation" (p. 65). Researching this specific group of patients, she reflects: "A person may sit passively during traditional qualitative talking interviews, waiting for guidance on how to answer questions. I looked to find if there was another option that would allow the client participants to engage in a way that was familiar to them, and would not put undue pressure on them to speak continuously. I came across the walking interview." This description shows, how the researcher tries to adapt her method of inquiry to the group and the topic she wants to study—"walking alongside a participant in a familiar environment the researcher can gain insight into a sense of alienation or connection the participant has with their community. Because the researcher is observing the participant while also interviewing them, it is possible to gather information about how the mental health client interacts with both their physical and social environment" (p. 80). By connecting oneself with the usual environment of the interviewee, the researcher might get an idea and a feeling from "inside," how this situation affects the everyday life of the interviewed person. That means of course exposing oneself to the researched world, becoming ethnographic, for grasping the researched topic in a more complete, both rational and sensual way—at least to a certain extent.

A special mode of doing ethnography, i.e., autoethnography, is constructing a position of being both object and subject of the research, as done by Carla Willig in this book (Chap. 5). Her research aim is "to shed light on the lived experience of cancer in contemporary Western culture" to "understand the nature and quality of the distress that can be generated by a cancer diagnosis" (p. 84). She points out, that "subjective experience is, at least in part, mediated and shaped by available discursive resources" and the active engagement with these resources is a way to create meaning for this experience (ibid.). This is also the starting point of the above-mentioned study by Challenor et al. (Chap. 6) named "Listening to what is not said." The authors exchange the foreground with the background: using different discourse analytic approaches, they are concerned with "in whose interest it might be that certain discourses or discursive repertoires are *not* heard" (p. 105, italics by M.B.) and "what function is served by the absence of alternative ways of speaking, thinking and doing" (p. 106). This creates an extraordinary position of the respective research, as the analysis not only gives voice to the researched (be it oneself or someone else) but shows also, that adopted discourses are always only *one* option of making sense of one's experience. Other, alternative discourses are marginalized or even excluded and these exclusions follow certain functions: the not-listened-to becomes a self-disciplining not-said, thus stabilizing existing power structures.

Power Issues and Ethical Considerations

Mariya Lorke, Carolin Schwegler, and Saskia Jünger show and explain in Chap. 7, how differently people make sense of being confronted with health risks; what does it mean to "be at risk" for a person, either to develop dementia (in their chapter: study 1) or psychosis (study 2)? The authors state: the "probabilistic form of medical risk factors leaves the individual unclear concerning their relative effect, and without certainty about the future. Notwithstanding this, the 'power of definition' with respect to health risks predominantly lies with professionals, i.e. scientists or health professionals, implying that there is one appropriate way of understanding and interpreting risk-related information, and transforming it into health-promoting behaviour" (p. 137 in this book).

As mentioned, reflexivity is a central concept and tool in qualitative research. Seeing research itself as social practice, qualitative research is usually more concerned with power issues than traditional quantitative approaches following a biomedical perspective. In addition to the analysis of the research interviews from both studies, Chap. 7 also presents ethical considerations around how to do research with vulnerable groups; intervision might be a format of choice to keep reflection on the research process ongoing, with positive outcomes both for the researched individuals and for the research goal.

Accumulating Knowledge

Two chapters in this book (Chaps. 3 and 5) use and explain their work with meta-synthesis of existing qualitative research, "Due to its commitment to a detailed exploration of meanings, qualitative research tends to use data from relatively small numbers of participants. This means that it can be difficult to draw wider conclusions from an individual piece of research. Metasynthesis is a methodology that provides us with an opportunity to integrate findings from several qualitative studies to produce a conceptually more robust account of the meaning and significance of an experiential phenomenon than would have been possible on the basis of a single qualitative study alone" (Willig, p. 96 in this book). Krivzov et al. explicate: "While being comparable with the better-known quantitative meta-analysis, metasynthesis can and should go beyond the mere question of treatment efficacy, which is often the focus of quantitative meta-analysis. Instead, metasynthesis can address more complex process-related questions" (p. 38). In their chapter, Juri Krivzov, Dewi Hannon, and Reitske Meganck refer to the Single Case Archive (www.singlecasearchive.com), an online database bringing together over 3000 psychotherapy case studies, collected by an international team of researchers (for more information see Chap. 3). This database is a unique opportunity for conducting metasyntheses, especially on process themes, as case studies have the advantage of reporting on therapy processes in naturalistic settings. Krivzov et al. invite us to witness sophisticated methodological innovations like the creation of timelines of therapeutic events.

Understanding Systems on Different Levels and Feeding Knowledge Back

The concrete interaction between the so-called service users and practitioners might be the level of concern in discursive research; we can frame the construction of this interactional arrangement as the therapeutic system in a narrower sense (see Chap. 8). As mentioned above, process research in naturalistic settings requires innovative methods. In their study on systemic couple therapies, Borcsa and Janusz implement Interpersonal Process Recall, also known as Stimulated Recall Interviews. "IPR/SRI has been developed as a method of reviewing a video recording to recall thoughts and feelings that occurred during the time of the recording. Hence, with regard to psychotherapy research, IPR as an interview approach was designed to access a therapy participant's experiences as close as possible to the moment of the original interaction" (p. 172 in this book). The aim of the presented analysis is to study the mutual dynamic between the couple therapists' references to their professional practice and to their personal experiences during the interview. To achieve this aim, two methodological approaches are employed: dialogical analysis to investigate the distinction between the therapist's professional and personal selves, and the narrative storytelling approach in order to describe the therapist's positioning in terms of his or her discursive identities being displayed in the IPR/SR interview.

The concrete interaction between any service user and professional is at all times embedded in an institutional situation. Fiorella Bucci, Rosa Maria Paniccia, Felice Bisogni, Stefano Pirrotta, Francesca Romana Dolcetti, Giulia Marchetti, and Katia Romelli make us acquainted with Emotional Textual Analysis (ETA). Chapter 9 describes ETA as a psychoanalytically informed method of text and discourse analysis, "to enable psychological research and intervention with social groups, institutions and organizations" (p. 201), aiming at researching the culture of the institution in question (in the authors' first study being a school, in the second study a healthcare organization providing services for adult disability). Focusing on emotions expressed in language, ETA states that they are a fundamental organizer of relationships, i.e., also in the relationship between clients and practitioners. The chapter transcends the structure of this book in two ways: ETA understands itself explicitly as an intervention-research tool, informing concrete training activities with staff as well as clients. Further, it is a mixed-method, as statistics are used in a second step of analysis (for further details, see Chap. 9).

Jäntti et al. (Chap. 10) draw our attention to the socio-historical aspects of mental health, giving us insight into Finnish psychiatric practice from 1930 onwards, which at that time was heavily based on psychiatric hospitals and institutionalization. The multidisciplinary research group comprising of a language and communication scientist, an art historian and cognitive scientist, an artist-researcher, a poetry therapy instructor and psychiatric nurse as well as two academics in history and ethnology, investigated how experiences in mental asylums are remembered today, analyzing writings by patients, relatives, personnel, and their children. This work gives us an extraordinary insight into the fruitfulness of a multidisciplinary approach, an approach which furthermore becomes interventive by creating artistic events and discussions with the audience following their research.

All this research sheds light on the social construction of mental health phenomena on the micro-interactional and macro-institutional level and makes us aware that historical change is possible and needed, locally and globally.

The Book Structure

The book structure follows the two main formats, which were included at the QRMH7 conference: individual presentations on the one hand and symposia on the other. All chapters refer to concrete research questions and present their respective results.

Part I of this book is dedicated to specific research studies, submitted as individual papers to the conference—they mirror different levels of academic work, some originating in Master theses, others conducted by Ph.D. candidates, yet others by experienced academics. Some of the chapters deriving from these presentations are more focused on data collection; others put their emphasis more on data analysis (for a detailed methodological reflection on the chapters of this book, see concluding Chap. 11).

The chapters in Part II are resulting from symposia where researchers had united beforehand for a larger cooperative research project, working on these projects in their respective home countries like Lorke et al. in Germany (Chap. 7) or Bucci et al. in Italy (Chap. 9) or Jäntti et al. in Finland (Chap. 10). Another group of papers has their commonalities in using similar research methods or methodologies, but in different studies: Challenor et al. (Chap. 6) present three different studies with the unifying feature of using discourse analytic approaches. Maria Borcsa has been working with Stimulated Recall Interviews in a couple therapy research project in Germany, while independently, Bernadetta Janusz has been using the same method in couple therapy research in Poland. In Chap. 8, they join their perspectives.

Recent individual, collaborative, or institutional endeavors mirror an increasing interest in studying mental health phenomena from more than one perspective and furthermore, bringing together existing qualitative research, as is done in metasynthesis. In view of that, the chapters in Part II of this book demonstrate clearly, how the combination of more than one methodological perspective can enrich data collection and analysis.

Hence, the uniqueness of this book is that it explicates innovative qualitative research methods, i.e., in terms of both data collection and analysis, and at the same time increases our insight into the mental health field by presenting the results of respective studies from different countries. Overall, the studies originate from Belgium, Finland, Germany, Italy, Malta, New Zealand, Poland, and the United Kingdom, raising our awareness of the mental health field within diverse cultural and discursive, organizational and institutional as well as legislative contexts. Each study is grounded in a defined epistemology; the area of interest informs the chosen methodological approach. Following the tradition of qualitative research as an intervention in science and society by giving voice to minorities like vulnerable populations, most chapters seek to promote social justice and empowerment. The position of the researcher in the research is reflected on and is mirrored also in the style in which the chapter is written (e.g., from an I-perspective); we as editors have promoted this diversity and refrained from requesting standardization.

References

Banks, M. (2001). *Visual methods in social research.* London: Sage.

Cohen, A., Patel, V., & Minas, H. (2014). A brief history of global mental health. In V. Patel, H. Minas, A. Cohen, & M. J. Prince (Eds.), *Global mental health: Principles and practice* (pp. 3–26). Oxford, UK: Oxford University Press.

Coskun, B. (2017). Mental health priorities around the world. In Bährer-Kohler, S. & Carod-Artal, F.J. (Eds) *Global mental health: Prevention and promotion* (p. 9–20). Cham, CH: Springer International.

Di Nicola, V. (2019). "A person is a person through other persons": A social psychiatry manifesto for the 21st century. *World Social Psychiatry, 1,* 8–21. https://doi.org/10.4103/WSP.WSP_11_19.

Flick, U. (2014). *An introduction to qualitative research* (5th ed., pp. 479–507). Thousand Oaks: Sage.

Giardina, M. D., & Donnelly, M. K. (Eds.). (2018). *Physical culture, ethnography and the body: Theory, method and praxis.* London: Routledge.

Gugutzer, R. (2006). *Body turn: Perspektiven der Soziologie des Körpers und des Sports.* Bielefeld: transcript Verlag.

Kromrey, H. (2005) *"Qualitativ" versus "quantitativ"—Ideologie oder Realität?* Symposium „Qualitative und quantitative Methoden in der Sozialforschung: Differenz und/oder Einheit?" auf dem 1. Berliner Methodentreffen. Online: http://www.berliner-methodentreffen.de/archiv/texte/texte_2005/kromrey.pdf.

Loewenthal, D., & Avdi, Evrinomy. (2017). Is research in psychotherapy and counselling a waste of time? *European Journal of Psychotherapy & Counselling, 19*(1), 1–5. https://doi.org/10.1080/13642537.2017.1291078.

Loewenthal, D., & Avdi, E. (2018). *Developments in qualitative psychotherapy research.* London: Routledge.

Mey, G., & Dietrich, M. (2016). From text to image—Shaping a visual grounded theory methodology. In: *Forum Qualitative Sozialforschung/Forum: Qualitative Social Research*, 17(2), Art. 2, Online: http://dx.doi.org/10.17169/fqs-17.2.2535.

Pauwels, L. (2000). Taking the visual turn in research and scholarly communication: Key issues in developing a more visually literate (social) science. *Visual Studies, 15*(1), 7–14.

Petersen, I., Barry, M., Lund, C., & Bhana, A. (2014). Mental health promotion and the prevention of mental disorders. In V. Patel, H. Minas, A. Cohen, & M. J. Prince (Eds.), *Global mental health: Principles and practice* (pp. 224–251). Oxford: Oxford University Press.

del Rio Carral, M., & Tseliou, E. (2019). Mapping qualitative research in psychology across Europe: Contemporary trends. *Qualitative Research in Psychology, 16*(3), 325–335. https://doi.org/10.1080/14780887.2019.1605276.

Strauss, A., & Corbin, J. (1998). *Basics of qualitative research: Techniques and procedures for developing grounded theory* (2nd ed.). Thousand Oaks: Sage.

Strübing, J., Hirschauer, S., Ayaß, R., Krähnke, U., & Scheffer, T. (2018). Gütekriterien qualitativer Sozialforschung. *Ein Diskussionsanstoß. Zeitschrift für Soziologie, 47*(2), 83–100.

United Nations, Human Rights Council. (2017). Report of the Special Rapporteur on the right of everyone to the enjoyment of the highest attainable standard of physical and mental health. https://ap.ohchr.org/documents/dpage_e.aspx?si=A/HRC/35/21. Retrieved 26 January 2021.

Wahlström, J. (2017). The researcher in the field: Some notes on qualitative research in mental health. *European Journal of Psychotherapy & Counselling, 19*(1), 97–109.

World Health Organization (WHO). (2019). Retrieved 22 April 2020. https://www.who.int/news-room/facts-in-pictures/detail/mental-health.

Part I
Illustrating Innovation in Qualitative Mental Health Research

Chapter 2
Psychiatrists' Perceptions
of Schizophrenia and Its Recovery:
A Thematic Analysis

Janice Sargent and Angela Abela

Abstract Through the lenses of critical realism and contextualism, this study is about how psychiatrists perceive schizophrenia and its recovery. Semi-structured interviews with six participants were conducted and analysed using thematic analysis. The findings were organized into four overarching themes: the psychiatrists' perceptions of schizophrenia; ways of working with individuals with schizophrenia; the relational aspect of working with individuals with schizophrenia; and psychiatrists' perceptions of recovery. All participants viewed schizophrenia as an illness with biological basis and based their diagnosis largely on clinical experience. Medication was seen as occupying a central role in treatment. Complete recovery was defined as being asymptomatic and being able to function without the use of medication; however, living in the community on medication was also seen as a form of recovery. Only one psychiatrist defined recovery according to the recovery model, viewing individuals as a whole with the potential of living a meaningful life despite having schizophrenia. The study concludes that psychiatrists' perceptions of schizophrenia and its recovery are influenced by a mental health system which is largely hospital-based and lacks adequate community support and are reflected in the way psychiatrists interact with the patient and the treatment decisions they take on the journey of recovery.

Keywords Psychiatrist · Schizophrenia · Recovery model · Mental health · Thematic analysis

J. Sargent (✉) · A. Abela
University of Malta, Msida, Malta
e-mail: Janice.Sargent.10@um.edu.mt

A. Abela
e-mail: Angela.abela@um.edu.mt

© Springer Nature Switzerland AG 2021
M. Borcsa and C. Willig (eds.), *Qualitative Research Methods in Mental Health*,
https://doi.org/10.1007/978-3-030-65331-6_2

Introduction

Schizophrenia is and is not a thing in the world. (Luhrmann, 2016, p. 1)

In a sentence, the above quote captures the complexity involved in defining schizophrenia which in a way has guided the conceptual framework of this study. Schizophrenia is a thing in the world in that "there certainly is a real and terrible disorder, the most devastating of all the psychiatric illnesses, that at its most severe has clearly recognizable features and is found in nearly every corner of the world" (Luhrmann, 2016, p. 1). However, at the same time, the true meaning of schizophrenia as a diagnosis and a disease seems to be quite difficult to capture. Given that the sense we make as professionals can have "major consequences in people's lives" (Geekie, Randal, Lampshire, & Read, 2012, p. 2), this situation calls for further research into the area, especially with regard to the diagnosis and the view of recovery by psychiatrists who are primarily involved in the diagnosis and treatment of schizophrenia.Qualitative research that looks into these perceptions would be best suited to capture their viewpoints. Such research is even more pertinent in the context of the current gap in the literature. To our knowledge, no recent qualitative research has been carried out on both psychiatrists' perceptions of schizophrenia and its recovery while keeping in mind the professional's medical training and work experience, as well as, the current mental health system in which they operate. This chapter will attempt to demonstrate what contextualist thematic analysis guided by contextualism and critical realism can achieve by using the topic of this study as an example.

The topic of schizophrenia has captured the interest of the first author ever since, as an adolescent, she was told that her grandmother, whom she had never met, had this diagnosis. Stories of men in white coming for her grandmother and taking her to the asylum in a white van in spite of her resistance instilled in the author a sense of curiosity and unease. Later on as a mental health recovery officer working for a local mental health NGO, the first author met Sebastian, the first client who carried the same diagnosis as her grandmother. Sebastian challenged her perceptions and made her question the nature of schizophrenia in the light of the treatment available and the local mental health system. In her work as a clinical psychologist, the second author also struggled at times with the diagnoses and the treatment on offer.

The Complexity Involved in Capturing Schizophrenia

The latest version of the ICD-11 *Classification of Mental and Behavioural Disorders* (ICD-11; WHO, 2018) marked a number of changes in the diagnosis of schizophrenia from the ICD-10 (WHO, 1992). Through these changes, the diagnosis of schizophrenia in the latest version of the ICD-11 became more similar to the diagnosis of schizophrenia in the fifth edition of the *Diagnostic and Statistical Manual of*

Mental Disorders (DSM-5, APA, 2013) which requires the presence of two or more of delusions, hallucinations, disorganized speech, grossly disorganized behaviour and negative symptoms, one of which must be any one of the first three symptoms. While both classification systems view particular symptoms as being more clinically significant and that cognitive impairment might also be present, they also note that this disorder has no pathognomonic symptoms and is highly heterogeneous, not only in symptom presentation, but also in duration and course of illness (Jablensky, 2013). However, the ICD and the DSM disagree in terms of duration of illness and functional disability. Highlighting the changes between revisions and drawing out the differences between the two major classification systems draws one's attention to the continuously changing nature of the meaning we attribute to schizophrenia.

Moreover, one cannot help but further question the validity of the diagnosis of schizophrenia when one considers that there seem to be phenomenological, biological and genetic overlaps between schizophrenia and autism spectrum disorder (e.g., Kincaid, Doris, Shannon, & Mulholland, 2017; McCarthy et al., 2009; Toal et al., 2009), and schizophrenia, bipolar disorder and schizoaffective disorder (e.g., Cosgrove & Suppes, 2013; Hamm et al., 2014; Keshavan, Nasrallah, & Tandon, 2011).

The perception of schizophrenia as a "progressive brain disease" (van Haren, Cahn, Pol, & Kahn, 2008), which appears to be gaining momentum within the psychiatric community (e.g., Lieberman & First, 2007; Miller, 2015; Naidoo, 2015), seeks to root the disorder in biology. Firstly, brain imaging studies have found clear differences in brain abnormalities between those who experienced their first episode of psychosis and those diagnosed with chronic schizophrenia (Ellison-Wright, Glahn, Laird, Thelen, & Bullmore, 2008; Meyer-Lindenberg, 2010; Shepherd, Laurens, Matheson, Carr, & Green, 2012). However, while abnormalities in certain brain regions at the early stages of psychosis are thought to have a genetic component, abnormalities found in other regions as the illness progresses are argued to be a result of medication (Ellison-Wright et al., 2008). Moreover, it must be said that these differences are only moderate and to a certain extent, are also found in controls (Meyer-Lindenberg, 2010). Secondly, functional studies have found that information is processed differently in persons with first-episode psychosis and schizophrenia, particularly in the domains of attention, memory, executive functioning, and emotion regulation (Aleman & Kahn, 2005; Callicott et al., 2000); however, these can in part be attributed to ongoing psychotic symptoms, early-onset and long-term institutionalization (Tamminga & Medoff, 2000). Lastly, genetic factors are said to contribute greatly to the aetiology of schizophrenia (e.g., APA, 2013). Recently, a genome-wide association study (GWAS; Schizophrenia Working Group of the Psychiatric Genomics Consortium, 2014) found 108 distinct loci involving around 350 genes which are thought to be implicated in the risk of developing schizophrenia, yet the specific variants of these loci which carry inherited risk are still to be identified (Need & Goldstein, 2014).

Although schizophrenia nowadays seems to belong to the realm of medicine, not all psychiatrists construct its meaning in the same way. The way psychiatrists perceive schizophrenia appears to be dependent on personal prejudices and clinical experiences, as well as, the culture in which the psychiatrist lives and its prevalent classification system (Cape, Antebi, Standen, & Glazebrook, 1994; van Os, Galdos, Lewis, Bourgeois, & Mann, 1993). There appears to be some disagreement when it comes to the usefulness of diagnosis, the classification of schizophrenia as a unitary disorder and the aetiology of schizophrenia. Although most psychiatrists tend to agree with the use of medication in treatment (Cape et al., 1994; Jorm, Korten, Jacomb, Christensen, & Henderson, 1999), the psychiatrist's belief about the aetiology of schizophrenia seems to impact the degree to which psychosocial interventions are used and the duration of medical treatment prescribed (Cape et al., 1994). This shows how psychiatrists' perceptions of schizophrenia impact treatment, and therefore, recovery.

Competing Viewpoints on the Recovery of Schizophrenia

A scientific, objective definition of recovery in schizophrenia generally relies on the subsidence of symptoms and return to psychosocial functioning (Bellack, 2006). That is, full recovery in schizophrenia is said to require the absence or reduction of symptoms to a point where they no longer meet the criteria for diagnosis alongside the return to functioning in terms of social activity and part or full-time employment or education (e.g., Harrow, Grossman, Jobe, & Herbener, 2005; Liberman, Kopelowicz, Ventura, & Gutkind, 2002; Torgalsbøen & Rund, 2002). By such definitions, recovery from schizophrenia was found to be rare (Torgalsbøen & Rund, 2002), with as few as one in seven experiencing full recovery in terms of symptom reduction and social functioning (Jääskeläinen et al., 2012).

First-hand accounts by service user-activists paint a more optimistic picture of recovery claiming that recovery in schizophrenia is quite a common occurrence (Bellack, 2006). Although such accounts have been criticized for lacking representation and on the basis that the majority of those making up the movement consist of service users who have had negative experiences of the mental health system and tend to be motivated by anger (Wallcraft, Read, & Sweeney, 2003), they do highlight that objective definitions based on the disease model of schizophrenia largely ignore the subjective experience of the individual (Davidson, Schmutte, Dinzeo, & Andres-Hyman, 2007).

What seems to be of consensus now is that the definition of recovery in the context of schizophrenia needs to incorporate both objective and subjective terms (Lysaker, Ringer, Maxwell, McGuire, & Lecomte, 2010). A systematic review of the literature on service users' perspective on recovery in schizophrenia shows that for them recovery is viewed as an outcome achieved only when medication is stopped; however, while being symptom-free is considered significant, understanding the illness and learning how to live with its aftermath is also seen to be a central part of recovery (Jose, Lalitha, Gandhi, & Desai, 2015). In addition, recovery is also seen by service users as a continuous battle and a gradual, nonlinear process towards building a meaningful life despite having schizophrenia. This is reflected in the position adopted by the American Psychiatric Association (2005) which encourages mental health professionals to build collaborative therapeutic relationships, restore hope and quality of life, as well as managing symptoms and supporting the reintegration of the service user within society.

Psychiatrists are more likely to adhere to the medical model of recovery in schizophrenia while service users tend to embrace the recovery-oriented approach (Zipursky & Agid, 2015) more willingly. However, some studies show that although psychiatrists tend to believe that recovery is only achieved when medication no longer needs to be prescribed, they also consider the patient's ability to live independently, engage in self-care and return to normal psychosocial functioning as being part of recovery. In saying this, only around 20% factor in subjective experiences such as regaining self-esteem as part of service users' process of recovery (Färdig, Lewander, Fredriksson, & Melin, 2011; Ng, Pearson, Chen, & Law, 2010; Tsang & Chen, 2007).

Mental health professionals including medical students, trainee psychiatrists and clinicians were found to hold a more pessimistic outlook on the possibility of recovery than patients (Gorwood et al., 2013; Ng et al., 2010; Noiseux & Ricard, 2008; Tsang & Chen, 2007), especially when positive symptoms were present (Klapheck, Lincoln, & Bock, 2014). Low expectations serve as a barrier to recovery (Liberman & Kopelowicz, 2002), and in itself, this viewpoint increases the stigma (Schlosberg, 1993), another barrier to recovery (British Psychological Society [BPS], 2013; Ng et al., 2010). This disagreement between patient and professional can cause difficulties within the therapeutic relationship because clients do not act on treatment goals which they do not perceive as important (Zipursky & Agid, 2015), which can in turn re-affirm the psychiatrist's belief that the possibility of recovery is minimal. This is problematic because psychiatrists give less importance to "patients who have a bad prognosis, who are chronic with relapses and where treatment is ineffective" (Schlosberg, 1993, p. 413).

In *Understanding Psychosis and Schizophrenia* (British Psychological Society [BPS], 2014), it is argued that, unlike medical diagnoses, psychiatric diagnoses do not explain aetiology, prognosis and treatment but merely classify them. Moreover, viewing psychosis as a symptom of schizophrenia stops the attempt to try and understand it further (Bracken & Thomas, 2005) and the use of medical language to refer to individuals' reactive experiences to overwhelming events gives the message that "people can do little to overcome their problems except to 'keep taking the tablets'" (BPS, 2014, p. 26). In discouraging the individual from taking an active role in the recovery process, the psychiatrist becomes the holder of expert knowledge, shifting the power within the therapeutic alliance away from the patient (Foucault & Gordon, 1980) and giving the message that "it is good to defer to medical authorities who know best" (Breeding, 2008, p. 490). This report has been criticized for downplaying the seriousness of schizophrenia and the suffering it causes patients and their relatives and for implying that the use of medication in the treatment of schizophrenia is not necessary (Carroll, 2015; Pierre, 2015; Pies, 2016). From this perspective, this notion can be dangerous especially when one considers that anti-psychotic medication was found to be more effective than placebo in preventing relapse and hospitalization, and improving quality of life (Leucht et al., 2012) and is considered to be the single-most consistent protective factor against the increased risk of suicide in those diagnosed with the disorder (Hor & Taylor, 2010).

The Research Questions

This study aims to address the research gap mentioned further above by asking a two-sided research question. First, in a context where the shift towards a recovery-oriented approach is being emphasized, where do psychiatrists locate themselves on the continuum between the biology-only perception of schizophrenia and its recovery and the biopsychosocial perspective of the disorder and its recovery? Second, how are such perceptions in turn manifested in their clinical practice?

Methodology

Epistemological Orientation

Before going further into the methodology for exploring the research questions, it is a must that the epistemological orientation of this study is made explicit as it is through the epistemological underpinnings that the questions "how, and what, can we know?" (Willig, 2013, p. 39) can be answered.

As shown in the introductory section, while a real and impactful disorder which seems to be found all over the world (Luhrmann, 2016, p. 1), an element of subjectivity seems to exist when attempting to capture the meaning of schizophrenia. Simultaneously, this study has also been influenced by Foucault's contention that the perception of madness as mental illness was born as a product of its time and culture (Foucault, 1972/2006). Taken together, this conceptual framework mirrors the epistemological underpinnings of this study; that is, on a continuum between naive realism and radical relativism, the orientation adopted in this research lies somewhere in between critical realism and contextualism.

Critical realism posits that although an ultimate reality exists, it can only be captured through the researcher's interpretation of the participants' explanation of their reality (Willig, 2013). That this study attempts to capture as truthfully as possible the meaning psychiatrists ascribe to schizophrenia and its recovery suggests that such perceptions do exist in reality. In this way, a realist position is adopted whereby "the role of the researcher in this situation is akin to that of a detective who uses his or her skills, knowledge and experience in order to uncover what is really going on" (p. 69). However, as opposed to the naive (direct) realist approach, which supposes that there is a direct relationship between what is said by participants and reality, a critical realist stance presumes that for the researcher to truly uncover reality, the underlying structures which support the participants' words must be uncovered (Willig, 2013).

As such, critical realism "combines the realist ambition to gain a better understanding of what is 'really' going on in the world with the acknowledgement that the data the researcher gathers may not provide direct access to this reality" (p. 60).

However, the interpretation of the meaning psychiatrists give to schizophrenia and its recovery does not sufficiently meet the conceptual framework of this study. Adopting only a critical realist stance on its own does not consider that the concept of mental illness is a constantly changing phenomenon dependent on time and culture. Therefore, to truly account for the underlying structures that lie beneath the meaning psychiatrists give to schizophrenia and its recovery, one must also consider that the meanings given themselves are dynamic and contextual. In essence therefore, the data gathered in this study must also be interpreted through a contextualist lens.

Contextualism is based on the idea that reality is constantly changing and that the meaning participants make must be considered in the light of the socio-historical and cultural context they find themselves in (Jaeger & Rosnow, 1988). Contextualism emphasizes that knowledge is relative because it only exists in relation to the context in which it is created and incomplete because the context itself is constantly transforming (Jaeger & Rosnow, 1988). The researcher, from a contextualist perspective, is viewed as a co-creator of the social context of human events within the wider system of time and culture (Jaeger & Rosnow, 1988). Contextualism, therefore, is "particularly concerned with the relationship between accounts and the situations in which they were produced" making it essential for the researcher to be mindful of his or her part in co-creating the context in which the knowledge is generated and cultural assumptions that are shared (Madill, Jordan, & Shirley, 2000, p. 10).

With regard to this study, this involves the awareness that both researchers and participants have experience of working with individuals with schizophrenia and are located within a hierarchical mental system which is currently in its initial phases of shifting towards a more recovery-oriented approach. Psychiatrists, who locally find themselves at the top of the hierarchical system, are asked, in an interview setting with a student of psychology and past mental health recovery officer, to relay information about the meaning they give to schizophrenia and its recovery. This could influence the way knowledge and assumptions are shared with the interviewer. However, although initially a sense of intimidation was created in the interviewer prior to the interviews, the power imbalance was not particularly experienced during the interviews.

The Research Design

The interview. Given that the aim of this study is to carry out an in-depth exploration of psychiatrists' perceptions of schizophrenia and its recovery, a semi-structured interview was chosen as the most suitable tool of data collection. This method of data collection is flexible, accessible, and allows for the collection of rich and detailed data (Braun & Clarke, 2013). Although an interview guide was created for the purpose of this study, its questions were not strictly adhered to during the interviews (refer to Appendix A). The place of the interview varied in accordance with the participants' availabilities and preference and was conducted over four weeks in May 2017 whereby each interview lasted approximately 40–50 min. Before each interview, the participants were asked to read the participant information sheet and to sign a consent form.

Participant recruitment and ethical considerations. Given the small size of the project and the small number of psychiatrists in Malta, only six participants were recruited for the purpose of this study. According to Braun and Clarke (2013), this number is sufficient to create a rich and detailed account of the social phenomenon under investigation. Following approval by the University Research Ethics Committee, permission was granted by the health department's clinical chairman of psychiatry to conduct the interviews. Twenty potential participants who showed initial interest in taking part in the study were contacted via e-mail. Ten potential participants responded with seven agreeing to take part. Interviews with six of these psychiatrists were eventually carried out.

Participant characteristics. Given the small number of psychiatrists on the island, preserving participant anonymity was given high priority in this study. Firstly, because female psychiatrists are largely underrepresented in the local mental health field, the gender of the participants remained hidden. Secondly, although the amount of experience working in psychiatry could potentially influence the psychiatrists' perceptions, stating the specific number of years can render the participant identifiable. Therefore, a range of years of experience was introduced with two psychiatrists having less than five years' experience following postgraduate specialization in psychiatry, two having between five and ten years of experience, and two having over ten years of experience. Finally, the protection of anonymity was also extended to the country of training, area of expertise, and place of employment.

Credibility checks. A contextualist framework assumes that reality is changeable and dependent on context, and "by implication, all accounts, whether those of participants or of researchers, are understood to be imbued with subjectivity and therefore not *prima facie*, invalidated by conflicting with alternative perspectives" (Madill et al., 2000, p. 9). Nonetheless, to ensure validity and reliability, a minimum of two validation strategies must be applied (Creswell, 2007). Firstly, rich descriptions of the results were provided in the write-up to enable readers to draw their own conclusions on transferability (Creswell, 2007); and the results were presented in the psychiatrists' own words to further help ground the findings (Tindall, 1994). Secondly, interpretations of the data were reviewed by peers and the second author to ensure the reliability of the study (Creswell, 2007). Finally, in stating our position on the view of schizophrenia and disclosing our personal and professional experiences at the outset together with the use of reflexivity in discussing the findings, the reader is allowed to reach his or her own conclusions about how the authors may have contributed in the co-creation of the context in which knowledge was generated (Creswell, 2007).

Thematic Analysis

The method of data collection chosen to reach the aims of this study is thematic analysis. In spite of its regular use in research, prior to its naming and claiming by Braun and Clarke (2006, 2013), thematic analysis was neither named as a type of analysis nor claimed as a method in its own right in the same way as other established methods such as grounded theory or Interpretative Phenomenological Analysis (IPA). Both grounded theory and IPA are examples of methodologies and are therefore governed by a "*theory* of how research needs to proceed, to produce valid knowledge about the psychological and social world" (Braun & Clarke, 2013, p. 31). Conversely, thematic analysis is "a method for identifying, analysing, and reporting patterns (themes) within data" (Braun & Clarke, 2006, p. 82) with no specific guiding theory towards knowledge and its attainment.

In spite of its flexibility however, thematic analysis still makes it possible for the researcher to attain rich and complex data and to gain analytic insight into the ways participants make meaning of a particular phenomenon. For this to work however, it is a must for the researcher to take a theoretical position with regard to the view of reality, knowledge and so on. This will make it possible for the researcher to be guided and directed as to what can be said about the knowledge gathered from data analysis. Specifically, the researcher must make active choices with respect to the type of analysis required to answer the research question "in a way that is theoretically and methodologically sound" (Braun & Clarke, 2006, p. 81).

First, a contextualist method of thematic analysis is chosen over an essentialist/realist or constructionist method to parallel the epistemological underpinnings of this study. Second, it was decided that through the analysis, themes will be identified in a deductive, top down manner rather than in an inductive, bottom up way as this would best answer the research question based on the literature reviewed. Lastly, the third decision revolves around whether themes are identified at a semantic, explicit level or a latent, interpretative level. Since themes at a latent level are usually associated with constructionist epistemologies, to match the contextualist method of thematic analysis, themes will be identified at a semantic level. In practice however, themes tend to have both explicit and interpretative elements within them (Braun & Clarke, 2013).

Transcription and data analysis. Following data collection, the interviews were transcribed and analysed. Because thematic analysis does not have the power to allow the researcher to make claims about the effects of language (Braun & Clarke, 2013), when transcribing the interviews, focus was placed on what was said rather than how it was said.

The six stages of analysis as described by Braun and Clarke (2006, 2013) were applied. Firstly, to familiarize ourselves with the data and to find patterns related to the subject of the study, the transcripts were read in an active manner. This was guided by the primary decision to identify themes on a semantic level and in a deductive manner based on the literature review. Therefore, rather than providing a rich description of the whole data set, a more detailed analysis of aspects of the data set, such as the meaning ascribed to schizophrenia and recovery, was actively looked for.

Secondly, initial codes, consisting of "a *word* or *brief phrase* that captures the essence of why you think a particular bit of data may be useful" (Braun & Clarke, 2013, p. 207), were generated. This was done in a complete as opposed to a selective way whereby "*anything* and *everything* of interest or relevance" to answer the research question across the entire data set was identified (Braun & Clarke, 2013, p. 206). While some data were coded using a number of initial codes, others were coded using a single code. Codes which were similar were then grouped together with their corresponding data.

Thirdly, the clusters of similar codes were further grouped into potential themes and sub-themes or "patterns across an (entire) data set" (Braun & Clarke, 2006, p. 84). At this point, it is important to draw one's attention to how themes did not simply emerge from the data set but rather, the researchers played an active part in identifying them (Braun & Clarke, 2006). This highlights the researchers' contribution to findings of the study, which fit with both the critical realist and the contextualist positions.

In the fourth phase, themes were reviewed and refined. This involved the merging of some themes into overarching themes, the taking apart and the discarding of others. In doing so, sub-themes making up the overarching themes became more coherent and meaningful, and more clearly distinguished from each other (Braun & Clarke, 2006, p. 96). Finally, while the fifth stage involved the defining and naming of the final themes (see Table 2.1), the sixth entailed the writing up of the results.

Findings and Discussion

Following the data analysis stage, the findings are presented and discussed in this section. Overarching themes and sub-themes were primarily identified at a semantic level using a deductive method based on the literature review (refer to Table 2.1). They are taken to a new level of meaning in the discussion in the light of the literature and the conceptual and epistemological framework of this study. The findings selected for discussion in this section best demonstrate what thematic analysis can achieve by stating its strengths and limitations in comparison to other methodologies.

Perceptions of Schizophrenia

The strength of thematic analysis lies in its capacity to identify patterns across the whole data set. At the same time, it gives the possibility to account for differences in what participants say. These differences were also taken into account by eliciting all points of view even if contrasting ones as is evident hereunder.

Table 2.1 Overarching themes and sub-themes

Overarching theme	Sub-themes
The Psychiatrists' Perceptions of Schizophrenia	Schizophrenia as a set of symptoms leading to a diagnosis Schizophrenia as a syndrome not a condition Schizophrenia as heterogeneous and something that can develop into other disorders Psychosis as an extension of normality A biological view of schizophrenia The seriousness of schizophrenia The prognosis of schizophrenia Changes in perceptions through experience Schizophrenia as a stigmatising illness Psychiatrists as stigmatizers and as professionals who are stigmatized
Ways of working with individuals with schizophrenia limited by available local structures	Making a diagnosis of schizophrenia Medication as a form of treatment The possibility of involuntary hospitalization in the treatment of schizophrenia Community support is close to zero in Malta and everything is still hospital-based Addressing all aspects of the patient's life and working as part of a team Involving the family in treatment
The relational aspect of working with individuals with schizophrenia	Addressing psychotic symptoms Techniques used by psychiatrists to engage the patient in treatment Finding the right timing for sharing the diagnosis Educating and encouraging the patient Coping with the suffering
Psychiatrists' Perceptions of Recovery in Schizophrenia	Defining recovery in schizophrenia The possibility of recovery Factors influencing recovery The illness itself and/or response to treatment The impact of substance misuse on recovery The individual's background and social support and its impact on recovery The doctor-patient relationship

The participants in this study were found to view schizophrenia as a biological disease described as a set of symptoms, an illness and a "chronic brain disorder" (psychiatrist 1). It was frequently discussed through its comparison with physical illnesses ranging from the common cold and diabetes to Huntington's and Parkinson's disease. A number of psychiatrists said they believe that individuals diagnosed with schizophrenia are likely to have a genetic predisposition for the disorder which then manifests itself gradually or suddenly following triggers such as stress, substance misuse, trauma and upbringing.

Although the participants noted that factors other than genetics do play a role in the development of schizophrenia, the general sense was that the main culprit remains biological in nature (Boyle, 2013). In keeping with a contextualist position, this pattern immediately highlights the participants' background in medicine which seems to be the primary position through which the perspective of schizophrenia is developed. This came out most clearly in psychiatrist 5's argument on the difference between disease and being diseased.

> *There's a difference between saying somebody is unwell and diseased and what is the disease.*
> *The disease is eh the biological cause. We don't know it... When you see somebody who's*
> *diseased, you can say, tell it from a hundred miles. You know people with schizophrenia, you*
> *can tell something is wrong... I think in medicine we're used to this idea.*

As we shall discuss in the Implications for Clinical Practice, it might also be due to their medical background that the psychiatrists in this study were found to view medication as a primary and essential part of treatment, a perception that influences the techniques they use to engage their patients in treatment. At the same time, the participants also highlighted the impact the limitations of the mental health system have on the choices they make with respect to treatment.

Although the frequency of similar answers given by participants is telling, thematic analysis is about "meanings, rather than numbers" (Braun & Clarke, 2013, p. 223). That is, while it is important to note the general meaning given by the participants, it is also important to report nuances which might further help to answer the research question. For example, it was interesting to find that psychiatrist 5 held two apparently contradictory views when it came to ascribing meaning to schizophrenia. Apart from the perception of schizophrenia as a diagnosable illness with a genetic component, this psychiatrist simultaneously viewed psychosis as an extension of normality. This is in line with the continuum model of abnormality which rejects the idea of classification systems altogether based on the assumption that there is no definitive line between sanity and madness and that psychosis is "just part and parcel of human variation, rather than as an illness" (Bentall, 2003, p. 96).

We noted that this psychiatrist was quite careful not to minimize the pathology as though doing so would minimize the functional disability and distress that often accompany schizophrenia. Indeed, as was found in the literature, all participants in this study stressed the seriousness of the disorder, with some mentioning the elevated risk of suicide either as a result of the disorder or upon finding out about the disorder (Carroll, 2015; Pierre, 2015; Ucok, Polat, Sartorius, Erkoc, & Atakli, 2004). While some participants took into account that schizophrenia varies within itself and between individuals and that other mental illnesses can be equally disabling, it is schizophrenia that was perceived as "one of those which most devastatingly takes a downward spiral" (psychiatrist 1).

The heterogeneity of schizophrenia was brought up by a number of participants. Psychiatrist 1 in particular spoke about the implications of this in his practice. He criticized classification systems for not being inclusive of the diverse patient populations diagnosed with schizophrenia. He argued that if the classification of schizophrenia was better streamlined, the psychiatrist would be better able to prescribe more specific treatment for patients with different sub-disorders. Instead,

> *all of them* [patients] *will get what happens to be my favourite anti-psychotic and then* [if] *that fails, go for the second one and then da da da da go for clozapine.*

The view of schizophrenia as a heterogenous disorder was also found in the literature. In a quantitative study by Cape and colleagues (1994), which looked at experienced psychiatrists' perceptions of the aetiology and prognosis of schizophrenia and how these in turn influence clinical practice, 85% of the sample believed the nature of schizophrenia to be heterogeneous. Yet, on its own, this quantitative study was unable to capture the frustration psychiatrists may experience when it comes to the apparent heterogeneity of schizophrenia. Therefore, findings such as this demonstrate how qualitative research can supplement quantitative research by adding texture to numbers.

Perceptions of Recovery

All participants in this study believed that schizophrenia can be a long-term illness which is likely to be chronic with recurring relapses. In saying this, only two participants claimed that recovery in schizophrenia is rare or unlikely (psychiatrists 1 & 3), going against findings in the literature which claim that most psychiatrists hold a negative outlook on the prospect of recovery (Gorwood et al., 2013; Klapheck et al., 2014; Ng et al., 2010; Ucok et al., 2004). Moreover, although studies using the objective definition suggest that the prospect of recovery is bleak (e.g., Harrow et al., 2005; Jääskeläinen et al., 2012; Torgalsbøen & Rund, 2002), adopting this perspective did not necessarily translate into having a negative outlook of recovery for the participants in this study. However, it was those who fully or partially adopted concepts from the recovery model that had the most positive outlook on the possibility of recovery.

The psychiatrists' perceptions of recovery in schizophrenia appeared to be influenced by the context in which they worked and their experiences. In terms of the nature of their work, some psychiatrists noted their increased exposure to individuals who do not recover rather than to those who do. In this regard, psychiatrist 4 claimed that it is this which could have led to his skewed perception of the prognosis of schizophrenia. As it were, Cohen and Cohen (1984) argue that as a result of being exposed to that segment of the population who remain ill, professionals develop what is known as the "clinician's illusion", or "the attribution of the characteristics and course of those patients who are currently ill to the entire population contracting the illness" (p. 1180).

Because the qualitative study by Ng and colleagues (2010) looked into medical students' and trainee psychiatrists' perceptions of recovery, it could not bring out the impact of work experience on changing perceptions. In this study, psychiatrists 2 and 3 spoke about how starting their training in psychiatry in a rehabilitation ward at the local mental health hospital shaped their initial perception of schizophrenia as a chronic illness with little possibility of recovery, as was the case for the trainees in the study by Ng and colleagues. However, although the two psychiatrists in this study shared similar experiences, the way their perceptions changed over time is somewhat different. While psychiatrist 3 chose not to work with individuals with schizophrenia following his experience, psychiatrist 2 claimed that the more experience he gained, the more he started "seeing people at different stages of the disease" and concluded that, particularly during the early stages, there were many psychosocial interventions that could be used to mitigate the impact and severity of schizophrenia. It must be said however, that although experience has the potential of shaping one's perceptions, this change also seems to be influenced by the professional's personal disposition. At this point, it is important to note however that this conclusion is only tentative and could have been better reached using other methodologies such as narrative analysis which would have allowed for the participants' narratives to remain intact rather than split into themes.

Lastly, the psychiatrists' perception of recovery also seems to be affected by their view of the individual carrying the label and the effectiveness of medication. An interesting finding in this study is that those participants who defined recovery in strictly scientific terms and held the belief that recovery in schizophrenia is unlikely (psychiatrists 1 & 3), it was the negative symptoms' resistance to medication that elicited in them the greatest sense of hopelessness. As claimed by psychiatrist 1, "in a condition like schizophrenia, chances are nothing's going to work 100%". In a way, this shows that these participants' focal point was the illness itself rather the person behind the disorder. This point can be substantiated by the fact that psychiatrist 3 often referred to individuals diagnosed with schizophrenia as "schizophrenics" during the interview. Such claims may have been better substantiated through discourse analysis given that it would have allowed further insight into the therapeutic relationship and psychiatrist-patient interactions.

Conversely, those participants who felt most optimistic about the prospect of recovery (psychiatrists 2 and 6) did not seem to focus on the condition and on the response to medication as much as they gave consideration to the importance of working on all aspects of the individual's life. As psychiatrist 2 argued, "ultimately because you have schizophrenia, you're not schizophrenic. But there's more to you than that". Therefore, despite all participants holding a medical view of schizophrenia, those who focused more on the disease and its medical treatment as opposed to viewing the person as a whole and incorporate diverse interventions, appeared to develop a more pessimistic view of recovery in schizophrenia.

Implications for Clinical Practice

In keeping to a contextualist framework, when it comes to the manifestations of the participants' perceptions in their clinical practice, one must consider the context in which they operate. First, perhaps due to their medical training and their perception of schizophrenia as a disease, the psychiatrists in this study seemed to perceive medication as the primary and necessary form of treatment. When working with individuals with schizophrenia, refusing medication was seen as a "big issue" (psychiatrist 4), to the extent that two psychiatrists noted that they at times feel the need to resort to white lies and manipulation in order to encourage compliance. Similarly, the importance of having the family on board to help the psychiatrist convince the patient to take the medication was noted by a number of participants. This shows how the patient's voice is sometimes somewhat lost in the planning of his or her treatment, thereby discouraging the individual from taking an active role in the recovery process and shifting the power within the therapeutic alliance away from the patient (Foucault & Gordon, 1980).

It is not only the psychiatrists' perceptions of the use of medication that carries implications for treatment options however. The mental health system in which psychiatrists operate seems to greatly influence their decisions when it comes to treating individuals diagnosed with schizophrenia. Although the mental health act (2012) states that treatment should primarily take place in the community, the participants claimed that community support is lacking, with psychiatrist 3 again noting that "our community support is close to zero" and that the mental health system in Malta is still hospital-based. This psychiatrist further claimed that moving towards a more community-based system is dependent on the pressure placed on psychiatrists to prevent hospitalizations as much as possible, in part by reducing the number of beds in mental health hospitals. However, according to psychiatrist 3, in Malta, "bed availability just happens" which is in agreement with research which shows that Malta has 185 beds per 100,000, a figure which is quite high when compared to the average of 72 beds per 100,000 across the European Union (World Health Organization, 2017). These factors, together with the high caseload, lack of resources such as professionals and multidisciplinary teams (psychiatrists 1, 2, 3, 4 and 5), appear to make it more likely for individuals diagnosed with schizophrenia to receive treatment in hospital rather than in the community which can be traumatic for the patient (Galea, 2009) and ultimately acts as a barrier to recovery (Jacobson & Greenley, 2001).

Limitations of the Study and Recommendations for Future Research

Firstly, using a semi-structured interview to gather the data meant that the participants were free to discuss what they felt was relevant for them. Because of this, not all participants were given the opportunity to discuss all issues brought up in this study. Also, the presence of the interviewer in face-to-face interviews may have influenced the way participants responded to certain questions. Secondly, this study could not draw conclusions on gender differences when it comes to perceptions of schizophrenia and its recovery, which could be an interesting topic for future research. Thirdly, although in this study it seems that psychiatrists' past experiences may shape current perceptions, this could not be confirmed by using thematic analysis as this method does not allow one to "retain a sense of continuity and contradiction through any one individual account" (Braun & Clarke, 2006, p. 27). Lastly, the use of thematic analysis could not make it possible to make claims about the use of language to substantiate findings on the power imbalance between the psychiatrist and the patient as would have other qualitative methodologies such as discourse analysis.

This study has looked into psychiatrists' perceptions of schizophrenia and its recovery and the implications these have on their clinical practice. It would be interesting if future research focused specifically on the idiosyncratic narratives of psychiatrists to gain insight into how their perceptions are shaped by experiences over time. Conversely, perhaps a large-scale quantitative study on psychiatrists' perceptions of schizophrenia and its recovery across Europe can serve as a starting point to understanding how these have changed over time since the study conducted by Cape and colleagues in 1994.[1]

Conclusion

The qualitative study presented in this chapter highlights the need for policy makers to become sensitive to the influences of the mental health system on the psychiatrists' choices with regard to treating the individual diagnosed with schizophrenia. A number of psychiatrists mentioned that they had never had the opportunity to reflect on what schizophrenia truly means to them and on how working with individuals with this diagnosis impacts their well-being. These statements, which are typical following in-depth interviews, reflect the impact of qualitative research on the participants (Sammut Scerri, Abela, & Vetere, 2012). They also suggest that perhaps, providing a space where psychiatrists can discuss their experiences and dilemmas through clinical or peer supervision might support them in their work with service users.

---

[1] Through the use of a questionnaire, this quantitative study looked at experienced psychiatrists' (n = 119) views on aetiology, diagnosis and treatment of schizophrenia. The majority of psychiatrists in this sample rated clinical impression as being more useful for diagnosis than Schneider's first-rank symptoms, the ICD 9 or the DSM III. With regard to aetiology, the psychiatrists in this study gave the highest ratings to biological factors, followed by life events, which in turn was followed by psychosocial factors. The prescription of medication was significantly higher when compared to other interventions. Interestingly, while those who believed schizophrenia to be the result of biological causes were more likely to choose medication over other forms of interventions, those who believed schizophrenia to be a product of psychosocial factors were found to be more likely to choose psychological treatments.

Appendix

Appendix A: Revised Interview Guide

General Introduction

1. How many years of experience do you have working as a psychiatrist?
2. During this time, approximately how many cases of schizophrenia have you come across?

Perceptions of Schizophrenia as a Disease and as a Diagnosis, Possible Stigmatising Attitudes, Therapeutic Relationship

3. What is schizophrenia?
4. If you had to come up with a metaphor to describe schizophrenia, what would it be?

   How would you compare schizophrenia to other mental illnesses?

5. What was your impression of schizophrenia when you first started working with individuals with mental health problems? Has this changed over time?
6. Have you worked with a patient with schizophrenia in the past week? What was this like for you? How do you relate to a patient with schizophrenia? How does a patient who presents with symptoms of schizophrenia make you feel? What would be going through your mind at that moment? What would your main concerns be? How do you address hallucinations, delusions, and lack of insight?
7. Can you take me through your experience of working with a particular patient with schizophrenia? What stuck with you the most with this client?
8. What informs you the most when you are making a diagnosis of schizophrenia?

   Do you and if so, how, do you inform patients and their families about the diagnosis? Why or why not? Does this differ from other diagnoses?
   Would you like to share any thoughts on the DSM-5 or the ICD-10?

Recovery in Schizophrenia

8. In your line of work, have you ever observed recovery in schizophrenia?
9. Based on your experience, do you think full recovery in schizophrenia is possible?

   If so, how do you define recovery? If not, why not? What would be helpful? What usually serves as a hindrance or a barrier?

10. Is there a particular patient that comes to mind when I ask this question? Can you tell me a bit more about this patient? How did the patient recover? Were there any other professionals involved? What treatment was the patient offered? In your opinion, what was particularly helpful for this patient? Were there any obstacles?

Possible Hierarchy

11. May I ask what your initial reactions to being asked to take part in a study on schizophrenia were?
12. Do you have any other thoughts you would like to share? What was the interview like for you?

References

Aleman, A., & Kahn, R. S. (2005). Strange feelings: do amygdala abnormalities dysregulate the emotional brain in schizophrenia? *Progress in Neurobiology, 77*(5), 283–298. http://doi.org/10.1016/j.pneurobio.2005.11.005.

American Psychiatric Association. (2005). *Position statement on the use of the concept of recovery.* Washington, DC: American Psychiatric Association.

American Psychiatric Association. (2013). *Diagnostic and statistical manual of mental disorders: DSM-5.* Washington, DC: American Psychiatric Association.

Bellack, A. S. (2006). Scientific and consumer models of recovery in schizophrenia: Concordance, contrasts, and implications. *Schizophrenia Bulletin, 32*(3), 432–442. https://doi.org/10.1093/schbul/sbj044.

Bentall, R. P. (2003). *Madness explained: Psychosis and human nature.* London, UK: Penguin Books.

Boyle, M. (2013). The persistence of medicalisation: Is the presentation of alternatives part of the problem? In S. Coles, S. Keenan, & B. Diamond (Eds.), *Madness contested: Power and practice.* Ross-on-Wye, UK: PCCS Books.

Bracken, P., & Thomas, P. (2005). *Postpsychiatry: Mental health is a postmodern world.* Oxford, UK: Oxford University Press.

Braun, V., & Clarke, V. (2006). Using thematic analysis in psychology. *Qualitative Research in Psychology, 3*(2), 77–101. https://doi.org/10.1191/1478088706qp063oa.

Braun, V., & Clarke, V. (2013). *Successful qualitative research: A practical guide for beginners.* Thousand Oaks, CA: Sage.

Breeding, J. (2008). To see or not to see "schizophrenia" and the possibility of full "recovery". *Journal of Humanistic Psychology, 48*(4), 489–504. https://doi.org/10.1177/0022167808316942.

British Psychological Society. (2013). *Classification of behaviour and experience in relation to functional psychiatric diagnoses: Time for a paradigm shift: DCP position statement.* Retrieved from http://www.bps.org.uk/system/files/Public%20files/cat-1325.pdf.

British Psychological Society. (2014). *Understanding psychosis and schizophrenia: Why people sometimes hear voices, believe things that others find strange, or appear out of touch with reality, and what can help.* Retrieved from http://www.bps.org.uk/system/files/Public%20files/rep03_understanding_psychosis.pdf.

Callicott, J. H., Bertolino, A., Mattay, V. S., Langheim, F. J., Duyn, J., Coppola, R., … Weinberger, D. R. (2000). Physiological dysfunction of the dorsolateral prefrontal cortex in schizophrenia revisited. *Cerebral Cortex, 10*(11), 1078–1092. http://doi.org/10.1093/cercor/10.11.1078.

Cape, G., Antebi, D., Standen, P., & Glazebrook, C. (1994). Schizophrenia: The views of a sample of psychiatrists. *Journal of Mental Health, 3*(1), 105–113. https://doi.org/10.3109/09638239409003784.

Carroll, B. (2015, March 18). *Reply to Professor David Pilgrim* [Online forum comment]. Message posted to https://www.psychologytoday.com/comment/755248#comment-755248.

Cohen, P., & Cohen, J. (1984). The clinician's illusion. *Archives of General Psychiatry, 41*(12), 1178–1182. https://doi.org/10.1001/archpsyc.1984.01790230064010.

Cosgrove, V. E., & Suppes, T. (2013). Informing DSM-5: Biological boundaries between bipolar I disorder, schizoaffective disorder, and schizophrenia. *BMC Medicine, 11*(1), 127–133. https://doi.org/10.1186/1741-7015-11-127.

Creswell, J. W. (2007). *Qualitative inquiry & research design: Choosing among five approaches* (2nd ed.). Thousand Oaks, CA: Sage.

Davidson, L., Schmutte, T., Dinzeo, T., & Andres-Hyman, R. (2007). Remission and recovery in schizophrenia: Practitioner and patient perspectives. *Schizophrenia Bulletin, 34*(1), 5–8. https://doi.org/10.1093/schbul/sbm122.

Ellison-Wright, I., Glahn, D. C., Laird, A. R., Thelen, S. M., & Bullmore, E. (2008). The anatomy of first-episode and chronic schizophrenia: An anatomical likelihood estimation meta-analysis. *American Journal of Psychiatry, 165*(8), 1015–1023. https://doi.org/10.1176/appi.ajp.2008.07101562.

Färdig, R., Lewander, T., Fredriksson, A., & Melin, L. (2011). Evaluation of the illness management and recovery scale in schizophrenia and schizoaffective disorder. *Schizophrenia Research, 132*(2), 157–164. https://doi.org/10.1016/j.schres.2011.07.001.

Foucault, M. (2006). *History of madness* (J. Murphy & J. Khalfa, Trans.). Abingdon, OX: Routledge (Original work published 1972).

Foucault, M., & Gordon, C. (1980). *Power/knowledge: Selected interviews and other writings, 1972–1977.* Broadway, New York: Pantheon Books.

Galea, R. (2009). *Living outside mental illness—The subjective experience of recovery from mental illness: A qualitative study.* Unpublished master's dissertation, University of Malta, Malta.

Geekie, J., Randal, P., Lampshire, D., & Read, J. (2012). *Experiencing psychosis: Personal and professional perspectives.* New York, NY: Routledge.

Gorwood, P., Burns, T., Juckel, G., Rossi, A., San, L., Hargarter, L., & Schreiner, A. (2013). Psychiatrists' perceptions of the clinical importance, assessment and management of patient functioning in schizophrenia in Europe, the Middle East and Africa. *Annals of General Psychiatry, 12*(1), 8–15. http://doi.org/10.1186/1744-859x-12-8.

Hamm, J. P., Ethridge, L. E., Boutros, N. N., Keshavan, M. S., Sweeney, J. A., Pearlson, G. D., … Clementz, B. A. (2014). Diagnostic specificity and familiality of early versus late evoked potentials to auditory paired stimuli across the schizophrenia-bipolar psychosis spectrum. *Psychophysiology, 51*(4), 348–357. http://doi.org/10.1111/psyp.12185.

Harrow, M., Grossman, L. S., Jobe, T. H., & Herbener, E. S. (2005). Do patients with schizophrenia ever show periods of recovery? A 15-year multi-follow-up study. *Schizophrenia Bulletin, 31*(3), 723–734. https://doi.org/10.1093/schbul/sbi026.

Hor, K., & Taylor, M. (2010). Suicide and schizophrenia: A systematic review of rates and risk factors. *Journal of Psychopharmacology, 24*(4), 81–90. https://doi.org/10.1177/1359786810385490.

Jääskeläinen, E., Juola, P., Hirvonen, N., McGrath, J. J., Saha, S., Isohanni, M., … Miettunen, J. (2012). A systematic review and meta-analysis of recovery in schizophrenia. *Schizophrenia Bulletin, 39*(6), 1296–1306. http://doi.org/10.1093/schbul/sbs130.

Jablensky, A. (2013). Schizophrenia in DSM-5: Assets and liabilities. *Schizophrenia Research, 150*(1), 36–37. https://doi.org/10.1016/j.schres.2013.07.037.

Jacobson, N., & Greenley, D. (2001). What is recovery? A conceptual model and explanation. *Psychiatric Services, 52,* 482–485.

Jaeger, M. E., & Rosnow, R. L. (1988). Contextualism and its implications for psychological inquiry. *British Journal of Psychology, 79*(1), 63–75. https://doi.org/10.1111/j.2044-8295.1988.tb02273.x.

Jorm, A. F., Korten, A. E., Jacomb, P. A., Christensen, H., & Henderson, S. (1999). Attitudes towards people with a mental disorder: A survey of the Australian public and health professionals. *Australian and New Zealand Journal of Psychiatry, 33*(1), 77–83. https://doi.org/10.1046/j.1440-1614.1999.00513.x.

Jose, D., Lalitha, K., Gandhi, S., & Desai, G. (2015). Consumer perspectives on the concept of recovery in schizophrenia: A systematic review. *Asian Journal of Psychiatry, 14,* 13–18. https://doi.org/10.1016/j.ajp.2015.01.006.

Keshavan, M. S., Nasrallah, H. A., & Tandon, R. (2011). Schizophrenia, "Just the Facts" 6. Moving ahead with the schizophrenia concept: From the elephant to the mouse. *Schizophrenia Research, 127*(1–3), 3–13. https://doi.org/10.1016/j.schres.2011.01.011.

Kincaid, D. L., Doris, M., Shannon, C., & Mulholland, C. (2017). What is the prevalence of Autism Spectrum Disorder and ASD traits in psychosis? A systematic review. *Psychiatry Research, 250,* 99–105. https://doi.org/10.1016/j.psychres.2017.01.017.

Klapheck, K., Lincoln, T. M., & Bock, T. (2014). Meaning of psychoses as perceived by patients, their relatives and clinicians. *Psychiatry Research, 215*(3), 760–765. https://doi.org/10.1016/j.psychres.2014.01.017.

Leucht, S., Tardy, M., Komossa, K., Heres, S., Kissling, W., & Davis, J. M. (2012). Maintenance treatment with antipsychotic drugs for schizophrenia. *Cochrane Database Systematic Reviews, 16*(5). https://doi.org/10.1002/14651858.cd008016.

Lieberman, J. A., & First, M. B. (2007). Renaming schizophrenia. *British Medical Journal, 334*(7585), 108. https://doi.org/10.1136/bmj.39057.662373.80.

Liberman, R. P., & Kopelowicz, A. (2002). Recovery from schizophrenia: A challenge for the 21st century. *International Review of Psychiatry, 14*(4), 245–255. https://doi.org/10.1080/095402602 1000016897.

Liberman, R. P., Kopelowicz, A., Ventura, J., & Gutkind, D. (2002). Operational criteria and factors related to recovery from schizophrenia. *International Review of Psychiatry, 14*(4), 256–272. https://doi.org/10.1080/0954026021000016905.

Luhrmann, T. M. (2016). Introduction. In T. M. Luhrmann & J. Marrow (Eds.), *Our most troubling madness: Case studies in schizophrenia across cultures* (pp. 1–25). Oakland, CA: University of California Press.

Lysaker, P. H., Ringer, J., Maxwell, C., McGuire, A., & Lecomte, T. (2010). Personal narratives and recovery from schizophrenia. *Schizophrenia Research, 121*(1–3), 271–276. https://doi.org/10.1016/j.schres.2010.03.003.

Madill, A., Jordan, A., & Shirley, C. (2000). Objectivity and reliability in qualitative analysis: Realist, contextualist and radical constructionist epistemologies. *British Journal of Psychology, 91*(1), 1–20. https://doi.org/10.1348/000712600161646.

McCarthy, S. E., Makarov, V., Kirov, G., Addington, A. M., McClellan, J., Yoon, S., … Krause, V. (2009). Microduplications of 16p11.2 are associated with schizophrenia. *Nature Genetics, 41*(11), 1223–1227.

Mental Health Act. (2012). Chapter 525. *Laws of Malta.* Retrieved from http://www.justiceservi ces.gov.mt/DownloadDocument.aspx?app=lom&itemid=11962&l=1.

Meyer-Lindenberg, A. (2010). From maps to mechanisms through neuroimaging of schizophrenia. *Nature, 468*(7321), 194–202. https://doi.org/10.1038/nature09569.

Miller, B. (2015, July, 28). *The 2015 international congress on schizophrenia research.* Retrieved from http://www.psychiatrictimes.com/schizophrenia/2015-international-congress-schizophrenia-research.

Naidoo, Y. (2015, June, 1). *Schizophrenic disorders: Is there an elephant?* Retrieved from http://www.psychiatrictimes.com/schizophrenia/schizophrenic-disorders-there-elephant.

Need, A. C., & Goldstein, D. B. (2014). Schizophrenia genetics comes of age. *Neuron, 83*(4), 760–763. https://doi.org/10.1016/j.neuron.2014.08.015.

Ng, R. M., Pearson, V., Chen, E. E., & Law, C. W. (2010). What does recovery from schizophrenia mean? Perceptions of medical students and trainee psychiatrists. *International Journal of Social Psychiatry, 57*(3), 248–262. https://doi.org/10.1177/0020764009354833.

Noiseux, S., & Ricard, N. (2008). Recovery as perceived by people with schizophrenia, family members and health professionals: A grounded theory. *International Journal of Nursing Studies, 45*(8), 1148–1162. https://doi.org/10.1016/j.ijnurstu.2007.07.008.

Pierre, J. (2015, March 5). *Psychosis sucks! Antipsychiatry and the romanticization of mental illness.* Retrieved from https://www.psychologytoday.com/comment/755248#comment-755248.

Pies, R. W. (2016, June 1). *How antipsychotic medication may save lives.* Retrieved from http://www.psychiatrictimes.com/schizophrenia/how-antipsychotic-medication-may-save-lives/page/0/2.

Sammut Scerri, C. S., Abela, A., & Vetere, A. (2012). Ethical dilemmas of a clinician/researcher interviewing women who have grown up in a family where there was domestic violence. *International Journal of Qualitative Methods, 11*(2), 102–131. https://doi.org/10.1177/160940691201100201.

Schizophrenia Working Group of the Psychiatric Genomics Consortium. (2014). Biological insights from 108 schizophrenia-associated genetic loci. *Nature, 511*(7510), 421–427.

Schlosberg, A. (1993). Psychiatric stigma and mental health professionals (stigmatizers and destigmatizers). *Medical Law Journal, 12*(3–5), 409–416.

Shepherd, A. M., Laurens, K. R., Matheson, S. L., Carr, V. J., & Green, M. J. (2012). Systematic meta-review and quality assessment of the structural brain alterations in schizophrenia. *Neuroscience and Biobehavioral Reviews, 36*(4), 1342–1356. https://doi.org/10.1192/bjp.188.6.510.

Tamminga, C. A., & Medoff, D. R. (2000). The biology of schizophrenia. *Dialogues in Clinical Neuroscience, 2*(4), 339–348. Retrieved from https://europepmc.org/articles/pmc3181617.

Tindall, C. (1994). Issues of evaluation. In P. Banister, E. Burman, I. Parker, M. Taylor, & C. Tindall (Eds.), *Qualitative methods in psychology: A research guide* (pp. 142–159). Buckingham: Open University Press.

Toal, F., Bloemen, O. J., Deeley, Q., Tunstall, N., Daly, E. M., Page, L., … Murphy, D. G. (2009). Psychosis and autism: Magnetic resonance imaging study of brain anatomy. *The British Journal of Psychiatry, 194*(5), 418–425.

Torgalsbøen, A. K., & Rund, B. R. (2002). Lessons learned from three studies of recovery from schizophrenia. *International Review of Psychiatry, 14*(4), 312–317. https://doi.org/10.1080/0954026021000016950.

Tsang, H. W., & Chen, E. Y. (2007). Perceptions on remission and recovery in schizophrenia. *Psychopathology, 40*(6), 469. https://doi.org/10.1159/000108128.

Ucok, A., Polat, A., Sartorius, N., Erkoc, S., & Atakli, C. (2004). Attitudes of psychiatrists toward patients with schizophrenia. *Psychiatry and Clinical Neurosciences, 58*(1), 89–91. https://doi.org/10.1111/j.1440-1819.2004.01198.x.

van Haren, N. E., Cahn, W., Pol, H. H., & Kahn, R. S. (2008). Schizophrenia as a progressive brain disease. *European Psychiatry, 23*(4), 245–254.

Van Os, J., Galdos, P., Lewis, G., Bourgeois, M., & Mann, A. (1993). Schizophrenia sans frontieres: Concepts of schizophrenia among French and British psychiatrists. *BMJ, 307*(6902), 489–492. https://doi.org/10.1136/bmj.307.6902.489.

Wallcraft, J., Read, J., & Sweeney, A. (2003). *On our own terms.* London, UK: The Sainsbury Centre for Mental Health. Retrieved from http://www.nsun.org.uk/assets/downloadableFiles/on-our-own-terms.pdf.

WHO. (2017). *Data and statistics.* Retrieved from http://www.euro.who.int/en/health-topics/non communicable-diseases/mental-health/data-and-statistics.

Willig, C. (2013). *Introducing qualitative research in psychology* (3rd ed.). New York, NY: Open University Press.

World Health Organisation. (1992). *The ICD-10 classification of mental and behavioural disorders: Clinical descriptions and diagnostic guidelines* [PDF file]. Available from http://www.who.int/classifications/icd/en/bluebook.pdf.

World Health Organization. (2018, December). *ICD-11 for mortality and morbidity statistics.* Retrieved from https://icd.who.int/browse11.

Zipursky, R. B., & Agid, O. (2015). Recovery, not progressive deterioration, should be the expectation in schizophrenia. *World Psychiatry, 14*(1), 94–96. https://doi.org/10.1002/wps.20194.

Chapter 3
Approaching Psychotherapy Case Studies in a Metasynthesis: Deficit vs. Conflict in Treatment of Medically Unexplained Symptoms

Juri Krivzov⊙, Dewi Hannon⊙, and Reitske Meganck⊙

Abstract *Metasynthesis* is currently considered one of the most promising directions for qualitative research, as it can contribute to the generalizability of qualitative findings and increase their impact. At the same time, *single case studies* gain attention in the field of psychotherapy research, as they offer unique insights into psychotherapy process and promote theory building. In the following, we will elaborate on a worked example of a metasynthesis of published psychotherapy case studies. Thereby, we investigated the psychotherapeutic process in ten case studies of patients with medically unexplained symptoms (MUS), while focusing on the theoretical concepts of *deficit* and *conflict*. The reader will be guided through the dilemmas and choices in research design and data analysis. First, the theory-building approach toward metasynthesis will be discussed. Then, a novel search engine, the Single Case Archive, will be introduced as an easy way to access and systematically search for psychotherapeutic case studies in a database with over 3000 cases. Furthermore, we will share our experience of adapting data analysis procedures for the purpose of a metasynthesis of case studies. As case studies describe the psychotherapy process in its complexity unfolding over time, they cannot be approached in the same manner as interview material, thus asking for methodological innovations. Through the creation of timelines of therapeutic events, process-oriented themes could be detected that would not have been found when only using line-by-line coding. Finally, limitations of the metasynthesis are discussed.

Keywords Single Case Archive · Case study · Metasynthesis · Qualitative meta-analysis · Timeline · Medically unexplained symptoms · Functional Somatic Syndromes · Psychosomatics · Alexithymia · Mentalization

J. Krivzov (✉) · R. Meganck
Department of Psychoanalysis and Clinical Consulting, Ghent University, Ghent, Belgium
e-mail: Juri.Krivzov@UGent.be

D. Hannon
Department of Experimental-Clinical and Health Psychology, Ghent University, Ghent, Belgium

© Springer Nature Switzerland AG 2021
M. Borcsa and C. Willig (eds.), *Qualitative Research Methods in Mental Health*,
https://doi.org/10.1007/978-3-030-65331-6_3

Introduction

Metasynthesis (Thomas & Harden, 2008), also referred to as *qualitative meta-analysis* (Timulak, 2009) aims at aggregating and interpreting the results of qualitative studies in order to establish overarching findings and to enhance theory-building. Metasynthesis is currently considered one of the most promising directions for qualitative psychotherapy research, as it can contribute to its generalizability and increase its impact (Timulak & Elliott, 2019). Further, metasynthesis can also contribute to the sustainability of qualitative research, as it can prevent researchers from "reinventing the wheel" (Paterson, 2012, p. 3) and protect vulnerable populations from unnecessary research interventions (Dickson-Swift, James, Kippen, & Liamputtong, 2007). While being comparable with the better-known quantitative meta-analysis, metasynthesis can and should go beyond the mere question of treatment efficacy, which is often the focus of quantitative meta-analysis. Instead, metasynthesis can address more complex process-related questions (Thorne, 2019).

In the area of psychotherapy research, the crisis of current methodological and theoretical approaches[1] drives more and more researchers toward alternative methodologies (Toomela, 2008). Thereby, first-person accounts of subjective experience of therapists and patients come back to the spotlight after almost one hundred years of being rejected as "unscientific" (Desmet, 2018). In the last two decades, especially *single case studies* become increasingly recognized in the field of psychotherapy research, as they can offer unique in-depth insights into psychotherapy process and further promote theory building (McLeod & Elliott, 2011). The creation of two specialized journals (Clinical Case Studies in 2002 and Pragmatic Case Studies in Psychotherapy in 2005), numerous special issues on single case research, as well as the construction of the Single Case Archive (SCA; Desmet et al., 2013) reflect the increasing importance of case study research. In the following, we will elaborate on an example of a metasynthesis applied to published psychotherapy case studies, thus combining these two promising approaches.

Whereas metasynthesis is usually concerned with published qualitative studies and focuses mainly on their results sections (e.g., on the 'themes' retrieved by the original research teams; Timulak, 2009), a metasynthesis of *psychotherapy case studies* might consider the whole study as an object of investigation and source of data. For example, *clinical case studies* (Iwakabe & Gazzola, 2009) are usually written by therapists themselves and represent their first-person accounts of the therapy process; they may also contain patients' quotes or partial transcripts of the sessions. On the other hand, *systematic case studies* (Iwakabe & Gazzola, 2009) may be conducted by large research teams and contain qualitative or mixed-method analyses, which implement rigorous reflective procedures like the Hermeneutic Single-Case Efficacy

---

[1]The notion of the crisis in modern-day psychology refers to multiple issues, such as poor replicability of published findings (Open Science Collaboration, 2015), problematic validity of psychological measurement instruments (Desmet, 2018), conceptual problems of variable construction (Toomela, 2008), as well as disproportional focus on neurobiological instead of essentially psychological phenomena (Derksen, 2012).

Design (HSCED; Elliott, 2002) or Consensual Qualitative Research for Case Studies (CQR-C; Jackson, Chui, & Hill, 2011). Such case studies produce themes, reflections, and abstractions that are the result of a rigorous research process by the primary research team and provide a sophisticated 'results section'. Many case studies fall in between these two prototypes, containing first-person accounts of the therapist, as well as some quantitative and qualitative data and the author's (usually therapist's) secondary elaboration of the case. This brings the challenge that a metasynthesis must deal with both aspects of primary narrative and higher-order interpretations and at the same time critically reflect on the quality of both.

Aggregative vs. Interpretative Approaches in Metasynthesis

The answer to the challenge of such diverse data could be a movement toward a strict formalization of the metasynthesis process as described by the Cochrane Collaboration guidelines (Morton, Berg, Levit, & Eden, 2011). This logic strives for a certain uniformity of reporting results and attempts to provide tools for rigorous quality assessment of the primary studies (Lockwood et al., 2017). The general direction of such an approach leans more toward meta-aggregation (Hannes & Pearson, 2011) and to a lesser extent toward interpretation or theory-building. While this approach is being criticized for a potential loss of richness of the primary qualitative results, it can satisfy the need for transparency of qualitative meta-studies and increase trust in the research findings, particularly among those who are critical and/or suspicious of qualitative research (Hannes & Pearson, 2011; Thorne, 2019). However, a byproduct of such an approach could be the creation of artificially simplified themes taken out of context, thus sacrificing possible interconnection between them. In the spirit of qualitative research, such loss of holistic understanding of the psychotherapy process could lead to throwing the baby away with the bathwater (Thorne, 2019).

An alternative answer to the diverse materials that we encounter in the case studies is to explicitly rely on *theory-building*. This means that the research question should be explicitly guided by a pre-existing theoretical interest, the material should be treated in an interpretative manner and the discussion part should gain prominence in the publication. The advantages of such an approach are that diverse case material (therapist's reports, patient's quotes, themes from qualitative data analysis, and even bits of quantitative data) could be appraised from the theoretical point of view and set in relation to each other, like a puzzle. Thereby, such theory-driven metasynthesis could be testing multiple theoretical notions at the same time, letting different theoretical concepts compete for the most satisfying explanation and allow for detecting theoretical inconsistencies (Stiles, 2015). As a result, theory-driven metasynthesis would produce a deeper-going analysis of clinical phenomena and not a mere superficial summary of themes (Timulak & Elliott, 2019).

Choosing the Research Question: Process vs. Effectiveness

When choosing the theoretical framework and the research question we have to ask ourselves for which aims the material of the case studies is best suited. Case studies could give us direct and accessible descriptions of the therapeutic process. Case studies have the advantage that they report on the therapy process in a naturalistic setting, highlight 'tipping points' and significant events in therapy (Timulak, 2010), often describing the therapeutic process as it unfolds over time from the beginning of the therapy until follow-up (Hayes, Laurenceau, Feldman, Strauss, & Cardaciotto, 2007). Therapists and research teams often use audio recordings and session notes in order to maintain the continuity of assessment. This has major advantages compared to interviewing therapists or clients retrospectively. At the same time, case studies are always the product of the lens of the author, who is often also the therapist (in clinical case studies). Inevitably, the author's theoretical affiliation, education, and personal experience, as well as the journal policy, "marketing" considerations, and scientific spirit in the field could influence the presentation of the case a lot. From a qualitative research perspective, such influence of the researcher/therapist can however not be excluded (Denzin & Lincoln, 2005).

This does not mean that questions of treatment efficacy cannot be addressed within a metasynthesis of case studies. Indeed, the majority of the field of psychotherapy research is ultimately concerned with efficacy (Lambert, 2013) and case studies can and should make a valuable contribution to this (Elliott, 2002). However, in our view, the potential of case studies lies predominantly in studying processes and especially dynamic and interactive aspects of the therapy, thus leading us to choose process-oriented research questions.

In the study that we describe as an example in this chapter, we deliberately chose the psychodynamically inspired concepts of *deficit* and *conflict* in their application to the psychotherapeutic treatment of medically unexplained symptoms (MUS). In the following, we will demonstrate how these theoretical concepts give shape to and guide the process of metasynthesis. The current study emerged from our pilot metasynthesis (Hannon, 2018) based on case studies from the Single Case Archive (see also Willemsen et al., 2015). All authors participated in the Single Case Archive collaboration and were interested in the potential of the SCA for its application for meta-studies.

Incorporating Theory-Building into the Research Question: The Concepts of Deficit and Conflict in Psychotherapeutic Treatment of Medically Unexplained Symptoms

Medically Unexplained Symptoms (MUS) were chosen as an example for the current chapter as they confront us with multiple clinical and theoretical challenges that can be studied in-depth especially in the psychotherapeutic setting. MUS are somatic symptoms "for which no objective physical or pathological changes can be found" (Aggarwal, McBeth, Zakrzewska, Lunt, & Macfarlane, 2006, p. 468). A multitude of terms such as Functional Somatic Syndromes, Conversion Disorders, Psychosomatic Disorders, Somatic Symptom Disorder, etc. has been introduced to describe these conditions, while here we stick to the term MUS, which is considered a consensual umbrella term (Creed, 2016). MUS can range from pain, fatigue, and general malaise to gastrointestinal disfunction and pseudo-neurological complaints (Henningsen, Zipfel, & Herzog, 2007). The symptoms are often persistent (Carson et al., 2003; Kroenke & Mangelsdorff, 1989) and can have a severe impact on the patient's ability to carry out daily activities, social functioning, and mental health (Carson et al., 2003; De Waal, Arnold, Eekhof, & Van Hemert, 2004). Moreover, many patients risk unnecessary, and above all, potentially harmful diagnostic investigations and invasive treatments (olde Hartman et al., 2009). MUS also represent an important socioeconomic problem because of the considerable costs of frequent attendance in primary care (Barsky, Orav, & Bates, 2005; Zook & Moore, 1980). Patients with MUS use non-psychiatric healthcare facilities more often than other patients (Fink, Sørensen, Engberg, Holm, & Munk-Jørgensen, 1999) and often go through a large number of medical investigations (Reid, Wessely, Crayford, & Hotopf, 2002).

A rich tradition of psychotherapeutic treatment of MUS exists since Freud (Verhaeghe, 2004); currently, psychotherapy has been shown to be overall moderately successful (Henningsen et al., 2007). The treatment of MUS is considered to be challenging, as the patient and the therapist need to agree on common aims and on the understanding of the mind-body connection (olde Hartman et al., 2009). Further, the treatment of MUS is often dominated by illness behavior (Waller, Scheidt, & Hartmann, 2004) and low patient satisfaction (Salmon, Dowrick, Ring, & Humphris, 2004), while psychotherapists often experience the therapeutic relationship as troubled (Luyten, Van Houdenhove, Lemma, Target, & Fonagy, 2012).

From our literature review (Hannon, 2018), we identified two major approaches to psychotherapeutic treatment of MUS, based on the psychodynamic model by Bronstein (2011): the concepts of *deficit* and *conflict*.

The concept of *deficit* is defined as a deficiency in the capacity to experience internal states and regulate tensions by psychological means. Deficit models imply that patients prone to MUS lack the means to translate somatic arousal into verbal expression and are thus experiencing the arousal directly in the body (Verhaeghe, 2004). This persistent arousal could lead to chronic overactivation and subsequent breakdown of pain regulation mechanisms and cause chronic MUS (Luyten et al., 2012). Patients with MUS are consistently shown to have flat affect, poor fantasy life, and limited emotional vocabulary, a trait often referred to as *alexithymia* (Waller & Scheidt, 2004). Possibly, individuals with MUS grow up in a "culture of emotional avoidance" (Lind, Delmar, & Nielsen, 2014) and could thus lack the learned capacity to verbalize emotional distress. Deficit-oriented psychodynamic approaches typically aim at increasing the mentalizing capacity of the patients with MUS (Luyten et al., 2012) and improving the connections between bodily perceptions and mental states. Similarly, cognitive-behavioral approaches aim at correcting hyperfocused and biased perception of bodily stimuli and pain (Witthöft & Hiller, 2010), or aim at increased mindfulness, which results in more accurate perception of bodily signals (van Ravesteijn et al., 2013) and a better connection between body and mind (Röhricht, 2009).

The concept of *conflict* is defined as an unconscious psychic conflict, carrying symbolic meaning, which is projected onto the body due to psychic defense mechanisms. Thereby, the patient defends the self from consciously unacceptable, but unconsciously present ideas (Bronstein, 2011). The bodily symptoms might symbolically "express psychological distress without consciously acknowledging the psychic conflict responsible for it" (Brown, 2004, p. 797). Working with conflict may involve confrontation and uncovering of the conflicting, forbidden or shameful impulses and emotions, since the avoidance of conflict is considered to be on the root of MUS in this case (Abbass, Grantmyre, & Kay, 2013). Outside of psychoanalytic approaches, the idea of *identified patient* from the systemic family therapy could also be seen as an example of a conflict-oriented approach. For example, the child's MUS could serve to maintain "a delicate homeostasis in the family and is reinforced by the avoidance of conflict" (Husain, Browne, & Chalder, 2007, p. 3).

Importantly, *deficit* and *conflict* aspects do not have to be mutually exclusive (Bronstein, 2011), on the contrary, they could be present simultaneously in the treatment of the same patient (Dobersch, Grosse Holtforth, & Egle, 2018). It is the interplay between *deficit* and *conflict*-aspects in psychotherapy that could improve our understanding of the psychotherapeutic process in patients with MUS. In the spirit of the psychotherapy integration literature, we are going to investigate the role of these factors cross-theoretically, assuming that therapists in real-life experiment, discover, and use the techniques that work rather than blindly follow a certain dogma (Norcross & Alexander, 2019).

The aim of this study is to examine the process of therapeutic change in psychotherapy in patients with MUS. Hereby, our research questions are (RQ1): *How do therapists describe the psychotherapy process in patients with medically unexplained symptoms?* And (RQ2): *How is the approach of the therapist in his or her encounter with patients with MUS related to the concepts of deficit and conflict?* Thereby, we want to gain a deeper understanding of the interplay between the *deficit* and *conflict* aspects in therapy. Working with two research questions—a broad exploratory and a narrower theory-driven one allows for integrating a multitude of unexpected findings along the lines of the theoretical concepts.

Method

The Single Case Archive

The Single Case Archive (SCA; www.singlecasearchive.com) was used for the data collection. The SCA is a novel online database that currently contains over 3000 psychotherapy case studies collected by an international team of researchers by systematically screening peer-reviewed journals of various theoretical orientations from 1985 until recently (Desmet et al., 2013). Thereby, they obtained a collection of cases that covers considerable parts of the field and can claim to be representative, while also including cases that are not easily accessible with regular search terms in other search engines such as Web of Science. Each case study is coded according to the diagnosis, descriptive characteristics of patient and therapist, therapy modality, and outcome (Meganck et al., 2017). All diagnoses from various diagnostic systems are systematically translated into DSM-IV-TR categories for the sake of comparability. Author's own diagnostic formulations are additionally included into a separate search field. This allows for immediate search of sets of cases that are relevant for particular research questions via the in-built search engine.

The SCA hosts a multitude of case studies that focus on diverse topics, such as treatment efficacy, alliance rupture and repair, culturally sensitive interventions (e.g., with examples of Latino, Asian, and Native American cultures), therapist's personal experience, self-disclosure, supervision issues, etc. A variety of clinical phenomena of interest is mentioned in the database, such as transference (over 450 cases), dreams (over 160 cases), impact of certain historic events on patients and therapists (e.g., 14 cases dealing with 9/11), or patient's drawings (over 40 cases). The SCA also hosts over 30 publications on prominent classic and contemporary case studies such as *Anna O.* (Schonbar & Beatus, 1990), *Gloria* (Bohart, 1991) or *Amalia X* (Kächele et al., 2006).

Purposive vs Exhaustive Sampling Strategy

Although the SCA cannot claim to be an exhaustive database, as it does not contain every published case study in the world, it can still claim good enough representativity in the field due to its construction method. Furthermore, the SCA is currently the largest and most diverse online database for single case studies and could therefore be pragmatically used as the only source for data collection. Ideally, when searching for cases outside of the SCA, researchers should also always contribute the case studies to the SCA, thus making it to grow further.

Methodological guidelines would typically drive the researcher toward strictly exhaustive sampling in a metasynthesis (Benoot, Hannes, & Bilsen, 2016). An exhaustive sampling implies "funneling" when items from a multitude of databases are first broadly assessed and then systematically excluded after reading titles, abstracts, and full texts. However, this view is more and more questioned within the field. Besides pragmatic arguments of being unnecessarily time consuming, "[…] exhaustive sample risks to produce rather superficial synthesis findings, with a large number of studies that fail to go beyond the level of description" (Benoot et al., 2016, p. 2). Running contrary to the idea of ideographic investigation, exhaustive samplings often produce too much information that will be reduced in too superficial a manner, devoid of context and texture (Thorne, 2019). If one was to conduct a thematic analysis on all the cases from the SCA, one would probably end up with themes like 'adhering to the protocol', 'symptomatic improvement' and 'alliance'—a boring summary probably merely repeating the research questions and as such reflecting a common flaw of qualitative research (Timulak & Elliott, 2019).

We therefore decided for a *purposive sampling* strategy in the current study, as illustrated in Fig. 3.1. We first used the descriptive category 'diagnosis' in the search engine of the SCA. Thereby, we could retrieve all cases in which the complaints were labeled under the broad DSM-IV-TR category 'somatoform disorders', since this is the closest definitional approximation of MUS. This search provided 119 results (state of the SCA on 17.02.2018). Then, titles and abstracts were examined for their relevance to the research question. Articles excluded during this first reading

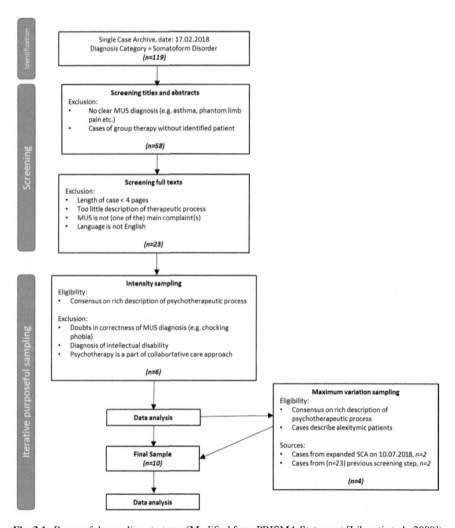

Fig. 3.1 Purposeful sampling strategy (Modified from PRISMA Statement [Liberati et al., 2009])

were mostly articles where no clear MUS was described (e.g., stress-related asthma, phantom limb pain) and cases of group therapy without an identified patient. This resulted in 58 remaining articles. Then, case studies were evaluated by reading full texts. Subsequently, articles were excluded based on the following exclusion criteria: length of the case being too short (<4 pages); too little description of the therapeutic process; MUS not being (one of) the main complaint(s), and the language of the article being other than English. This step delivered 23 articles. Subsequently, we followed the guidelines suggested by Benoot et al. (2016) for purposive sampling in a metasynthesis. We first retrieved the core 6 studies which constituted an *intensity sampling* and later added 4 studies for the purpose of *maximum variation sampling*.

Intensity Sampling

Both the first and the second author evaluated the remaining 23 articles. Only those articles where a consensus was reached on the *rich description of the psychothera-peutic process* were included. It should be noted that case studies differ widely with respect to the amount and quality of process description. Some cases consist of mere treatment protocol illustrations, some focus on narrow aspects of treatment, some cases only include a description of outcome (Desmet et al., 2013). These types of cases are potentially useful for other research questions but were excluded for the current study.

The last steps of the selection process in a metasynthesis will often produce *ad hoc exclusion and eligibility criteria* that were not foreseen at the beginning. For example, at this stage we still encountered studies where the somatic symptoms described did not clearly belong to the diagnostic category of MUS (e.g., a case of choking phobia by Connor-Greene, 1993) and were excluded. We further excluded cases concerning patients with an intellectual disability and cases where psychotherapy was a part of a collaborative care approach. Eventually, we maintained six studies with a rich description of the psychotherapeutic process (Baslet & Hill, 2011; Ciano-Federoff & Sperry, 2005; Holland, 1997; Küchenhoff, 1998; Martínez-Taboas, 2005; Milrod, 2002). These cases represent the *intensity sample* of our data analysis as rich and representative examples of the phenomenon of interest (Benoot et al., 2016).

Maximum Variation Sampling

After conducting data analysis on the first six cases, we concluded that the sample contained many cases with the characteristics of conversion disorder and that these cases felt rather 'dramatic and eventful' to us. The concept of *conflict* could be studied in-depth there (we were approaching saturation), whereas the concept of *deficit* appeared less nuanced in these cases. Therefore, we decided to expand our sample with four additional studies (Jacobs & Dinoff, 2012; Shapiro, 2003;

Vranceanu et al., 2008; Weaver, Nishith, & Resick, 1998) as part *of maximum variation sampling*. Thereby, we opted for cases that tended to describe more alexithymic patients, whereby the therapy is considered rather slow and 'uneventful' in the literature (Vanheule, Desmet, Meganck, & Bogaerts, 2007). This provided us with a more heterogeneous and balanced sample allowing for detecting themes that were disconfirmatory to the preliminary findings of the first six studies. Such a sample could also better reflect the clinical reality of working with patients with MUS who are often restricted in emotional expression (Lind et al., 2014). These four additional case studies are also available on the Single Case Archive. Two cases (Jacobs & Dinoff, 2012; Shapiro, 2003) were already taken into consideration during the previous selection. Another two cases (Vranceanu et al., 2008; Weaver et al., 1998) were retrieved from the Single Case Archive on 10.06.2018 since the amount of cases in the SCA was still increasing at the time of our research. Hereby we obtained a heterogenous sample that included cases with a variety of psychotherapeutic approaches (Cognitive-behavioral, psychodynamic, and mindfulness-based), patients of different age groups, and various MUS conditions (see Appendix A).

Figure 3.1 illustrates how the straightforward sampling idea as expressed in the PRISMA statement collides with the purposive iterative sampling and how it *cannot* be easily illustrated in the PRISMA flowchart. Whereas PRISMA guidelines (Liberati et al., 2009) suggest a linear "funneling" from large to small samples via successive exclusion of records (Benoot et al., 2016), we actually increased our sample size in the last stage.

Furthermore, in the last stages, the presented sampling process is *iterative* and inseparable from the data analysis, in line with qualitative approaches which are more focused toward theory-building and conflicting with quantitative approaches where standardization and hypothesis testing are central.

Data Analysis: Critical Realism as Epistemological Position

Dealing with pre-interpreted case material requires the researchers to be clear on their own epistemological position and theoretical premises from the very beginning of the research process. We believe that the psychotherapy process as reported by the authors of case studies could be pre-selected and influenced by their theoretical orientation, training, personal experience, journal policy and other factors. However, we also believe that practitioners generally produce accounts of a certain empirical "reality", that could be studied cross-theoretically and that is not a mere social construction/discourse or a mere product of the theoretical school (Sims-Schouten, Riley, & Willig, 2007). We also do not share current cognitive psychology's focus on therapists as a "source of bias" (Shedler, Mayman, & Manis, 1993; Spaanjaars, Groenier, van de Ven, & Witteman, 2015). Currently, within the culture of publishing case studies, practitioners are more and more encouraged to report on their own personal, educational, and theoretical background and to reflect on possible biases (Fishman, 2013; Jackson et al., 2011). Our epistemological position therefore leans mostly toward *critical realism*. Including cases from various theoretical backgrounds and reflecting on the potential bias of the authors appears to us to be the golden middle way instead of dismissing the practitioner perspective altogether or viewing the case data as pure social construction.

Data Analysis: Case Level as Primary Level of Analysis; Creating Process Themes

In conducting this metasynthesis, we followed the suggestions outlined by Thomas and Harden (2008) on methods for thematic synthesis of qualitative research: (1) line-by-line coding resulting in 'descriptive codes'; (2) the construction of 'descriptive themes' and (3) the development of 'analytical themes'. Hereby, each case was considered as a unit of analysis, since it seemed difficult to investigate a therapeutic process if data would be extracted from the case and merged without the contextual information (Hoon, 2013). Therefore, it was decided to first read and analyze each case separately, and to search for overarching themes in later stages. In addition, we decided to create a mind map and a timeline of significant events for every case. This way we could detect additional process-related themes that would not be found by solely conducting line-by-line coding. Visualizing psychotherapy process by means of a timeline also allowed us to detect temporal interdependences between themes, i.e., how processes unfold over time. We understand psychotherapy process as a complex dynamic system (Desmet, 2018) and believe that conducting qualitative analysis as if we were dealing with a static phenomenon will not meet the goal.

For the current chapter, we conducted a secondary analysis of our pilot study (Hannon, 2018), which initially had a broader scope (i.e., including the research question on therapist's explanatory models) and focused now on process and intervention domains.

Results

We could identify three main process themes: '*Breaking the vicious circle of medical interventions*', '*From physical pain to psychological pain*', and '*MUS not in the focus anymore*'. The themes that described interventions of the therapists were subsumed under conflict and deficit themes. We identified two conflict-related themes: '*Postponing conflict-interventions*' and '*Working through the conflict*' and two deficit-related themes: '*Linking body and mind*' and '*Teaching healthy coping*'. The themes that could not be adequately categorized within our framework of deficit and conflict were handled as nuancing and disconfirmatory themes: '*Focus of treatment on underlying psychopathological condition instead of MUS*' and '*Focus of treatment on trauma*'.

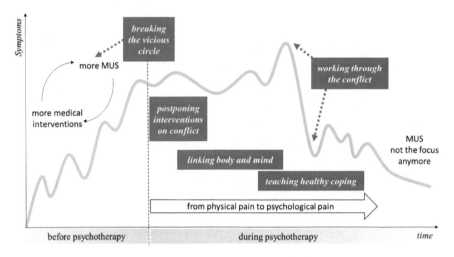

Fig. 3.2 Hypothetical timeline of the therapeutic process in patients with MUS

Reporting results of qualitative studies is a challenge of a special kind, as it should be both methodologically rigorous and at the same time the themes should be illustrative and appealing to the reader (Timulak & Elliott, 2019). While reporting the results of the metasynthesis of psychotherapy case studies, one could choose from different options, instead of reporting a mere code list/tree, since our ambition is to describe an unfolding dynamic process. An appealing solution could be the creation of an ideal-typical case story out of multiple cases as chosen by Keogh and Timulak (2015, June). In line with this idea, we decided to shape our report in the form of an ideal-typical/hypothetical timeline of the treatment, along which the themes unfold (see Fig. 3.2). The presented themes are not necessarily present in each case, but the overall pattern reflects our holistic understanding of the psychotherapy process unfolding over time in the sample.

Breaking the Vicious Cycle of Medical Interventions

Patients with MUS often seek multiple unnecessary medical investigations before they start psychotherapy. Thereby, the interventions sometimes become quite invasive and dramatic, and subsequently, the symptoms may worsen, or new (more dramatic) symptoms may emerge, leading to new and more invasive investigations [2, 4, 6],[2] as illustrated in the following example:

> During summer vacation […], his symptoms became markedly aggravated, and Niccolo complained of searing pain in his right ear and began to scream and moan in pain (from both of his ears) loudly and continuously while he was awake. Not even the slightest ear pathology could be identified. His anxious parents had him seen by multiple Italian and American

---

[2]The numbers in square brackets indicate the number of the case study in which the theme has been found from Appendix A.

specialists, but his endless moaning and complaints only worsened. He was admitted to a hospital in Milan, where he was treated with general anaesthesia (!)[3] in order to stop his moaning. Family anxiety ran high. When he awoke several days later, Niccolo's pain had worsened and he could no longer walk, despite having a normal neurological examination. He was discharged from the hospital in a wheelchair. (Milrod, 2002, pp. 624–625)

As a reaction, therapists may actively encourage stopping medical investigations and interventions, in order to break the vicious circle, and to prepare the ground for the psychotherapy [4, 6, 7, 8].

From Physical Pain to Psychological Pain

The grand trajectory of the psychotherapy process in our sample can be formulated as an *evolution from physical pain to psychological pain* (visualized as the big arrow in Fig. 3.2). During the therapy, patients who are initially focused on physical symptoms and resist linking their emotional state to MUS begin to discover feelings, and previously hidden conflicts become visible. Gradually, the focus shifts away from physical symptoms and the pain becomes a psychological one. This process may be accompanied by (sudden) changes in MUS.

At the beginning of the treatment patients may be exclusively focused on the physical symptoms, which constitutes the central point of their narrative and therapeutic request [2]. Patients initially refuse to link their emotional state to physical symptoms [4, 5, 7, 8]. In the course of the therapy, an almost ubiquitous pattern is the emergence of feelings [1, 3, 4, 5, 6, 7, 8, 10]. It is remarkable how many times the words 'feeling', 'emotion', and 'affect' are used in the narrative of the case studies. Feelings are often experienced by the patient for the first time in a long while. They cry for the first time in therapy [3] or feel angry for the first time [4]. Several therapists stress the value of undisturbed experiencing of emotion:

> […] interventions involved directly discussing her feelings using principles of acceptance. Hence, she learned how to accept her feelings for what they are, sit with her emotions, and mindfully and nonjudgmentally observe them dissipate. (Vranceanu et al., 2008, p. 249)

Talking about one's feelings may lead to a sudden increase in MUS [1, 5, 7]:

> In the next session, while talking about her regret for not doing anything that fateful night, Nayda immediately had a psychogenic convulsion. (Martínez-Taboas, 2005, p. 8)

At the same time, there are reports of a decrease in MUS after patients start to talk about their feelings [5]. It seems that changes in MUS in either direction can go along with the emergence of feelings [2, 5, 10]. Next to the emergence of feelings, the underlying conflict may emerge as the focus of the psychotherapy [1, 4, 7, 10].

---

[3]Punctuation by the author of the original paper.

At the end of the treatment, patients are better able to link their behavior, feelings and MUS [4, 5, 6, 7, 9].

Postponing Conflict Interventions

Several therapists decide to wait with conflict-oriented interventions at the start of treatment, in order to bypass the patient's resistance, to build the therapeutic alliance and trust, or to work on the deficit first [3, 4, 6, 7, 8]. Therapists often presume that a preparatory phase or a supportive approach might be necessary at the begin of the treatment:

> Key aspects of the preparatory phase with Kai included respecting the mind–body split as a primary defense, avoiding premature confrontation, listening and speaking the language of the body as well as the language of the mind [...]. (Shapiro, 2003, p. 448)

Validating the MUS experience could be seen as a crucial intervention to build rapport [9]. The therapist may choose to halt deeper-going interventions even despite the patient's wish and first give space and show respect to the symptom itself:

> [...] although she herself had indicated at the start that she wanted to understand the links between her physical symptoms and her psychological state, I accepted the actuality, the awfulness, of the bodily experiences in their own right, rather than diminishing them by hasty associations, or dynamic interpretations. (Holland, 1997, pp. 221–222)

Instead of confrontation, therapists may decide to stay close to patient's own illness attribution and explanatory model of the MUS [1, 2, 3, 4, 6, 7, 8, 9]. Only in one case the therapist decided for a conflict intervention at the beginning of the treatment, exploring an intense guilt conflict [1].

Working Through the Conflict

The majority of the authors see an (unconscious) internal conflict at the root of MUS [1, 2, 3, 4, 5, 6, 7] and some authors additionally search for a symbolic meaning to the MUS that represents this conflict [1, 4, 5, 6], as in the following example:

> Niccolo came from a musically focused family in which hearing and listening were highly valued (cathected) activities. It is not surprising that his conversion symptoms were aurally focused. (Milrod, 2002, p. 629)

Interestingly, on one occasion the authors do not report on the symbolic meaning of the MUS, although to our research group symbolic meaning appears present (persistent hand pain in a patient who has been raped, while her hands were bound) [5, p. 60].

During the treatment, patients become less defensive [1, 3, 5, 6] which gives space for the intervention on conflict. Working through the conflict happens as a confrontation or as a gradual discovery of the (unconscious) conflict [1, 4, 7] as in the following example:

I wish I could push the clock back to being a baby—maybe to last year when I was sick …
I hated being sick, but it was just me and my family … I felt protected, close, like a baby
would feel. [She abruptly looked at me, eyes wide and stunned.] You don't think that's why
I'm having trouble? (Shapiro, 2003, p. 554)

Subsequently, confrontation with conflict may go along with an increase in MUS, as
at the end of the session cited above:

Walking toward the door she slouched more, her face crumpled, she looked down and grabbed
her stomach. 'My stomach hurts', she whisper-wailed as she walked out the door. (Shapiro,
2003, p. 554)

Furthermore, five case studies describe a decline in MUS following conflict resolution. [1, 3, 4, 5, 6]. Overall, working through the conflict may be connected to both
increase and decrease in MUS (as indicated by arrows in Fig. 3.2).

Linking Body and Mind

The initial disconnection between body and mind is broadly addressed in the case
studies while using terms such as minimal symbolization [3] or alexithymia [2]. The
authors describe various ways in which linking body and mind is encouraged [3, 4,
7, 9]. For example, the therapist may use psychoeducation to explain that emotions
are common correlates of pain and can influence it [9], or point out to the patient
how he or she expresses feelings through the body [4]. The therapist may even use
writing tasks so as to teach the patient to express vague sensations ("I am smoking")
in a more concrete way:

For example, the therapist would type out several incomplete sentences for her to complete
and she would type several answers to each statement. Specifically, when asked how she
would express intense anger, she stated she would say, "I'm smokin'.[4]" As a result, several
lines that said, "I'm smokin'" were put on the computer and she completed the unfinished phrases. Her first response, for example, was I'm smokin' "because my life is being
destroyed" and her second was, "because my family didn't care to keep me home with them
and to find out or ask me what had happened." […] She eventually completed 45 "I'm
smokin'" statements without difficulty. (Ciano-Federoff & Sperry, 2005, p. 65)

The therapist may also introduce physical therapy next to psychotherapy in order
for the patient to get to a new way of relating to their own body, hence building a
mental picture of the body [7]. During the treatment, the body may also become
more present in the fantasies of the patient [6].

Teaching Healthy Coping

Several authors believe that MUS are influenced by maladaptive ways of coping, and
avoidance is often named as an important contributor to (the reinforcement of) MUS

---

[4]Spelling by the author of the original paper.

[9]. Teaching healthy coping may be then considered crucial intervention and lead to more empowerment:

> Jean also learned to cognitively reframe her pain-related negative thoughts. For example, when she noted thinking that 'pain is awful and overwhelming,' she learned to replace that thought with a more adaptive one: 'I can do many things in spite of pain.' This was a key session for Jean, as it changed the manner in which she construed herself. Instead of 'a victim of her pain,' Jean began to experience herself as someone who was learning and employing strategies to cope with her pain. (Vranceanu et al., 2008, p. 248)

Change in coping is considered a critical moment in the therapy in two cases [9, 10], but teaching different coping strategies is also widely described in the sample [1, 5, 8, 9, 10].

MUS Not the Focus Anymore

In line with the theme '*From physical pain to psychological pain*', talking about physical symptoms becomes less important for the patients at the end of the therapy [2, 3, 5, 7, 8, 9]. Instead, patients shift the focus toward current feelings, fantasies, relationships, and conflicts:

> While she still complained about her headaches, during this appointment, Anne's discussion was centered on her plans to transition her life after the divorce. Her headaches were not the main focus of the discussion. (Baslet & Hill, 2011, p. 105)

Even if the symptoms do not disappear completely, the patient may be less frightened of them or show more acceptance [9] and start focusing on other matters.

Disconfirmatory Findings as Facilitators of Theory-Building: Deficit, Conflict and Trauma

Contrary to our initial assumption, we could not interpret the material of case studies in the sample-based solely on our framework of *deficit* and *conflict*. In several passages, we encountered the logic of treating an 'underlying' mental condition instead of deficit or conflict, whereby MUS were considered 'side effects' of the comorbid condition [2, 10]. This was especially striking in the case of trauma.

While conducting qualitative analyses, the concept of *trauma* appeared so prominent in the narrative of several case studies that in our view it deserved a separate thematic category alongside *deficit* and *conflict*. In five case studies, we found a description of a traumatic event at the onset of the MUS, such as guilt-provoking suicide of a relative [1], prolonged adverse life events [3], rape and assault [5, 10] and war-related PTSD [8]. Therapists described implementing trauma-specific interventions such as exposure [1], which could not be directly categorized as deficit- or conflict-oriented. These findings are however very well in line with the current literature on MUS–trauma link (Van der Kolk, 2014). At this point, the research team

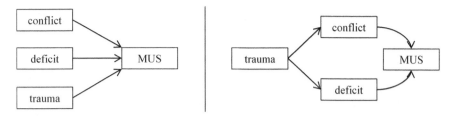

Fig. 3.3 Trauma as a third category alongside deficit and conflict vs. trauma underlying both deficit and conflict

can stop and go back to the initial research question, and for example, re-consider the categorization into *deficit*, *conflict* and *trauma* and re-analyze the data.

Another option would be to use this finding to deepen the theory-building on MUS by proposing possible connections between these categories for discussion. On the one hand, trauma could be seen as a third major component, contributing to the emergence of MUS alongside deficit and conflict (Fig. 3.3, left). On the other hand, trauma in itself may lead to both deficit (i.e. alexithymia; Zlotnick, Mattia, & Zimmerman, 2001) and conflict (PDM Task Force, 2006), as illustrated in Fig. 3.3, right. Although the question of causality cannot be answered within our research design, formulating new and sharpening old research questions may be a worthwhile aim to strive for in a theory-building metasynthesis.

Discussion

This chapter focused first of all on the decisions researchers can make during the stages of a metasynthesis of psychotherapy case studies. In our worked example, we decided to follow a non-exhaustive purposive sampling procedure and to focus on themes that are process-oriented. We used an explicit theoretical framework of deficit and conflict instead of 'allowing the material to speak for itself'. Thus, we mostly opted for 'unorthodox' decisions, which may be justified for the current research question, but not suitable for other research questions.

Our findings reflect the spirit of current integrative guidelines for psychotherapy for MUS, especially on themes such as postponing conflict interventions, encouraging healthy coping and mentalization (Dobersch et al., 2018; Roenneberg et al., 2018). Further, our findings emphasize the role of trauma in MUS that should be studied in-depth by means of qualitative research.

The major limitation of the current metasynthesis is that it included only successful or mixed-outcome cases, which is partially due to the publication bias in the field of single case studies (Desmet et al., 2013). Including cases with failure outcome could enrich our understanding of psychotherapy process and show different facets of deficit and conflict in the treatment of MUS.

In accordance with the recommendations by Jackson and colleagues (2011), our research team consisted of members with different backgrounds and levels of clinical expertise. The first author has been socialized in the clinical tradition of the German psychosomatic school and was previously working at a psychodynamic- and mindfulness-oriented clinic. While conducting the metasynthesis, the second author had not yet been exposed to clinical practice but shared the interest in psychodynamic approaches. The third author had an extensive experience as a Freudian-Lacanian psychoanalyst and supervisor. Thus, despite differences in background, all authors shared general psychodynamic/psychoanalytic spirit, which could have influenced the results. For example, it appeared that we approached cases of CBT treatment from the point of view of interpersonal dynamics first, and only then from the genuine perspective on learning processes, which lead to discovering the theme *'Teaching healthy coping'* rather later in the course of the project. Inclusion of an external team member from a cognitive-behavioral background could have promoted this insight at an earlier stage. In the absence of such a member, we tried to create as much alternative hypotheses and themes as possible to test the trustworthiness of out themes. Presenting the preliminary results on two interdisciplinary conferences and a workshop on MUS helped us to get more external input. Also, based on our experience, we strongly agree with Flyvbjerg (2006) on his point that case study research, by virtue of its rich material, is especially apt to disconfirm preconceptions of the researchers.

Our general experience of working in team was that of "convergence" toward the end of the process. Whereas initially the first and the second author had different ideas on handling the (theoretical) interpretations of the therapists, during the first year of work they reached consensus based on *critical realism* paradigm described earlier in this chapter. If discussions came up, they often centered around the issue of trustworthiness of therapist's selective rapportage. In one case, we decided to elaborate in our results section on such an (apparent to us) inconsistency in author's presentation, indicating that the authors of the case study missed to report symbolic/traumatic meaning of patient's MUS (Ciano-Federoff & Sperry, 2005, p. 60). Thereby, reaching consensus on an "anomaly" was something that appeared valuable in our eyes to test the overall replicability of our results. For researchers who attempt a metasynthesis on published cases studies, we would encourage alternating between being an "empathic reader" of the therapist/author (i.e., "How would I feel if I were in your skin as a therapist?") and an "advocatus diaboli", who would actively propose different explanations and mistrust the primary narrative of the therapist (Elliott, 2002).

Finally, we would like to point out that our experience of conducting the metasynthesis was very enriching from a professional perspective. We feel that while dealing with case material, one gains a more active and lively grip on the theories and findings in the field as compared to conducting a more traditional literature review. We would thus encourage young qualitative researchers to start approaching their subject by conducting a metasynthesis, before moving on to developing their own empirical studies.

Acknowledgements This work was supported by the German National Academic Foundation and the Hercules Foundation; the authors declare no conflict of interest.

Appendix A: List of Selected Studies with Characteristics of Patients

The numbers in square brackets [ ] in the text of the manuscript refer to the order in which the case studies were analyzed. The cases were analyzed in the following order: [1] Martínez-Taboas (2005); [2] Baslet and Hill (2011); [3] Holland (1997); [4] Milrod (2002); [5] Ciano-Federoff and Sperry (2005); [6] Küchenhoff (1998); [7] Shapiro (2003); [8] Jacobs and Dinoff (2012); [9] Vranceanu et al. (2008); [10] Weaver et al. (1998).

Study	Country	Patient Name	Age	Sex	Somatic symptoms	Other symptoms	Onset of (somatic) symptoms	Period of symptom onset before therapy	Type of therapy	Inpatient/outpatient	Frequency and duration of therapy
1 Martínez-Taboas (2005)	Puerto Rico	Nayda	24	F	Psychogenic seizures	Memory loss	Traumatic event witnessing the house of her grandmother on fire without calling for help	>5 years	CBT; hypnosis	Outpatient	22 sessions
2 Baslet & Hill (2011)	USA	Anne	31	F	Conversion disorder: psychogenic seizures, headaches, paralysis, tremor; fibromyalgia	Depression, anxiety, dissociation	Onset in late childhood, but exacerbation after hysterectomy	>10 years	ACT; MBT	Outpatient and inpatient	/
3 Holland (1997)	UK	Ruth	adult	F	Chronic fatigue syndrome (CFS)/myalgic encephalomyelitis (ME): extreme fatigue, muscle pains, palpitations, insomnia		After developing influenza, being confronted with her father having a life-threatening illness and feeling abandoned by her mother		Psychodynamic psychotherapy	Outpatient	2–3 sessions a week/3 years

(continued)

(continued)

	Study	Country	Patient Name	Age	Sex	Somatic symptoms	Other symptoms	Onset of (somatic) symptoms	Period of symptom onset before therapy	Type of therapy	Inpatient/outpatient	Frequency and duration of therapy
4	Milrod (2002)	USA	Niccolo	9	M	Conversion disorder: tussis nervosa, pain in the ears, inability to walk		/	4 months	Psychoanalysis	Outpatient	4 sessions a week/4 years
5	Ciano-Federoff and Sperry (2005)	USA	Amy	36	F	Conversion disorder: hand pain, numbness in hand, sores from contact dermatitis	PTSD, dysthymia	/		CBT: Exposure-Based Therapy for PTSD	Outpatient	10 months + 19 sessions Exposure-Based Therapy
6	Küchenhoff (1998)	Germany	Mrs. X	adult	F	Diarrhea, expiratory bronchial spasm, allergic rhinitis		After moving in with boyfriend		Psychotherapy + psychoanalysis	Outpatient	1 year + 4 years
7	Shapiro (2003)	USA	Kai	13	F	Fibromyalgia: total body pain	Fatigue	/		Psychotherapy + psychoanalysis	Outpatient	1 session a week/3 years
8	Jacobs and Dinoff (2012)	USA	David	90s	M	Undifferentiated somatization disorder (USD): high blood pressure, muscle weakness, malaise, and locking knee joints	Anxiety, depression, dementia, PTSD?	After serving the country in World War II	>10 years	CBT, ACT	Inpatient (nursing home)	not mentioned

(continued)

(continued)

	Study	Country	Patient			Somatic symptoms	Other symptoms	Onset of (somatic) symptoms	Period of symptom onset before therapy	Type of therapy	Inpatient/outpatient	Frequency and duration of therapy
			Name	Age	Sex							
9	Vranceanu et al. (2008)	USA	Jean	40s	F	Idiopathic arm pain		Pain started when trying to put a 30-pound box on a shelf, but no fracture of dislocation was observed	2 months	CBT	Outpatient	8 sessions
			Laura	40s	F	Idiopathic arm and hand pain, mild headaches, fatigue		/	3 years	CBT	Outpatient	8 sessions
10	Weaver et al. (1998)	USA	Jane	34	F	Irritable bowel syndrome	Depression, anxiety attacks, PTSD	Multiple traumatic events	12 years	CBT: prolonged exposure	Outpatient	9 sessions

References

References marked with an asterisk indicate included in the metasynthesis.

Abbass, A., Grantmyre, J., & Kay, R. L. (2013). Anxiety related to sexual abuse: A case of recurrent priapism. *Canadian Urological Association Journal, 7*(1–2), 48–50. https://doi.org/10.5489/cua j.233.

Aggarwal, V. R., McBeth, J., Zakrzewska, J. M., Lunt, M., & Macfarlane, G. J. (2006). The epidemiology of chronic syndromes that are frequently unexplained: Do they have common associated factors? *International Journal of Epidemiology, 35*(2), 468–476. https://doi.org/10.1093/ije/dyi265.

Barsky, A. J., Orav, E. J., & Bates, D. W. (2005). Somatization increases medical utilization and costs independent of psychiatric and medical comorbidity. *Archives of General Psychiatry, 62*(8), 903–910. https://doi.org/10.1001/archpsyc.62.8.903.

*Baslet, G., & Hill, J. (2011). Case report: Brief mindfulness-based psychotherapeutic intervention during inpatient hospitalization in a patient with conversion and dissociation. *Clinical Case Studies, 10*(2), 95–109. https://doi.org/10.1177/1534650110396359.

Benoot, C., Hannes, K., & Bilsen, J. (2016). The use of purposeful sampling in a qualitative evidence synthesis: A worked example on sexual adjustment to a cancer trajectory. *BMC Medical Research Methodology, 16*(1), 21–32. https://doi.org/10.1186/s12874-016-0114-6.

Bohart, A. C. (1991). The missing 249 words: In search of objectivity. *Psychotherapy, 28*(3), 497–503. https://doi.org/10.1037/0033-3204.28.3.497.

Bronstein, C. (2011). On psychosomatics: The search for meaning. *The International Journal of Psychoanalysis, 92*(1), 173–195. https://doi.org/10.1111/j.1745-8315.2010.00388.x.

Brown, R. J. (2004). Psychological mechanisms of medically unexplained symptoms: An integrative conceptual model. *Psychological Bulletin, 130*(5), 793–812. https://doi.org/10.1037/0033-2909.130.5.793.

Carson, A. J., Best, S., Postma, K., Stone, J., Warlow, C., & Sharpe, M. (2003). The outcome of neurology outpatients with medically unexplained symptoms: A prospective cohort study. *Journal of Neurology, Neurosurgery and Psychiatry, 74*(7), 897–900. https://doi.org/10.1136/jnnp.74.7.897.

*Ciano-Federoff, L. M., & Sperry, J. A. (2005). On "converting" hand pain into psychological pain: Treating hand pain vicariously through exposure-based therapy for PTSD. *Clinical Case Studies, 4*(1), 57–71. https://doi.org/10.1177/1534650103259673.

Connor-Greene, P. A. (1993). The therapeutic context: Preconditions for change in psychotherapy. *Psychotherapy, 30*(3), 375–382. https://doi.org/10.1037/0033-3204.30.3.375.

Creed, F. (2016). Exploding myths about medically unexplained symptoms. *Journal of Psychosomatic Research, 85,* 91–93. https://doi.org/10.1016/j.jpsychores.2016.02.007.

De Waal, M. W., Arnold, I. A., Eekhof, J. A., & Van Hemert, A. M. (2004). Somatoform disorders in general practice. *The British Journal of Psychiatry, 184*(6), 470–476. https://doi.org/10.1192/bjp.184.6.470.

Denzin, N. K., & Lincoln, Y. S. (2005). *The Sage handbook of qualitative research* (3rd ed.). Thousand Oaks, CA: Sage.

Derksen, J. J. L. (2012). *Bevrijd de psychologie uit de greep van de hersenmythe* [Free psychology from the brain mythos]. Amsterdam: Uitgeverij Bert Bakker.

Desmet, M. (2018). *The pursuit of objectivity in psychology.* Ghent: Owl Press.

Desmet, M., Meganck, R., Seybert, C., Willemsen, J., Van Camp, I., Geerardyn, F., … Kächele, H. (2013). Psychoanalytic single cases published in ISI-ranked journals: The construction of an online archive. *Psychotherapy and Psychosomatics, 82*(2), 120–121. https://doi.org/10.1159/000 342019.

Dickson-Swift, V., James, E. L., Kippen, S., & Liamputtong, P. (2007). Doing sensitive research: What challenges do qualitative researchers face? *Qualitative Research, 7*(3), 327–353. https://doi.org/10.1177/1468794107078515.

Dobersch, J., Grosse Holtforth, M., & Egle, U. T. (2018). Interaktionelle Gruppentherapie bei stressinduzierten Schmerzstörungen [Interactional group therapy for stress-induced pain disorders]. *Psychotherapeut, 63*(3), 226–234. https://doi.org/10.1007/s00278-017-0266-9.

Elliott, R. (2002). Hermeneutic single-case efficacy design. *Psychotherapy Research, 12*(1), 1–21. https://doi.org/10.1093/ptr/12.1.1.

Fink, P., Sørensen, L., Engberg, M., Holm, M., & Munk-Jørgensen, P. (1999). Somatization in primary care: Prevalence, health care utilization, and general practitioner recognition. *Psychosomatics, 40*(4), 330–338. https://doi.org/10.1016/s0033-3182(99)71228-4.

Fishman, D. B. (2013). The pragmatic case study method for creating rigorous and systematic, practitioner-friendly research. *Pragmatic Case Studies in Psychotherapy, 9*(4). https://doi.org/10.14713/pcsp.v9i4.1833.

Flyvbjerg, B. (2006). Five misunderstandings about case-study research. *Qualitative Inquiry, 12*, 219–245.

Hannes, K., & Pearson, A. (2011). Obstacles to the implementation of evidence-based practice in Belgium: A worked example of meta-aggregation. In K. Hannes & C. Lockwood (Eds.), *Synthesizing qualitative research: Choosing the right approach*. Hoboken, NJ: Wiley.

Hannon, D. (2018). *Deficit and conflict in the psychotherapeutic treatment of medically unexplained symptoms: A meta-synthesis of published case studies* (Unpublished master's thesis). Ghent University, Ghent, Belgium.

Hayes, A. M., Laurenceau, J.-P., Feldman, G., Strauss, J. L., & Cardaciotto, L. (2007). Change is not always linear: The study of nonlinear and discontinuous patterns of change in psychotherapy. *Clinical Psychology Review, 27*(6), 715–723. https://doi.org/10.1016/j.cpr.2007.01.008.

Henningsen, P., Zipfel, S., & Herzog, W. (2007). Management of functional somatic syndromes. *The Lancet, 369*(9565), 946–955. https://doi.org/10.1016/s0140-6736(07)60159-7.

*Holland, P. (1997). Coniunctio—In bodily and psychic modes: Dissociation, devitalization and integration in a case of chronic fatigue syndrome. *Journal of Analytic Psychology, 42*(2), 217–236. https://doi.org/10.1111/j.1465-5922.1997.00217.x.

Hoon, C. (2013). Meta-synthesis of qualitative case studies: An approach to theory building. *Organizational Research Methods, 16*(4), 522–556. https://doi.org/10.4135/9781473915480.n57.

Husain, K., Browne, T., & Chalder, T. (2007). A review of psychological models and interventions for medically unexplained somatic symptoms in children. *Child and Adolescent Mental Health, 12*(1), 2–7. https://doi.org/10.1111/j.1475-3588.2006.00419.x.

Iwakabe, S., & Gazzola, N. (2009). From single-case studies to practice-based knowledge: Aggregating and synthesizing case studies. *Psychotherapy Research, 19*(4–5), 601–611. https://doi.org/10.1080/10503300802688494.

Jackson, J. L., Chui, H. T., & Hill, C. E. (2011). The modification of consensual qualitative research for case study research: An introduction to CQR-C. In C. E. Hill (Ed.), *Consensual qualitative research: Practical resources for investigating social science phenomena* (pp. 285–303). Washington, DC: American Psychological Association.

*Jacobs, L., & Dinoff, B. (2012). War-related somatoform disorder in an older adult veteran. *Clinical Case Studies, 11*(5), 376–392. https://doi.org/10.1177/1534650112461848.

Kächele, H., Albani, C., Buchheim, A., Hölzer, M., Hohage, R., Mergenthaler, E., … Thomä, H. (2006). The German specimen case, Amalia X: Empirical studies. *The International Journal of Psychoanalysis, 87*(3), 809–826. https://doi.org/10.1516/17nn-m9hj-u25a-yuu5.

Keogh, D., & Timulak, L. (2015, June). *The process of emotional transformation in emotion-focused therapy treatments for depression and anxiety: A meta-synthesis of four single case-studies*. Paper presented at the 46th International Annual Meeting of the Society for Psychotherapy Research, Philadelphia, PA.

Kroenke, K., & Mangelsdorff, A. D. (1989). Common symptoms in ambulatory care: Incidence, evaluation, therapy, and outcome. *The American Journal of Medicine, 86*(3), 262–266. https://doi.org/10.1016/0002-9343(89)90293-3.

*Küchenhoff, J. (1998). The body and the ego boundaries: A case study on psychoanalytic therapy with psychosomatic patients. *Psychoanalytic Inquiry, 18*(3), 368–382. https://doi.org/10.1080/07351699809534198.

Lambert, M. J. (2013). Introduction and historical overview. In M. J. Lambert (Ed.), *Bergin and Garfield's handbook of psychotherapy and behaviour change* (6th ed., pp. 3–20). Hoboken, NJ: Wiley.

Liberati, A., Altman, D. G., Tetzlaff, J., Mulrow, C., Gøtzsche, P. C., Ioannidis, J. P. A., … Moher, D. (2009). The PRISMA statement for reporting systematic reviews and meta-analyses of studies that evaluate health care interventions: Explanation and elaboration. *PLoS Medicine, 6*(7), e1000100. https://doi.org/10.1371/journal.pmed.1000100.

Lind, A. B., Delmar, C., & Nielsen, K. (2014). Struggling in an emotional avoidance culture: A qualitative study of stress as a predisposing factor for somatoform disorders. *Journal of Psychosomatic Research, 76*(2), 94–98. https://doi.org/10.1016/j.jpsychores.2013.11.019.

Lockwood, C., Porrit, K., Munn, Z., Rittenmeyer, L., Salmond, S., Bjerrum, M., … Stannard, D. (2017). Chapter 2: Systematic reviews of qualitative evidence. In E. Aromataris & Z. Munn (Eds.), *Joanna Briggs Institute reviewer's manual*. The Joanna Briggs Institute. Retrieved from https://reviewersmanual.joannabriggs.org/.

Luyten, P., Van Houdenhove, B., Lemma, A., Target, M., & Fonagy, P. (2012). A mentalization-based approach to the understanding and treatment of functional somatic disorders. *Psychoanalytic Psychotherapy, 26*(2), 121–140. https://doi.org/10.1080/02668734.2012.678061.

*Martínez-Taboas, A. (2005). Psychogenic seizures in an espiritismo context: The role of culturally sensitive psychotherapy. *Psychotherapy: Theory, Research, Practice, Training, 42*(1), 6–13. https://doi.org/10.1037/0033-3204.42.1.6.

McLeod, J., & Elliott, R. (2011). Systematic case study research: A practice-oriented introduction to building an evidence base for counselling and psychotherapy. *Counselling and Psychotherapy Research, 11*(1), 1–10.

Meganck, R., Desmet, M., Inslegers, R., Krivzov, J., Notaerts, L., & Willemsen, J. (2017). *Inventory of basic information in single cases (IBISC) manual*. Retrieved January 21, 2019, from https://singlecasearchive.com/downloads/IBISC%20manual4.pdf.

*Milrod, B. (2002). A 9-year-old with conversion disorder, successfully treated with psychoanalysis. *The International Journal of Psychoanalysis, 83*(3), 623–631. https://doi.org/10.1516/1f8k-t4cj-vl37-uffl.

Morton, S., Berg, A., Levit, L., & Eden, J. (2011). *Finding what works in health care: Standards for systematic reviews*. Washington, DC: National Academies Press.

Norcross, J. C., & Alexander, E. F. (2019). A primer on psychotherapy integration. In J. C. Norcross & M. R. Goldfried (Eds.), *Handbook of psychotherapy integration* (2nd ed., pp. 3–27). Oxford: Oxford University Press.

olde Hartman, T. C., Borghuis, M. S., Lucassen, P. L., van de Laar, F. A., Speckens, A. E., & van Weel, C. (2009). Medically unexplained symptoms, somatisation disorder and hypochondriasis: Course and prognosis: A systematic review. *Journal of Psychosomatic Research, 66*(5), 363–377. https://doi.org/10.1016/j.jpsychores.2008.09.018.

Open Science Collaboration. (2015). Estimating the reproducibility of psychological science. *Science, 349*(6251), aac4716. https://doi.org/10.1126/science.aac4716.

Paterson, B. L. (2012). "It looks great but how do I know if it fits?": An introduction to meta-synthesis research. In K. Hannes & C. Lockwood (Eds.), *Synthesizing qualitative research: Choosing the right approach*. Chichester: Wiley.

PDM Task Force. (2006). *Psychodynamic diagnostic manual* (1st ed.). Silver Spring, MD: Alliance of Psychoanalytic Organizations.

Reid, S., Wessely, S., Crayford, T. I., & Hotopf, M. (2002). Frequent attenders with medically unexplained symptoms: Service use and costs in secondary care. *The British Journal of Psychiatry, 180*(3), 248–253. https://doi.org/10.1192/bjp.180.3.24.

Roenneberg, C., Hausteiner-Wiehle, C., Schäfert, R., Sattel, H., Henningsen P., et al. (2018). *S3 Leitlinie "Funktionelle Körperbeschwerden"* [S3 Guideline "Functional Somatic Complaints"].

Retrieved May 21, 2019, from https://www.awmf.org/uploads/tx_szleitlinien/051-0011_S3_Funk tionelle_Koerperbeschwerden_2018-11.pdf.

Röhricht, F. (2009). Body oriented psychotherapy: The state of the art in empirical research and evidence-based practice: A clinical perspective. *Body, Movement and Dance in Psychotherapy, 4*(2), 135–156. https://doi.org/10.1080/17432970902857263.

Salmon, P., Dowrick, C. F., Ring, A., & Humphris, G. M. (2004). Voiced but unheard agendas: Qualitative analysis of the psychosocial cues that patients with unexplained symptoms present to general practitioners. *British Journal of General Practice, 54*(500), 171–176.

Schonbar, R. A., & Beatus, H. R. (1990). The mysterious metamorphoses of Bertha Papenheim: Anna O. revisited. *Psychoanalytic psychology, 7*(1), 59–78. https://doi.org/10.1037/0736-9735. 7.1.59.

*Shapiro, B. (2003). Building bridges between body and mind: The analysis of an adolescent with paralyzing chronic pain. *The International Journal of Psychoanalysis, 84*(3), 547–561. https:// doi.org/10.1516/rm8h-aef8-galp-3m5n.

Shedler, J., Mayman, M., & Manis, M. (1993). The illusion of mental health. *American Psychologist, 48,* 1117–1131. https://doi.org/10.1037//0003-066x.48.11.1117.

Sims-Schouten, W., Riley, S. C., & Willig, C. (2007). Critical realism in discourse analysis: A presentation of a systematic method of analysis using women's talk of motherhood, childcare and female employment as an example. *Theory & Psychology, 17*(1), 101–124.

Spaanjaars, N. L., Groenier, M., van de Ven, M. O. M., & Witteman, C. L. M. (2015). Experience and diagnostic anchors in referral letters. *European Journal of Psychological Assessment, 31*(4), 280–286. https://doi.org/10.1027/1015-5759/a000235.

Stiles, W. B. (2015). Theory-building, enriching, and fact-gathering: Alternative purposes of psychotherapy research. In O. Gelo, A. Pritz, & B. Rieken (Eds.), *Psychotherapy research: General issues, process and outcome* (pp. 159–179). New York: Springer-Verlag.

Timulak, L. (2009). Qualitative meta-analysis: A tool for reviewing qualitative research findings in psychotherapy. *Psychotherapy Research, 19*(4–5), 591–600. https://doi.org/10.1080/105033008 02477989.

Timulak, L. (2010). Significant events in psychotherapy: An update of research findings. *Psychology and Psychotherapy: Theory, Research and Practice, 83*(4), 421–447.

Timulak, L., & Elliott, R. (2019). Taking stock of descriptive–interpretative qualitative psychotherapy research: Issues and observations from the front line. *Counselling and Psychotherapy Research, 19*(1), 8–15.

Thomas, J., & Harden, A. (2008). Methods for the thematic synthesis of qualitative research in systematic reviews. *BMC Medical Research Methodology, 8*(1), 45–54. https://doi.org/10.1186/ 1471-2288-8-45.

Thorne, S. (2019). On the evolving world of what constitutes qualitative synthesis. *Qualitative Health Research, 29*(1), 3–6.

Toomela, A. (2008). Variables in psychology: A critique of quantitative psychology. *Integrative Psychological and Behavioral Science, 42*(3), 245–265.

Van der Kolk, B. (2014). *The body keeps the score: Mind, brain and body in the transformation of trauma.* London, UK: Penguin Books.

van Ravesteijn, H., Grutters, J., olde Hartman, T., Lucassen, P., Bor, H., van Weel, C., ... Speckens, A. (2013). Mindfulness-based cognitive therapy for patients with medically unexplained symptoms: A cost-effectiveness study. *Journal of Psychosomatic Research, 74*(3), 197–205.

Vanheule, S., Desmet, M., Meganck, R., & Bogaerts, S. (2007). Alexithymia and interpersonal problems. *Journal of Clinical Psychology, 63*(1), 109–117.

Verhaeghe, P. (2004). *On being normal and other disorders: A manual for clinical psychodiagnostics.* New York, NY, USA: Other Press Llc.

*Vranceanu, A.-M., Ring, D., Kulich, R., Zhao, M., Cowan, J., & Safren, S. (2008). Idiopathic hand and arm pain: Delivering cognitive behavioral therapy as part of a multidisciplinary team in a surgical practice. *Cognitive and Behavioral Practice, 15*(3), 244–254. https://doi.org/10.1016/j. cbpra.2007.04.003.

Waller, E., & Scheidt, C. E. (2004). Somatoform disorders as disorders of affect regulation: A study comparing the TAS-20 with non-self-report measures of alexithymia. *Journal of psychosomatic research, 57*(3), 239–247.

Waller, E., Scheidt, C. E., & Hartmann, A. (2004). Attachment representation and illness behavior in somatoform disorders. *The Journal of Nervous and Mental Disease, 192*(3), 200–209.

*Weaver, T. L., Nishith, P., & Resick, P. A. (1998). Prolonged exposure therapy and irritable bowel syndrome: A case study examining the impact of a trauma-focused treatment on a physical condition. *Cognitive and Behavioral Practice, 5*(1), 103–122. https://doi.org/10.1016/s1077-722 9(98)80023-0.

Willemsen, J., Inslegers, R., Meganck, R., Geerardyn, F., Desmet, M., & Vanheule, S. (2015). A metasynthesis of published case studies through Lacan's L-schema: Transference in perversion. *International Journal of Psychoanalysis, 96*(3), 773–795.

Witthöft, M., & Hiller, W. (2010). Psychological approaches to origins and treatments of somatoform disorders. *Annual Review of Clinical Psychology, 6*(1), 257–283.

Zlotnick, C., Mattia, J. I., & Zimmerman, M. (2001). The relationship between posttraumatic stress disorder, childhood trauma and in an outpatient sample. *Journal of Traumatic Stress, 14*(1), 177–188.

Zook, C. J., & Moore, F. D. (1980). High-cost users of medical care. *New England Journal of Medicine, 302*(18), 996–1002. https://doi.org/10.1056/nejm198005013021804.

Chapter 4
Walking Interviews: A Novel Way of Ensuring the Voices of Vulnerable Populations Are Included in Research

Penelope Kinney

Abstract Including the voices of clients who live with major mental illness is paramount if researchers are truly trying to understand their worlds, however, there are challenges to overcome. Living with major mental illness often affects a person's ability to hold spontaneous conversation. A person may sit passively during a traditional talking interview, waiting for guidance on how to answer questions. To overcome these impediments alternative methods of data collection outside of the traditional qualitative interview should be used to facilitate dialogue while keeping the client safe. Walking interviews are a novel approach that can be used to overcome some of these challenges. The use of walking interviews (where the interviewer walks alongside the participant) as a method of collecting data is increasing. The walking interview also provides insights into the connections between the participant and their community. While sitting comfortably in a chair these connections may not easily be described. While walking alongside a participant in a familiar environment the interviewer can gain insight into a sense of alienation or connection the interviewee has with their community. Though mobile interviewing is still at the infant stage as a methodology, it does shed light on how individuals frame and understand the spaces and places they use in their lives. This chapter will explore the relevance of walking interviews when including vulnerable populations, such as clients within forensic mental health services, into qualitative research and provide insights into how this novel method can successfully be included into qualitative research.

Keywords Walking interview · Mobile interviewing · Forensic mental health · Vulnerable populations · Community connections

P. Kinney (✉)
School of Occupational Therapy, Otago Polytechnic | Te Kura Matatini ki Otago, Forth Street, Private Bag 1910, Dunedin Campus, Dunedin 9054, New Zealand
e-mail: Penelope.Kinney@op.ac.nz

© Springer Nature Switzerland AG 2021
M. Borcsa and C. Willig (eds.), *Qualitative Research Methods in Mental Health*,
https://doi.org/10.1007/978-3-030-65331-6_4

Introduction

It was during the development of the qualitative research project for my Ph.D. that I explored a range of possible data collection methods I might use with my client participants, who were within a regional forensic psychiatric service in New Zealand. I was aware, from my previous experience of working for six years as an occupational therapist within forensic psychiatric services, living with major mental illness often affects a person's ability to hold spontaneous conversation. A person may sit passively during traditional qualitative talking interviews, waiting for guidance on how to answer questions. I looked to find if there was another option that would allow the client participants to engage in a way that was familiar to them, and would not put undue pressure on them to speak continuously. I came across the walking interview. Walking interviews (where the researcher walks alongside the participant) are a novel approach that can be used to overcome some of the challenges experienced by clients of mental health services within the context of a research interview. The research discussed within this chapter focuses on forensic psychiatric clients' experience of transitioning from hospital to living in the community, and as this was their story, they needed to be part of the research. The research was based on the assumption that if forensic psychiatric clients' voices are to be part of research then the data collection methods used needed to be ones that they could engage with. Walking alongside a clinician was a familiar experience for the clients, as this was often the first way a person was able to access the world outside of the hospital ward. The choice to use walking interviews was based on this.

The chapter begins by providing a brief overview of the research that was conducted and why the walking interview was explored. The walking interview is then outlined, the strengths it brings to research, and then the three types of walking interviews, the go-along, bimbling and participatory walking interviews used are presented. The advantages and insights produced by these interviews, along with the challenges and limitations associated with the method, are also presented. The chapter finishes by overviewing a range of considerations that researchers must take into account if they are to use these types of interviews.

Transitioning from Hospital to the Community

The process of transition occurs throughout life for every human being. People transition from adolescence to adulthood, student to worker; they move geographical locations and adjust to a disease or accident. These transitions may be voluntary or be forced upon us; whichever way, it is a process to be gone through. Help with this process comes in many forms and is often sought by the person undergoing the change, especially if they recognise they are experiencing challenges while going through it.

People in forensic psychiatric services, like the majority of the population, undergo a variety of transitions. Many are forced upon them and their perception, often based on reality, is that they have limited control over these processes. Moving to the community after significant periods of time in psychiatric hospitals is challenging for the majority of those making this transition (Coffey, 2012b; Grusky, Tierney, Manderscheid, & Grusky, 1985). Leaving the support and structure of a ward, managing budgets and adapting to new accommodation are just a few of the process those leaving hospital have to make that can be challenging (Nolan, Bradley, & Brimblecombe, 2011). Transitioning from a hospital setting to the community requires a person to be aware of the changes occurring and to be able to adapt to the ways of doing a task, as well as to how they think about it. For example, in hospital, meals are usually selected from menus and eaten at times when the delivery truck arrives. When clients return to the community, they are required to budget to ensure they can afford the food for meals they will now need to plan and cook for themselves and eat at times that they choose.

Information relating to transitions for clients within a forensic psychiatric service is scarce. There is an acknowledgement by a range of authors that there is very little literature available regarding moving forensic psychiatric clients to the community. Focus of past research has centred on risk and recidivism and very little related to how forensic psychiatric clients attempted to adapt and transition towards a non-deviant lifestyle (Bjørkly, 2004; Coffey, 2012a; Jamieson, Taylor, & Gibson, 2006; Kaliski, 1997; Viljoen, Nicholls, Greaves, de Ruiter, & Brink, 2011).

There are many challenges when moving an individual from hospital to the community that confronts the clinical team. Needing to treat and return an individual to the community while protecting that community from potential harm can often cause conflict for health professionals (Kaliski, 1997). Successful transitions for those people within forensic psychiatric services into the community are important not only to ensure safety of the community but to ensure the individual themselves has a meaningful and productive life (Gerber et al., 2003; Gustafsson, Holm, & Flensner, 2012). The literature explored used the voice of the client sparingly. A number of challenges were identified by researchers who did attempt to include clients' voices and those authors called for future research that included clients' narratives (Coffey, 2006; Jamieson et al., 2006; Livingston, 2018; Völlm, Foster, Bates, & Huband, 2017). Therefore, the project that I completed, that explored how clients within forensic psychiatric services transitioned back into the community, needed to include the voice of the client (Kinney, 2018a). To ensure the clients' voice was included I utilised a data collection method that the client participants were able to engage with. This chapter is primarily focused on introducing and discussing a method of data collection that is suitable to use with mental health client participants, it will not discuss the method of data analysis used in the project.

The Walking Interview

The Mobilities Paradigm (Sheller & Urry, 2006) has developed over recent years, gaining support across multiple disciplines. With an increasing interest in aspects of life that are mobile and the desire to explore the link between self and place the new mobility paradigm is continuing to gain attention (Evans & Jones, 2011; Hein, Evans, & Jones, 2008). Located predominantly within geographical literature (Anderson, 2004; Evans & Jones, 2011; Holton & Riley, 2014) the use of walking interviews (where the researcher walks alongside the participant) as a method of collecting data has also increased over the past number of years by social scientists (Butler & Derrett, 2014; Carpiano, 2009; Clark & Emmel, 2010; Hall, Lashua, & Coffey, 2006; Jones, Bunce, Evans, Gibbs, & Hein, 2008; Kinney, 2018a; Kusenbach, 2003).

Though mobile interviewing could still be regarded as developing, it does show great potential for providing insight into how individuals structure and engage with the spaces they use in their lives (Jones et al., 2008). Interest is developing in methods that challenge the traditional sedentary nature of social research (Sheller & Urry, 2006) and the walking interview helps address that challenge.

Walking alongside the participant, the researcher can gain insights into the participants' connection to their world, both physical and social (Evans & Jones, 2011). The walking interview provides the researcher with an opportunity to gain access to the participants' attitudes and knowledge about their environment and the connection or alienation they have to the social networks they have within it (Clark & Emmel, 2010). The walking interview can be an iterative process. The participants' narratives regarding their experiences of place can be challenged and restructured, thus making the walking interview an opportunity to explore how experiences are altered and re-constructed over time (Holton & Riley, 2014), making engaging with the participants' understanding of place easier. By walking alongside a participant in a familiar environment, engaging in a usual routine, the researcher can gain insight into the participants' physical capacity, where a description in a sit-down interview may not sufficiently represent their reality (Butler & Derrett, 2014), for example, observing a person's fitness level when walking to and from an appointment, rather than taking the bus. The walking interview provides opportunities to explore issues the participant may have in relation to the space (Jones et al., 2008), for example, access and mobility concerns or lack of opportunity for social connection.

Participants within sedentary interviews can drift from a topic when their knowledge on the given area has been exhausted. Participants, during walking interviews, tend to talk more spontaneously about the place they are walking through. More specific information regarding place is produced as the researcher can ask specific questions in response to the participants' engagement during the walking interview (Evans & Jones, 2011). By being outside of the traditional formal research format, the walking interview can also improve the participants' comfortability with taking part in research, the power imbalance is reduced because the researcher is walking alongside a participant, rather than sitting looking at the person (Trell & Van Hoven, 2010). Talk often becomes easier when walking, the natural occurrences when walking replace the unnatural pauses that happen in a sedentary interview. Participants are not required to maintain constant conversation and pauses are an expected part of the walking interview. Crossing the road, walking up a hill, turning a corner are natural pauses that allow the conversation to be brought back to the everyday (Hall et al., 2006).

Three types of walking interviews are outlined below. Each was used within the research conducted. They are the go-along interviews, bimbling interviews and the participatory interviews.

Go-Along Interview

The go-along is regarded as a mix between an interview and participant observation. During the outing, the researcher is asking questions, listening and observing the participant as they go about their usual routines (Kusenbach, 2003). The go-along interview has been identified as a unique qualitative method that can be used to study health issues in the local environment (Carpiano, 2009). The go-along is a distinctive tool that can be used to meet a number of challenges that are present within health and place literature. It can be used to examine the physical, social and emotional dimensions of place and how they interact with each other for an individual over time (Carpiano, 2009).

The go-along interview occurs when the researcher accompanies a participant on an outing that would normally occur, even if the researcher was not there. It is important that during these go-alongs the researcher is following participants in their natural environment, completing their normal routines and ensuring these are occurring on the usual day, at the usual time and following the usual route they would normally take (Kusenbach, 2003). The go-along can be conducted via walking (walk-along) or by driving (ride-along) or a mixture of both (Kusenbach, 2003).

"Unusual" walks have been used with participants in the past where the walk is not based on what the participant would normally do however, the process of just walking with the participant was found to be useful. The action of walking promoted a connection with the surrounding environment, it allowed an understanding of place by exploring the route participants took and it enabled the creation of social connections (Hein et al., 2008). However, Kusenbach (2003) views these types of go-alongs as contrived social situations as the researcher is disrupting the normal pattern of how the participant interacts with the environment.

The interview structure of the go-along can follow a similar structure to that of a sit-down interview. An open-ended format allows participants the freedom to speak about what they would like to say. Only little direction regarding points to discuss is offered by the researcher, such as pointing out a nearby feature so as to hear the participant's thoughts on that feature. A semi-structured format comprises of both prepared and ad hoc questions. The researcher heads out on the go-along with a list of prepared questions they want to ensure they will get answered. As the interview progresses, further questions will be identified. This format is thought to be more conversational (Carpiano, 2009).

The go-along interview is viewed as a more inclusive process (as opposed to the sit-down interview) because the participant engages in the interview, which is more of a partnership rather than just being a subject who is being interviewed (Carpiano, 2009). The go-along works to reduce the power imbalance, especially in marginalised populations, as the participant works as a tour guide, deciding what is important and should be shared with the researcher (Carpiano, 2009). The go-along interview also works well with Photovoice (Wang & Burris, 1997) as it can help bring about community change. The use of photos and subsequent narratives can have powerful effects when shown to policy makers. The photos can be either taken by the participant or taken by the researcher but at the direction of the participant. It is always preferable to have the participant take the photo however there are times when this may not be possible or appropriate. Whenever a photo is taken, the participant should be asked to explain why that particular object was the focus of the photo (Carpiano, 2009).

Bimbling Interview

Evans (1998) has described the practice of going for a walk to blow off steam as bimbling, that is, walking or wandering with no clear aim. Bimbling has now been used as a method for collecting data in qualitative research, mainly when exploring environmental activism and when there is a need to remove the participant away from an environment which is politicised due to protests taking place (Anderson, 2004; Hein et al., 2008). Anderson (2004) explained by walking or wandering with no clear aim, offered protesters an opportunity to have a break from the stress of being on a protest site. It also allowed protestors an opportunity to reconnect to the environment and landscape that they were attempting to protect. Walking alongside a protestor in this manner prompted that person to reminisce about why they were attempting to protect the given environment and it also often triggered other life-course memories associated with the person's connection to place.

This "talking while walking" interview is conducted in a similar fashion to the other walking interviews; however, the route taken is not necessarily known by either the researcher or participant and, in fact, is not important. The act of walking provides the opportunity for the participant to recollect experiences about the topic being discussed and to articulate them (Anderson, 2004; Moles, 2008) rather than being concerned about the specific location (Jones et al., 2008). The bimbling interview is useful when the researcher wants to encourage conversation with the participant and is aware of the potential intimidation the participant may feel being in a traditional qualitative interview. The location being used in the walking interview is not necessarily important, but the act of walking encourages conversation.

Participatory Walking Interview

The purpose of the participatory walking interview is to gain an understanding of the participants' sense of place and neighbourhood attachment (Clark & Emmel, 2010). The difference from the go-along interview is, rather than following a participant on an outing that would have occurred if the researcher was not present this interview takes place while walking around a route that the participant has determined which is in their familiar neighbourhood (Clark & Emmel, 2010). The routes used for the participatory walking interview are not to be considered representative of people's actual everyday routines and habits but rather indicative of how the participant thinks about their neighbourhoods (Clark & Emmel, 2010; Emmel & Clark, 2009). Clark and Emmel (2010) have developed a toolkit which future researchers can use as guides for the participatory walking interviews. Participants determine the route, the length of time the walking interview goes on for and what they want to show the researcher. A camera can be taken on the walking interview to record specific information. The toolkit also provides an interview schedule for the duration of the walking interview and also includes the questions asked during the walk.

The Advantages of the Walking Interview

There are a number of advantages to using any of the three walking interviews outlined above with mental health client participants. The walking interview allows the researcher to access the participant's attitudes and knowledge about the surrounding environment. By walking with a participant, the researcher is able to gain insights into both place and self (Evans & Jones, 2011). The walking interview allows insight into how the participant locates their social networks in relation to place (Clark & Emmel, 2010). This is especially important with forensic psychiatric clients as Gerber and colleagues (2003) outline the difficulties clients can have in connecting to the community they have moved to from hospital. The walking interview can help challenge a participant's narrative regarding their experience of place. For example, a participant, in a sit-down interview, may describe their lack of confidence in completing everyday activities, such as grocery shopping, thus verbalizing their reluctance to access the supermarket. While accompanying and observing a participant completing this activity, a researcher may ask clarifying questions that prompts the participant to think about their experience of the supermarket in a different light. During the walking interview, the participants' experiences can be reframed over time (Holton & Riley, 2014). The walking interview can make engaging with the participants' understanding of place easier for the researcher (Evans & Jones, 2011). It provides insight into the connections between the participant and the community. While sitting comfortably in a chair, these connections may not easily be described. While walking alongside a participant in a familiar environment, the researcher can gain insight into a sense of alienation or connection the participant has with their community (Butler & Derrett, 2014).

The walking interview gives control to the participant, the person can then determine what they would like to show the researcher. Showing the researcher can be more powerful than attempting to articulate thoughts about a place (Clark & Emmel, 2010). The natural environment can provide prompts to elicit further detail that might not have happened had the interview been room based, and it provides opportunities for the unanticipated to occur (Clark & Emmel, 2010).

A strength of the walking interview as a data collection method is that it can be used within a number of epistemological understandings. For example, it can be used within a subjectivist epistemology which views reality as being unique to individuals. An individual places meaning on the world and then interprets it in a manner that makes sense to them (Mills, Bonner, & Francis, 2006). It can also be used within a constructivist epistemology which disputes the idea that there is one objective reality but rather an individuals' reality is constructed through their engagement in their world (Lincoln, Lynham, & Guba 2018). The walking interview allows the researcher to access the meanings an individual may hold in regard to the physical and social environment the participant may hold important. The walking interviews were appropriate for this research project as it explored the unique meaning transition held for each participant.

The Research Project

The research project (Kinney, 2018a) was guided by Constructivist Grounded Theory (Charmaz, 2014). Savin-Baden and Howell Major (2013) believe grounded theory should be used when a social process is being explored and Stanley (2006) argues grounded theory research often asks the "how" and "what" questions. The aim of the project was to explore the transition process of adapting to living in the community after spending extended time in hospital for clients within a forensic psychiatric service in Aotearoa/New Zealand. Three main questions guided the research:

- How do clients within a forensic psychiatric service adapt to living in the community?
- What influences the transition experiences of clients making this adaptation?
- What would a successful transition look like?

Both clients and staff from within the forensic psychiatric service were invited into the research. Two types of interviews were used within the research, non-standardised, intensive interviews and walking interviews. Charmaz (2014) describes intensive interviewing as a flexible technique which allows the participant and researcher to co-construct the interview dialogue; this type of interview was used with both the client and staff participants. The walking interview, as discussed earlier in the chapter, was conducted only with the client participants.

Constructivist grounded theory supports the researcher returning to the same participant many times as it allows the researcher to delve deeper into their experience (Charmaz, 2014). Because of this, the client participants were invited to three interviews. Interview 1, a non-standardised, intensive interview, focused on the client participant's own transition experience. Interview 2, a walking interview, looked to explore the significance of place in relation to the client participant's transition. Interview 3, a non-standardised, intensive interview, was an opportunity to check with the client participant the initial coding from their previous interviews, follow up on any areas needing further exploration, and to discuss the developing codes.

The client participant inclusion criteria included:

- Living in the community for no more than 12 months following discharge from the forensic psychiatric hospital or in the process of transitioning to the community from an inpatient ward; and
- Remained under the supervision of the forensic psychiatric service

The clinical team discussed the clients who met these criteria as to whether they would be suitable for the research. A number of clients were not put forward for the research due to the clinical teams' concern regarding my safety. For example, one client often drank alcohol and was unpredictable when under the influence of alcohol. When a client was identified as appropriate, the client's case manager approached that person with information about the research and asked if they would like to hear more. Because I lived over 370 kms away from the location, the case manager was the person who first approached the client. When the client advised they were happy to hear more, their case manager notified me with the clients contact details. I then contacted the client directly and travelled to meet with them to talk them through the information sheet. I always stayed for at least two days to allow the client participants a minimum of 24 h to decide whether they wanted to join the research. I then conducted the first interview once they had signed the consent form.

Six client participants participated in a total of 16 interviews. Five of the participants completed all three interviews while one client participant became mentally unwell soon after completing the first interview, and based on the clinical team's recommendations, I did not continue with the other interviews with that person. All clients were in different stages of their transition. Some were already living seven nights out of hospital while others were beginning their transition, staying between one and three nights a week out of hospital. The length of time in hospital ranged from almost five to 13 years, though one client participant had come through the corrections service so had been in some type of secure environment for a total of 19 years.

All interviews were transcribed in full by myself and analysed immediately, the analysis then informed the following interviews that were still to be conducted.

The Walking Interviews in Action

Though I inherently believed the use of walking interviews as a data collection method for the research was going to be useful I didn't truly appreciate how valuable they would be until I had used them with the client participants.

The following are overviews of my experience of using the walking interviews with a selection of the client participants. The overviews also include the subsequent insights developed, as a direct result of using the walking interview.

Participant A

The walking interview completed with participant A was closer to that of the participatory interview. Initially A had identified the beach as a place where he would like to walk for the interview. On the day of the interview, participant A made contact with myself and requested a change to the geographical location where his home was situated. The request was made due to a number of contextual factors, the weather was unsettled and he didn't want to be at the beach in the rain and, most importantly, A lived about a 20 min drive from the beach and he did not have petrol in his car and didn't have the finances to put any in at that point. We agreed to begin walking from his home. During the walk A spoke of why this area was important to him, he identified landmarks and spoke about their significance to him during his transition. It was during the walk that I asked A about the significance of the beach. A advised that the beach hadn't been significant in his transition, he just thought I might like to see it because he knew I had come from almost 370 kilometres away and he wasn't sure if I'd been there before. A had initially wanted the walking interview to be more like a tour guide however it resulted closer to the participatory interview.

A had been living six nights a week in the community for approximately 18 months. A was required to return to the hospital ward one night every week for monitoring. He was not allowed to stay seven nights a week in the community because he had not yet obtained the necessary leave approval required under the legislation according to which he was being held. A verbalised confidence about living in the community and was looking forward to the time his clinical team would apply for extended leave. He advised that it was important for him to demonstrate to his clinical team that he was ready to make this final increase in leave.

A selected a route around his local suburb, where he was currently living, for his walking interview. A advised the route that we walked for the interview was one he had completed numerous times soon after shifting into his current living accommodation, in fact, initially he would complete this walk multiple times during a day. A had used the walk as a way of taking time to think and manage his anxiety about being in the community. He reported he now very rarely completed this walk as he did not believe he needed the time out like he used to.

As we were walking the route our conversation was triggered by events that were happening around us. As a result, our conversation was spontaneous and generally continuous. There were pauses as we crossed the road or waited to pass others on the footpath, all during times where conversation would be expected to either cease or reduce. On one occasion, a white van full of people drove past us. This prompted A to speak about the group community outings he participated in while on the hospital ward. He advised that prior to coming to hospital he used to make fun of those vans full of people. He used to joke that the people in the vans were odd and incapable of living independently. After spending time in hospital, he stated he soon realised how important those van trips were to his mental well-being. Having an opportunity to leave the ward and be amongst the community helped him believe he was "normal". He stated that being allowed to attend the community outings proved to him that he was getting better and that there was hope. He stated he no longer made fun of the vans full of people but rather wanted to support the people within the van, letting them know they were getting better.

On another occasion on the walk, we passed a house which had a very tidy front garden, the grass was mowed, the garden weeded and the house looked well kept. As we walked past the house, A remarked "I want to live in a house like that one day". I asked him to clarify what it was about the house that he liked, that made him want to live in something similar. A remarked "see they have their shoes on the front porch, it means it is a safe area, they haven't been stolen". A also remarked how he believed the suburb we were walking through was not a "poor" area which also contributed to it being safe in his eyes. Our conversation was then able to progress to discussing what it meant to feel safe, and the importance of being able to afford to buy what A viewed as luxury items. These two examples from A's walking interview demonstrates how the unanticipated can occur during these types of interviews and A being able to show the house he would like to live in one day was more powerful than if he had attempted to just describe it (Clark & Emmel, 2010).

Participant B

The walking interview I completed with participant B was closer to a bimbling interview. He had selected walking through the local public gardens as his interview location. During the interview, I became aware that this specific place did not have any real connection to him and his transition process but rather it was a place he wanted to go that particular day. I found we ended up talking mostly about his transition experience rather than the geographical location we were in. For B, the location where we were walking was not as important as participating in the walking.

Participant B had only very recently moved to living six nights a week in the community. He was still becoming accustomed to making decisions about what he wanted to do during the days he was in the community and where he might like to go that was outside of his accommodation. B had chosen to walk around the local public gardens as it was a place he advised was important during his time when he was initially becoming used to being outside of the hospital environment. It was a place he was familiar with as ward outings would visit the gardens during the summer when the weather allowed.

B had been advised he would direct the walking interview, making decisions which paths to follow and if there were any specific areas within the gardens he would like to visit.

The walking interview commenced at what could be regarded as a regular walking pace. Conversation was easy to maintain as the pace was not so fast that it was difficult to speak, breathe and walk at the same time. B chose to follow the marked pathways throughout the public gardens.

As discussed earlier, participant observation, during a walking interview, also provides valuable information for the researcher (Kusenbach, 2003). The walking interview with B demonstrated this. Initially, we would be walking side by side along the marked paths. Over time B's pace slowed and he would end up being one or two paces behind me. I would then slow to allow us to walk side by side again. I had thought that perhaps B's fitness level meant he was struggling to keep to the pace we had started on. After a few more minutes, I noticed B slow even further. What I then realised was that we were coming to a junction in the pathway where a decision was needed to determine which direction we would go in. I wondered if B was waiting for me to make that decision. At that point, I reminded B he was to determine where we were to walk. At that point, B's pace increased and he selected the direction we would walk. B continued at the same pace until we came to another junction that meant another decision was needed. B again slowed and remained at the slower pace until he was reminded he could make the decision. B continued to look to me to initially make decisions during the walking interview, even after being reminded he could direct the walk.

The walking interview was a powerful tool to show the differences between participant B and participant A's transition process to adapting to living in the community, even though both were living in the community six nights a week. Both participants were confident to speak to me about their transition and how they were engaging in the community, during their sit-down interview. The difference in their confidence with initiating decision making was more evident during their walking interview, showing participant B was less confident to take the lead than participant A.

Participant C

The walking interview I completed with participant C was similar to the go-along walking interview. I accompanied C on a walk he routinely completed around the hospital grounds. Participant C acted as a tour guide, showing me the area where he normally walked. The route we followed was the one he would routinely take each day (Kusenbach, 2003).

Participant C was only just beginning to transition to the community when he joined the research. He was only spending days at his community accommodation and it was after his walking interview that he started spending overnights there. As a result, C's walking interview occurred within the grounds of the hospital ward where he was still living. C had selected to walk a route that he usually completed for exercise twice a day and that followed the boundary of the hospital grounds. Similar to B, observation was an important tool during C's walking interview. C set off at a fast pace for the walk and at times it was difficult to maintain both conversation and walking speed. C reiterated multiple times during the interview the route that we were following was one that he completed for exercise and so his focus in the interview was to remain on getting exercise.

The boundary of the hospital grounds, which we were following, was often fenced and at times the fence ran in front of car parks which had cars parked within them. When we got to these areas instead of walking around the cars where there was plenty of room, C elected to walk between the cars and the fence. Often there was very little room and required us both to walk sideways to squeeze past the cars. When I questioned C why he had elected to walk, there he replied "that is where the boundary is and I walk the boundary". The walking interview reinforced the concrete and literal nature of C's thinking. It provided an opportunity to gain insight into C's connection to his world (Evans & Jones, 2011).

Participant D

The walking interview I completed with participant D was also similar to the go-along walking interview. I accompanied D on a walk he routinely completed within the hospital grounds. The route we followed was the one he would routinely take and he also acted as a tour guide, showing me areas he thought might interest me.

Participant D was commencing his transition so was not staying overnight in the community. The walking interview with D was conducted within the hospital grounds as well. D also liked to walk the boundary if possible, however, he was not as literal as C and deviated away from the boundary if there was a need to, such as limited room to walk beside the boundary. He preferred to walk the boundaries because in some of the areas there were no fences demarcating exactly where the boundary was. However, D was very aware of where the boundary was and always ensured he stayed within the hospital grounds. D's walking interview provided two unanticipated insights into the importance of place to D which would not have been readily accessible to if the walking interview had not been conducted (Clark & Emmel, 2010).

On part of the walk, where there was no fence, there was a seat that was on the hospital grounds and faced out towards the wider city. D advised he often sat on the seat looking out towards the city. He advised it was an opportunity to reflect on the fact he wanted to be out in the expanse that was in front to him. He would sit and look out and know that was his goal for his future that was where he wanted to be; all that he was doing as part of his treatment was about getting to be back in the community. The act of showing the expanse in front of him was more powerful than merely talking about it in a sedentary interview (Clark & Emmel, 2010).

The second unanticipated insight of D's walk occurred while we were walking close to the boundary of the hospital grounds, again, where there was no fence to demarcate where the boundary was. We were walking on the grass, beside which there was a footpath. When I asked why we weren't walking on the footpath, D advised the footpath was outside of the hospital grounds and he was not allowed to be there. He was concerned that members of the public might catch him outside of the grounds and then report him to either the media or his clinical team. D was aware that if he was caught outside of the hospital grounds, outside of where he had approved unaccompanied leave, he would likely have his leave rescinded and his move to the community would be slowed down. Though there was no structure to stop D from leaving the hospital grounds, D ensured he followed all expectations even though staff were not present. Foucault (1977) explains this behaviour through his social theory called Panopticonism. A metaphor that asserts humans are able to be controlled through subtle and unseen forces, i.e., by turning the disciplinary gaze upon themselves.

Considerations When Completing Walking Interviews

Gaining access to clients within forensic psychiatric services was a challenging obstacle to overcome; especially when the novel approach of a walking interview was being used. The safety concerns that were raised by the ethics committee and the service were manageable and were addressed to ensure this inclusive research with vulnerable populations could go ahead. The range of ethical considerations that were addressed have been addressed in detail in another publication and can be sourced there (Kinney, 2018b) and are only briefly covered here.

Confidentiality can't be assured due to the fact the general public can see the participant in the presence of the researcher and potentially hear the conversation. Discussions also need to occur regarding what should happen if the participant bumps into a person they know and who wants to know what is happening. Participants should be encouraged to decide how they would like to handle this potential conflict before the interview begins (Kinney, 2018b). Two of the client participants within my research met people they knew, one introduced me to them and told that person what we were doing while the other participant cut the person they knew off citing he was in an "interview" with me. He then kept walking. A walking interview may not be recommended for a participant if the topic of conversation is regarded as sensitive and could lead to the person becoming distressed. This is especially relevant in an environment that is densely populated with multiple people having the ability to overhear the conversation.

There are a number of conditions that are out of the control of the researcher that will impact on whether the walking interview will occur. Mother Nature, which includes the weather (such as rain and wind), and the participants' physical health both have the capacity to impact on the walking interview. Changing the interview from walking to driving may solve some of the problems but it also creates a number if the researcher is the lone researcher. Trying to conduct the interview while driving in high traffic areas or during conditions that are icy or heavy rain can pose a number of safety issues. Decisions on contingency plans need to be made before the walking interview is scheduled. I travelled over 370 km to the location where the participants lived. I was unable to reschedule easily so I had discussions with each client participant prior to finalising a time we would conduct the interview about what we would do if there were factors that meant the walking interview may not go ahead. This took a lot of pressure off the client participants as they knew what the plan was.

The time of day can potentially pose challenges. Depending on the availability of the participant it may not be appropriate for the researcher to be accompanying the participant on a walking interview in a particular geographical location due to safety reasons for both the researcher and participant, in fact a walking interview may not be recommended in these cases. For example, bars, due to the possibility of meeting intoxicated patrons, in or around the participants' home, especially if the participant has had concerns raised by their clinical team or secluded alleyways or other areas at dusk. Also, cultural considerations may deem certain spaces as not being appropriate for interviews to occur. It is important to have clarified these before the walking interview is scheduled.

I was clear with each client participant the walking interview was required to be completed during the hours of daylight. I was required to check in with each client participant's case manager regarding their current mental state and whether the walking interview could still go ahead. Though I did not know the exact route of each walking interview I did know the general location and I had advised the relevant case manager where the interview was going to occur, what time I was meeting the client participant and what time I anticipated being back. I then advised the relevant staff when the interview was completed. I also carried a cell phone in case of an emergency (Kinney, 2018a).

A good quality voice recorder is needed for the interview and the researcher should record the route taken. This can be completed by either using a street map or by using technology such as a Global Positioning System (GPS). When interviews are transcribed the linking back to the route is important (Clark & Emmel, 2010). Making decisions on how to record these interviews can take time. What type of recorder is used will depend on a range of factors including finances to purchase recorders, whether the researcher wants the recorder to be invisible, where the interviews will occur, and who will carry the recorder. I decided to test a number of different combinations with people I knew prior to making a decision. In the end I went with using a lapel microphone attached to the collar of my jacket. The digital recorder had a function I could select that reduced background noise and only picked up sound within 1–2 metres. I decided I wasn't going to try and get the participants to wear the microphone for multiple reasons including invading their personal space, concern about wearing the recording device and it looking out of place for them. This method worked well, though not all of each interview was easily heard when attempting to transcribe the interviews. Researchers should anticipate missing some of the interviews because of the conditions in which the interview is occurring (Clark & Emmel, 2010).

Conclusion

The walking interview shows great potential for research which includes the voice of the mental health client. It provides insight into the connections between the participant and their community. Walking alongside a participant in a familiar environment the researcher can gain insight into a sense of alienation or connection the participant has with their community. Because the researcher is observing the participant while also interviewing them, it is possible to gather information about how the mental health client interacts with both their physical and social environment. For example, the researcher can observe if a participant is walking with their head up, scanning their surroundings or walking with their head bent to focus on the footpath in front of them. The researcher can observe as to whether the participant notices an oncoming pedestrian and what reaction the participant may take. If walking in a built-up area the researcher can observe whether the participant is aware of any traffic in the surrounding area and whether the participant engages with the appropriate safety steps. These observations can then direct the researcher to follow up questions they might like to explore. The power of the walking interview is that it provides opportunities for the unanticipated to occur that would not have happened if a sedentary interview was being used (Clark & Emmel, 2010).

The walking interview can also help overcome the difficulty those living with enduring mental illness can have in regards to spontaneous verbal communication.

Within this chapter, I have presented three types of walking interviews and showed how they have been successfully used within research that has included the voices of forensic psychiatric clients. The walking interview does have a number of ethical considerations, which must be addressed to ensure the safety of mental health clients, however, these are manageable and able to be overcome.

Ensuring the voices of mental health clients are included in future research, especially research that is about them, is paramount. The use of walking interviews may very well help to ensure their voices are heard.

References

Anderson, J. (2004). Talking whilst walking: A geographical archaeology of knowledge. *Area, 36*(3), 254–261. https://doi.org/10.1111/j.0004-0894.2004.00222.x.

Bjørkly, S. (2004). Risk management in transitions between forensic institutions and the community: A literature review and an introduction to a milieu treatment approach. *International Journal of Forensic Mental Health, 3*(1), 67–76. https://doi.org/10.1080/14999013.2004.10471197.

Butler, M., & Derrett, S. (2014). The walking interview: An ethnographic approach to understanding disability. *The Internet Journal of Allied Health Sciences and Practice, 12*(3), Article 6. Retrieved from http://nsuworks.nova.edu/ijahsp/vol12/iss3/6/.

Carpiano, R. M. (2009). Come take a walk with me: The "go-along" interview as a novel method for studying the implications of place for health and well-being. *Health Place, 15*(1), 263–272. https://doi.org/10.1016/j.healthplace.2008.05.003.

Charmaz, K. (2014). *Constructing grounded theory* (2nd ed.). London: Sage.

Clark, A., & Emmel, N. (2010). Using walking interviews. *Realities, 13,* 1–6.

Coffey, M. (2006). Researching service user views in forensic mental health: A literature review. *The Journal of Forensic Psychiatry & Psychology, 17*(1), 73–107. https://doi.org/10.1080/147 89940500431544.

Coffey, M. (2012a). Negotiating identity transition when leaving forensic hospitals. *Health: An Interdisciplinary Journal for the Social Study of Health, Illness and Medicine, 16*(5), 489–506. https://doi.org/10.1177/1363459311434649.

Coffey, M. (2012b). A risk worth taking? Value differences and alternative risk constructions in accounts given by patients and their community workers following conditional discharge from forensic mental health services. *Health, Risk & Society, 14*(5), 465–482. https://doi.org/10.1080/ 13698575.2012.682976.

Emmel, N., & Clark, A. (2009). *The methods used in connected lives: Investigating networks, neighbourhoods and communities.* Retrieved from http://eprints.ncrm.ac.uk/800/.

Evans, J., & Jones, P. (2011). The walking interview: Methodology, mobility and place. *Applied Geography, 31*(2), 849–858. https://doi.org/10.1016/j.apgeog.2010.09.005.

Evans, K. (1998). *Copse: Cartoon book of tree protesting.* Chippenham: Orange Dog Publications.

Foucault, M. (1977). *Discipline & punish: The birth of the prison* (A. Sheridan, Trans.). New York, NY: Vintage Books.

Gerber, G. J., Prince, P. N., Duffy, S., McDougall, L., Cooper, J., & Dowler, S. (2003). Adjustment, integration, and quality of life among forensic patients receiving community outreach services. *International Journal of Forensic Mental Health, 2*(2), 129–136. https://doi.org/10. 1080/14999013.2003.10471184.

Grusky, O., Tierney, K., Manderscheid, R. W., & Grusky, D. B. (1985). Social bonding and community adjustment of chronically mentally ill adults. *Journal of Health and Social Behavior, 26*(1), 49–63. https://doi.org/10.2307/2136726.

Gustafsson, E., Holm, M., & Flensner, G. (2012). Rehabilitation between institutional and non-institutional forensic psychiatric care: Important influences on the transition process. *Journal of Psychiatric and Mental Health Nursing, 19*(8), 729–737. https://doi.org/10.1111/j.1365-2850. 2011.01852.x.

Hall, T., Lashua, B., & Coffey, A. (2006). Stories as sorties. *Qualitative Researcher, 3*(Summer), 2–4.

Hein, J., Evans, J., & Jones, P. (2008). Mobile methodologies: Theory, technology and practice. *Geography Compass, 2*(5), 1266–1285. https://doi.org/10.1111/j.1749-8198.2008.00139.x.

Holton, M., & Riley, M. (2014). Talking on the move: Place-based interviewing with undergraduate students. *Area, 46*(1), 59–65. https://doi.org/10.1111/area.12070.

Jamieson, L., Taylor, P. J., & Gibson, B. (2006). From pathological dependence to healthy independence: An emergent grounded theory of facilitating independent living. *The Grounded Theory Review, 6*(1), 79–108.

Jones, P., Bunce, G., Evans, J., Gibbs, H., & Hein, J. R. (2008). Exploring space and place with walking interviews. *Journal of Research Practice, 4*(2), Article D2. Retrieved from http://jrp. icaap.org/index.php/jrp/article/view/150/161.

Kaliski, S. Z. (1997). Risk management during the transition from hospital to community care. *International Review of Psychiatry, 9*(2–3), 249–256. https://doi.org/10.1080/09540269775466.

Kinney, P. (2017). Walking interview. *Social Research Update, 67,* 1–4. Retrieved from http://sru. soc.surrey.ac.uk/SRU67.pdf.

Kinney, P. (2018a). *Becoming an ex-forensic psychiatric client: Transitioning to recovery within the community.* Ph.D., University of Otago, Dunedin, New Zealand. Retrieved from https://our archive.otago.ac.nz/handle/10523/8761.

Kinney, P. (2018b). Walking interview ethics. In R. Iphofen & M. Tolich (Eds.), *The SAGE handbook of qualitative research ethics* (pp. 174–187). Thousand Oaks, CA: Sage.

Kusenbach, M. (2003). Street phenomenology: The go-along as ethnographic research tool. *Ethnography, 4*(3), 455–485. https://doi.org/10.1177/146613810343007.

Lincoln, Y. S., Lynham, S. A., & Guba, E. G. (2018). Paradigmatic controversies, contradictions, and emerging confluences, revisited. In N. K. Denzin & Y. S. Lincoln (Eds.), *The SAGE handbook of qualitative research* (5th ed., pp. 108–150). Thousand Oaks, CA: Sage.

Livingston, J. D. (2018). What does success look like in the forensic mental health system? Perspectives of service users and service providers. *International Journal of Offender Therapy and Comparative Criminology, 62*(1), 208–228. https://doi.org/10.1177/0306624x16639973.

Mills, J., Bonner, A., & Francis, K. (2006). Adopting a constructivist approach to grounded theory: Implications for research design. *International Journal of Nursing Practice, 12*(1), 8–13. https://doi.org/10.1111/j.1440-172X.2006.00543.

Moles, K. (2008). A walk in thirdspace: Place, methods and walking. *Sociological Research Online, 13*(4), 2.

Nolan, P., Bradley, E., & Brimblecombe, N. (2011). Disengaging from acute inpatient psychiatric care: A description of service users' experiences and views. *Journal of Psychiatric and Mental Health Nursing, 18*(4), 359–367. https://doi.org/10.1111/j.1365-2850.2010.01675.x.

Savin-Baden, M., & Howell Major, C. (2013). *Grounded theory: Qualitative research: The essential guide to theory and practice* (pp. 182–194). London: Routledge.

Sheller, M., & Urry, J. (2006). The new mobilities paradigm. *Environment and Planning A, 38*(2), 207–226. https://doi.org/10.1068/a37268.

Stanley, M. (2006). A grounded theory of the wellbeing of older people. In L. Finlay & C. Ballinger (Eds.), *Qualitative research for allied health professionals: Challenging choices* (pp. 63–78). England: Whurr Publishers Ltd.

Trell, E.-M., & Van Hoven, B. (2010). Making sense of place: Exploring creative and (inter) active research methods with young people. *Fennia-International Journal of Geography, 188*(1), 91–104.

Viljoen, S., Nicholls, T., Greaves, C., de Ruiter, C., & Brink, J. (2011). Resilience and successful community reintegration among female forensic psychiatric patients: A preliminary investigation. *Behavioral Sciences & the Law, 29*(5), 752–770. https://doi.org/10.1002/bsl.1001.

Völlm, B., Foster, S., Bates, P., & Huband, N. (2017). How best to engage users of forensic services in research: Literature review and recommendations. *International Journal of Forensic Mental Health, 16*(2), 183–195. https://doi.org/10.1080/14999013.2016.1255282.

Wang, C., & Burris, M. A. (1997). Photovoice: Concept, methodology, and use for participatory needs assessment. *Health Education & Behavior, 24*(3), 369–387. https://doi.org/10.1177/109019819702400309.

Chapter 5
Using Researcher Reflexivity and Multiple Methods to Study the Experience of Cancer-Related Distress

Carla Willig

Abstract This chapter describes the evolution of a pluralistic qualitative research programme into the experience of cancer-related distress. Starting with an autoethnographic exploration of her own experience of being diagnosed with cancer, the author describes how the use of discourse analysis, hermeneutic phenomenology and qualitative metasynthesis in a series of related studies enabled her to shed light on, and begin to theorise, the production of cancer-related distress. The chapter demonstrates how the combination of methods used in the research programme facilitated insights into the ways in which subjective experience is mediated and shaped by available discursive resources, and how people actively engage with these resources as they find their own way of finding meaning in their experience. The chapter argues that a research programme that uses a range of qualitative methods can produce a more rounded understanding of a phenomenon than a mono-method study alone would be able to achieve. Here, the in-depth focus on one individual's subjective experience that characterises autoethnography is complemented by the wider lens applied through metasynthesis, whilst a discourse analytic focus on sociocultural situatedness of experience is complemented by phenomenology's concern with lived, embodied experience. Such an approach to research allows us to examine experience in the light of discourse whilst at the same time paying close attention to experience as it is lived by those who describe it. It is an approach that can examine how constructions of meaning around cancer can have a detrimental effect on the quality of life of people who are living with cancer, and, hopefully, contribute to creating a sociocultural context within which cancer is talked about in a way that is mindful of the impact of discourse on experience.

Keywords Pluralistic research · Autoethnography · Discourse analysis · Hermeneutic phenomenology · Qualitative metasynthesis · Cancer diagnosis · Cancer experience · Cancer-related distress

C. Willig (✉)
Department of Psychology, City, University of London, London, UK
e-mail: c.willig@city.ac.uk

© Springer Nature Switzerland AG 2021
M. Borcsa and C. Willig (eds.), *Qualitative Research Methods in Mental Health*,
https://doi.org/10.1007/978-3-030-65331-6_5

Introduction

This chapter tells the story of how the emotionally challenging experience of being diagnosed with cancer led me to embark upon a methodological journey. As such, the chapter constitutes an exercise in researcher reflexivity as well as offering an account of how a combination of qualitative research methods can be used to study subjective experience within its social context. In this chapter, I describe how my initial reflections on my own experience led me to write an autoethnographic paper in which I raised questions about the social context within which my experience was taking place. In an attempt to answer these questions, I then conducted discourse analytic research into the ways in which cancer diagnosis is talked and written about. This, in turn, raised questions for me about the phenomenological repercussions of being positioned in dominant cancer discourses particularly for people living with cancers that cannot be cured and I conducted a phenomenological study into the experience of living with advanced cancer. Finally, to address questions about the extent to which the experiences identified in the small-scale phenomenological study might be shared among a wider population of cancer patients, I carried out a qualitative metasynthesis of studies of the experience of living with a terminal cancer diagnosis. Together these four qualitative studies can help to shed light on the lived experience of cancer in contemporary Western culture and they can help us understand the nature and quality of the distress that can be generated by a cancer diagnosis.

Since increasing numbers of people are being diagnosed with cancer and, thanks to improvements in available treatments, patients can live with the disease for relatively long periods of time, it is important to further our understanding of the psychological and social challenges inherent in this situation. Living with cancer can give rise to mental health issues and research consistently finds clinically significant levels of anxiety and depression in a large proportion (around 30%) of those diagnosed with cancer (e.g. Roy-Byrne et al., 2008; Sellick and Crooks, 1999). There is also evidence suggesting that being diagnosed with cancer constitutes a form of traumatisation (Propper, 2007). It is clear that coming to terms with a terminal cancer diagnosis constitutes a significant psychological challenge which has implications for the individual's mental health and well-being. The research presented in this chapter seeks to contribute to the literature by deepening our understanding of the ways in which cancer-related distress is produced, with a view to developing social and psychological interventions which can reduce such distress (see also Willig & Wirth, 2019, for more on this).

This chapter demonstrates how one researcher can use a range of qualitative methods in the pursuit of knowledge about a particular experiential phenomenon. It shows how shedding light on an experiential phenomenon can be a process of asking a series of questions, each of which requires the use of a different qualitative method, and so demonstrates how knowledge and understanding are built up over time by continuing to ask questions and choosing methods to answer them. Thus, pursuing a series of evolving research questions, each of which requires a different research

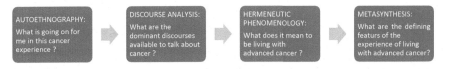

Fig. 5.1 Evolving research questions and methods

method, produces a pluralistic research programme which can generate topical as well as methodological insights (see Fig. 5.1).

Researcher reflexivity plays an important role in all forms of qualitative research. Researcher reflexivity involves attending to the context within which a piece of research has been conceived, designed and conducted, including the researcher's own motivation and their personal and epistemological commitments (Finlay & Gough, 2003; Gough & Madill, 2012; Willig, 2013). The starting point for the research programme discussed in this chapter was the experience of a traumatic interruption to the researcher's own sense of self and the thoughts and feelings that this generated. Even though the first piece of work (the autoethnography) was the most obviously personal and was based upon an explicit engagement with researcher reflexivity, the three studies that followed (the discourse analysis, the phenomenological study, and the metasynthesis) were also predicated upon the researcher's own experience of being diagnosed with cancer[1] and, as such, necessarily shaped by this experience. Perhaps most importantly, I am aware that the personal motivation that fed and sustained the investment of time and energy into the research programme was generated by my own experience.

The Experience of Being Positioned Within Dominant Cancer Discourses: An Autoethnographic Exploration

Following my own cancer diagnosis with a malignant melanoma in 2007, I became painfully aware that one of the many challenges of being diagnosed with cancer is that it requires us to make sense of our changed circumstances and to find meaning in an unwanted experience whilst being confronted with the meanings that other people attribute to this experience. My attention was drawn to the power of words when my own felt sense of myself was changing as a result of being positioned within cancer discourses. I wrote about my experience in a journal throughout the process of being diagnosed with cancer and its aftermath, and eventually published an autoethnographic paper in which I reflect on my experience of the struggle for meaning within the context of existential uncertainty during this time (see Willig, 2009).

---

[1]My own cancer was successfully treated by surgery alone and, therefore, the experience of living with advanced cancer is not something I have experienced personally. However, my interest in this experience was informed by my engagement with the possibility of receiving a terminal diagnosis during the 3-week period that I waited for the results of my first biopsy.

Autoethnography

Autoethnography is a method of qualitative research that uses the researcher's systematic self-reflection through writing to explore the meaning of their own experience and to make connections between that experience and the wider sociocultural context within which the experience takes place. According to Ellis, Adams, and Bochner (2011) 'autoethnography is an approach to research and writing that seeks to describe and systematically analyze personal experience in order to understand cultural experience (…) A researcher uses tenets of autobiography and ethnography to do and write autoethnography. Thus, as a method, autoethnography is both process and product' (Abstract, p. 1). Autoethnography requires the researcher to engage in high levels of researcher reflexivity as they examine their own experience and its relationship with the various social, cultural and material settings that constitute its context and that, arguably, give rise to it. For a piece of work to qualify as an autoethnography (as opposed to autobiographical writing or story-telling, for example), it needs to demonstrate (i) that it is purposefully commenting on (or critiquing) cultural practices, (ii) that it makes a contribution to the literature in the field, (iii) that it embraces vulnerability with a purpose, and (iv) that it creates a reciprocal relationship with audiences in order to compel a response (see Holman Jones, Adams, & Ellis, 2013, p. 22).

There are different types of autoethnography including analytic autoethnography and evocative autoethnography (see Ellingson & Ellis, 2008). The former is concerned with developing a theoretical understanding of how experience is produced within its social context whereas the latter seeks to have an emotional impact on readers which has a transformative effect of some kind.

My approach to autoethnography was analytic rather than evocative as my aim was to better understand and to make sense of an experience which I found deeply disturbing. Although I also wanted to give expression to my experience and its unsettling quality and therefore make it visible to other people, my primary motivation was to increase my own understanding of how and why my experience had come about. My approach to autoethnography was characterised by the five characteristics of analytic autoethnography outlined by Anderson (2006): complete member researcher status (I was myself diagnosed with cancer); analytic reflexivity (I attempted to reflect on my own experience through a critical, social scientific lens); narrative visibility of the researcher's self (I write about myself and use quotations from my personal journal to illustrate analytic insights); dialogue with information beyond the self (I draw on concepts from existential philosophy and discourse studies to make sense of my experience); and commitment to an analytic agenda (I aim to increase understanding of how and why my experience had come about). Having kept a journal throughout the process of being diagnosed with cancer, I was able to systematically review the journal entries that I had made over the course of the experience and to identify themes that captured the meanings around cancer which I encountered and grappled with as I tried to find my place in the world as a person with cancer. I identified themes by highlighting those patterns of meaning around cancer which impacted me emotionally and which I reflected on and problematised in my journal entries. These themes included 'the hard work involved in the struggle for meaning', 'constructions of death as unacceptable', 'constructions of cancer as the product of risky behaviour' and 'foregrounding the biochemical processes associated with cancer'. Each theme will be described and illustrated below.

Theme 1: 'The Hard Work Involved in the Struggle for Meaning'

During the course of the experience of being diagnosed with cancer, I became aware of the hard work involved in constructing and holding on to a 'serviceable narrative' which I felt could see me through the experience of confronting my own mortality. I experienced the struggle for meaning as physically exhausting and observed:

> For once, meaning-making – something which had always seemed more or less effortless, even playful at times- felt like hard physical labour involving my whole body in the struggle against the black hole of meaninglessness. (Journal entry, cited in Willig, 2009, ibid., p. 183)

> The last few days have continued in a similar vein, with me experiencing relatively short periods of intense anxiety during which I cannot help but hurl myself mentally into a projected future of horror and suffering. At such times I am not in the present but I leap into the future. It feels like in order to return to 'the other place', I need to laboriously swim against the stream, pulling various parts of myself back to the stable (and only 'real') point in the present. Once I have done that and dragged all the parts of me back into the present moment, I can feel myself relax and settle there (for the time being). (Journal entry, cited in Willig, 2009, p. 184)

I discovered that the adoption of a stance of acceptance of whatever was going to happen to me and the attempt to 'be there' and engage with whatever life was going to bring (including death) was helpful in alleviating my anxiety and bringing me a sense of peace. I wrote:

> I realise that the only way I can deal with this is by engaging with the experience and by confronting my mortality – and not to pretend that it isn't happening or to try to escape from it in some way. Attempts to avoid or escape from the experience only increase my anxiety and the sense of lurking horror. By contrast, the thought of embracing and fully entering this experience does not. If this is going to happen to me, I want to 'be there', and not try to be somewhere else. (Journal entry, cited in Willig, 2009, p. 184)

However, it was hard to maintain contact with this serviceable narrative and easy to lose myself in fearful projections and fantasies about my future with cancer. At the same time, as I was speaking with friends and relatives about my situation I realised that they had their own ways of making sense of cancer, and that other people's constructions of cancer often positioned me in ways that quickly removed my hard-earned serenity, my fragile sense of being 'at peace'. It was at this point that I was really struck by the power of discourse and its ability to determine how I felt about myself and my situation. I realised that since I was still in the process of trying to make sense of what was happening to me, I was particularly vulnerable to being unsettled by other people's constructions of meaning and the ways these positioned me as the person with cancer.

Theme 2: 'Constructions of Death as Unacceptable'

There were some ways of talking about cancer that I experienced as especially challenging to my own way of giving meaning to my situation and which I was confronted with repeatedly during the process of being diagnosed with and treated for cancer. One of these found expression in people reacting to my news by immediately giving me advice about how to avert the destructive effects of cancer by taking protective action (such as seeking private medical treatment or changing my diet). Whilst no doubt well-meant, these pieces of advice and their focus on evading the 'worst case scenario' (i.e. terminal illness) implicitly constructed death as a potential outcome of my encounter with cancer as unacceptable and not to be countenanced. This construction ruled out making peace with the prospect of death as a possible way of engaging with my situation and, as a result, made the idea of death appear more threatening to me. I wrote:

> I've also had a few more thoughts about 'living towards death' and how I would want to do this. I realise how easily other people can impose their own constructions, their sets of meaning about death, with very painful consequences. For example, I don't want to think of my life as a tragic abortion, just because there is an end in sight... I feel that thinking of death as something like an awful accident that could have been avoided (if the right protective actions had been taken) somehow devalues the life that still is and will be and which will finally come to an end in death. (Journal entry, cited in Willig, 2009, p. 185)

Theme 3: 'Constructions of Cancer as the Product of Risky Behaviour'

I also encountered a moral construction of cancer which took the form of questions about my lifestyle (did I smoke, drink, use sun protection, eat a healthy diet?). Here, people tried to make sense of my diagnosis by identifying a behavioural cause for it. Implicit in constructing cancer as the outcome of health-related behaviours is that it is potentially avoidable, a comforting thought for those who still have time to cut out risky behaviours but not so comforting for those who are made to feel responsible for inviting cancer into their lives through their own actions. I observed:

> My reaction to such questions was (...) a feeling of being used in someone else's struggle with the anxiety produced by encountering (someone with) cancer. I was reminded that, just like me, other people needed to construct a serviceable narrative in the face of anxiety and uncertainty (...) Understanding this, however, did not stop me from feeling isolated and excluded from the comfort zones that my questioners constructed for themselves. (Journal entry, cited in Willig, 2009, pp. 186–187)

Theme 4: 'Foregrounding the Biochemical Processes Associated with Cancer'

Finally, there was a way of talking about cancer which foregrounded bodily processes (such as cell division, the immune system, the process of metastasis) that had the effect of constructing the person with cancer (in this case, me) as inhabiting a damaged vessel which was self-destructing and which would take its inhabitant down with it. Such discourse interfered with my attempts to hold on to a sense of an experiential self that was whole and undamaged by the biochemical processes that were taking place at the level of the material body. I noted:

> My attempt to hold on to a sense of self that was whole and undamaged meant that I did not want to talk much about my body and what was happening to/within it. I felt uncomfortable when people showed a lively interest in biomedical aspects of my experience and wanted to talk about bodies as objects to be scrutinized. I remember a telephone conversation with a relative who discoursed about dividing cells, bodily defences and the process of metastasis, which left me feeling physically sick. (Journal entry, cited in Willig, 2009, p. 186)

My autoethnographic exploration led me to conclude that the emotional impact of being positioned in widely-used cancer discourses could be significant. Being diagnosed with cancer and finding myself in a situation that did not seem to make any sense, did not fit with the rest of my life, and over which I had little control, I found that a major effort was required on my part to re-build a sense of meaningfulness and agency, and to adopt a stance towards the situation that would make it bearable for me. In this situation, other people's comments had a powerful impact as they offered or even imposed meanings that often challenged or interfered with the fragile emerging meanings that I was able to construct for myself. I found my own experience echoed when I came across Stacey's (1997) cultural study of cancer, a book in which she explores:

> (…) some of the ways in which a person with cancer is subject to, if not bombarded with, powerful and contradictory discourses about the nature of their illness (…) As well as coping with the trauma and discomfort/pain of the illness, the person with cancer confronts a host of beliefs and practices which compete to define the meaning of the illness (…) Part of the experience of cancer in today's culture is suddenly confronting this excess of opinion about the meaning of disease and the logic of the cure. (p. 28)

Mapping the Language of Cancer: An Analysis of Cancer Discourse

From a social constructionist perspective, the meanings I encountered and grappled with during my experience of being diagnosed with cancer are constructed from the discursive resources available within one's culture. As a qualitative researcher with an interest in the role of language in shaping experience, I turned my attention to mapping the language of cancer so as to examine its social and psychological effects. I wanted to take a closer look at the dominant discourses surrounding cancer so that I could identify the discursive positions available to those diagnosed with cancer and to trace their implications for how cancer may be experienced and lived with. To this end, I identified recently published research papers concerned with how cancer is talked about in contemporary English-speaking societies (e.g. Mosher & Danoff-Burg, 2009; Williams Camus, 2009; Wray, Marcovic, & Manderson, 2007) as well as books about cancer discourse (e.g. Ehrenreich, 2009; Stacey, 1997), read them and extracted the authors' observations about how cancer is talked about and how such talk may impact on people living with cancer. I then published a paper reflecting on the social and psychological consequences of being positioned within dominant cancer discourses (Willig, 2011).

Discourse Analysis

There are many versions of discourse analysis and the researcher's choice of approach to this method will depend upon the research question that is driving the analysis. In this case, I was concerned with the discursive resources that are made available to people within a particular cultural and historical context (i.e. English-speaking Western industrialised countries around the turn of the twenty-first century) and I wanted to map out the most widely available subject positions for people who have been diagnosed with cancer. Therefore, I adopted an approach to discourse analysis that focused on the identification of discourses, defined by Parker (1994, p. 245) as 'systems of statements that construct objects and an array of subject positions' (rather than, for example, focusing on the contextual deployment of discursive strategies with specific conversational contexts, as seen in versions of conversational analysis as well as discursive psychology research). In other words, the aim of the analysis was to provide a systematic overview of the ways in which cancer and people with cancer are talked about (and, therefore, discursively constructed), and to identify how such talk positions people with cancer (e.g. as 'victim', as 'survivor', as 'fighter', etc.). The method used was informed by analytic guidance provided by Parker (1992) and Willig (2013). Textual material used to conduct the analysis included published first-person accounts of cancer experiences, and research papers on the subject. The selection of textual material was not systematic, and therefore not representative. It was driven by my interest in how cancer is talked about in contemporary English-speaking societies; it focused on books and papers that I had come across in my search for answers to my questions about the relationship between how cancer is talked about and how it is experienced, a search which had begun with my own cancer diagnosis in 2007, as outlined in the previous section on autoethnography. The analysis started from the premise that discourse constructs the objects and subjects of which it speaks. In particular, it involved scrutiny of the ways in which cancer and people who have been diagnosed with cancer are being constructed in and through discourse. The analysis began by delineating prevalent discursive constructions of meaning around cancer and people with cancer. This was done by identifying distinct interpretative repertoires used in the accounts. Such repertoires are characterised by the recurrent use of terms, expressions, stylistic and grammatical constructions, metaphors and figures of speech (see Potter & Wetherell, 1987). The use of metaphors constitutes a particularly powerful way of constructing versions of reality (see Lakoff & Johnson, 1980). The use of a particular repertoire informs the construction of meaning around the discursive object. For example, people with cancer are often described as 'victims of cancer'. Then, the possibilities for action contained within these constructions are mapped out. For example, the construction of people with cancer as 'victims' suggests a passive and object-like status. Finally, the analysis examines the consequences of being positioned within such constructions for a person's subjective experience of themselves and the world around them. For example, being positioned as 'victim' may produce feelings of helplessness and hopelessness.

Two discursive themes emerged from the analysis: (i) a cultural imperative to think positively and (ii) cancer as a moral concern. These two themes were derived from the dominant ways of constructing cancer and people with cancer identified in the texts, and they trace some of the implications for how cancer may be experienced when it is framed on the basis of these dominant ways of constructing cancer.

The 'cultural imperative to think positively' is based upon a construction of cancer as a problem that can, and must, be solved. As a result, talk about the possibility of death is constructed as morbid and defeatist and is contrasted with positive thinking which becomes mandatory and is presented as a healthy response to a cancer diagnosis.

The imperative to think positively encourages and rewards the construction of cancer as a 'wake-up call' or a 'gift' providing the person with cancer with an opportunity to make a fresh start and live a healthier, more self-aware life. The 'cultural imperative to think positively' positions the person with cancer as 'survivor' (rather than 'patient' or 'victim', for example) and expects the person with cancer to take responsibility for their health and well-being.

As part of the 'imperative to think positively', military metaphors are often employed which construct cancer as a war that must be fought and that can be won if fought hard enough and with enough determination. People with cancer are instructed to 'fight their cancer' which is constructed as a formidable enemy who must be fought by any means necessary. Military metaphors construct the patient's body as a battlefield upon which the battle between life and death is fought. Positioned as 'soldiers in the fight against cancer' patients are expected to display attributes of bravery and stoicism, and 'not giving up' is valued more highly than any other stance that might be taken within this context.

This discourse does not allow for the possibility of acceptance because from within this discourse cancer must be fought, solved or otherwise transformed into something else that makes it a positive experience. Staying with the experience and attempting to relate to it as it is experienced (with both its positive and negative dimensions) is not presented as a legitimate option, and the possibility of death is not acknowledged as a possible outcome.

For example, Lubbock (2012, pp. 76–77) describes his difficulties in communicating what it means to be living with terminal cancer when his interlocutor is seeking to give the experience a positive/hopeful inflection:

I meet someone who thinks I am now better. I explain that the treatment went well, but in fact I will never be better. Sooner or later I will get worse, and then even worse. It's very strange having to live in these spans, waiting at some point for the bad news to come. She says: I suppose you have to live in the present. I say that it is actually not a very encouraging thought. (...) the loss of a proper prospect is precisely what you miss – the 'one day', the open future, the possibility of relaxation that gives to life.

The second discursive theme, 'cancer as a moral concern', is based upon the construction of cancer as a disease that is 'home-grown' and 'occasioned by the self' (Stacey, 1997, p. 175) in that it is caused by the individual's behaviour and/or their physical constitution rather than having its cause outside the patient's body (as is the case, for example, when the cause of illness is a virus or some damage that is inflicted upon the body through an external agent). It is, therefore, seen as the result of their own inner weakness, be it via harmful lifestyles and risky behaviours, an ineffective immune system, or an unhealthy personality or outlook. A combination of beliefs about the aetiology of cancer (e.g. that it is the product of spontaneous cell growth and/or lifestyle and behavioural factors), popular mind-body metaphors that resonate with 'New Age' thinking (e.g. the idea that a healthy body is the manifestation of a healthy mind), and militarised immune system discourse (e.g. constructing the immune system as the body's army whose job it is to defend the body against foreign invasion and which, in the case of cancer, fails in this task, as cancer attacks the body from within) construct cancer as the product of the cancer patient's own failings and/or weakness. Here, the patient is positioned as responsible for their cancer and is expected to own 'their cancer' and learn from their mistakes, ideally by engaging in some lifestyle changes and moral reform. The cure of 'their' cancer, then, also becomes the patient's responsibility and, as such, evidence of the success (or otherwise) of their moral renewal. From within this discourse, dying from cancer constitutes another failure on the part of the patient. For example, Martin's (2000, p. 36) comments on her experience of being positioned as responsible for her recovery from cancer illustrate this:

(...) I often heard strong and sometimes rigid opinions from others about the attitudes of cancer patients and the how's and why's of whether we recover or not. Especially after metastatic growth it was all too easy for me to dip into an unhealthy level of self-doubt and confusion instigated by these all-knowing authorities who, for the most part, had not actually *had* cancer. Too often I felt guilty because I hadn't been able to cure myself.

Examining how cancer is constructed through discourse led me to conclude that the presence of two dominant ways of talking about cancer available in our culture (i.e. the imperative to think positively about cancer and cancer as a moral concern) can make life difficult for people who have been diagnosed with cancer. At a time when a person is confronted with the challenge of finding meaning in their encounter with cancer, when they are required to adjust or even modify their sense of self (e.g. by incorporating a stronger awareness of mortality, of physical and/or psychological vulnerability or by changing their relationship with their bodies), it can be a struggle to regain control of the story they can tell about themselves. And yet, the person with cancer must find a way to talk about their experience which renders it both meaningful and bearable. At such a time, being positioned in widely used cancer discourses can feel disempowering and alienating, especially in situations where popular constructions of what it means to have cancer do not, in fact, help to make sense of one's own actual experience. In particular, the dominance of the cultural imperative to 'think positively' about cancer means that being diagnosed with advanced (terminal) cancer makes it very difficult to find a meaningful position within dominant cancer discourse and to find a way of making sense of dying from cancer. This realisation led me to focus my attention on the experience of living with advanced cancer.

Living-with-Dying: A Phenomenological Study of the Experience of Living with Advanced Cancer

Having used autoethnography and discourse analysis to examine how dominant cancer discourses position those who have been diagnosed with cancer, I was struck by just how limiting the available repertoires were, particularly for those diagnosed with advanced forms of the disease. It seemed to me that 'positive thinking' and a preoccupation with a 'fight against cancer' do not offer meaningful positions for people who know that they cannot 'win' the fight against their cancer and who may feel the need to engage with the reality of their own mortality rather than wanting to focus on 'positive' thoughts instead. I wanted to know how people with advanced cancer made sense of their experience and live with the knowledge that they are very likely to die from their cancer. The next step in the research programme was, therefore, to conduct a phenomenological analysis of accounts of the experience of living with advanced cancer (Willig, 2015a).

Hermeneutic Phenomenology

Phenomenological research is concerned with accessing the meaning and quality of lived experience from the perspective of those who are undergoing the experience. There are different types of phenomenological research including descriptive phenomenology (e.g. Giorgi, Giorgi, & Morely, 2017), interpretative phenomenology (e.g. Smith et al., 2009), and hermeneutic phenomenology (e.g. Van Manen, 1990) (see also Langdridge, 2007). These differ in the way they approach data (e.g. a descriptive versus a more interpretative perspective) and in their aims (e.g. seeking to explore individual experience in all its complexity, versus seeking to extract an experiential essence from a series of accounts). The present study opted for an existentially informed hermeneutic phenomenological analysis (e.g. Van Manen, 1997; Willig & Billin, 2012) whose aim it is to obtain insight into the 'structure of the human lifeworld' (Van Manen, 1990, p. 101). Existentially informed hermeneutic phenomenological analysis seeks to make sense of what it means to be human, that is to say 'what it means to live as an embodied being in a (particular) physical and social world' (Willig & Billin, 2012, p. 118). Ultimately, this type of phenomenological analysis is concerned with fundamental human existential concerns such as the passing of time, our embodied nature (including mortality) and our being-in-the-world-with-others (see also Ashworth, 2003). Given the research question's focus on living with the prospect of one's own death from cancer occurring in the not-too-distant future, existentially informed hermeneutic phenomenological analysis seemed the most appropriate choice.

The study was conducted with two collaborators: Jacqui Farrants (City, University of London) and Catherine Nelson (Maggie's Cancer Centre, London). Data was collected on the basis of semi-structured interviews with 10 participants who were living with advanced (metastatic) cancer. The age range was mid-thirties to early eighties and all but one participant were female. Interviews were supported by the use of object elicitation (for more on this method, see Willig, 2017) whereby interviewees were invited to bring along objects that held special meaning for them during the current phase of their lives. The objects participants brought included photographs, books, jewellery, diaries, small household objects, items of clothing and recordings of music. Participants were invited to talk about each of the objects they had brought, explaining their meaning and significance and the role that they played in the participant's life at the present time. Interviews were conducted in a quiet room at a Cancer Centre or in the participant's home. They lasted between one and two hours and were audio-recorded and later transcribed verbatim.

Each interview transcript was analysed individually before an attempt at an integration of analytic observations across the ten interviews was made. Following Van Manen's (1997) guidance, each transcript was subjected to three readings: a *holistic* reading whereby the text and its message as a whole are attended to, a *selective* reading whereby segments of the text that appear particularly revealing or significant are interrogated, and a *detailed* reading whereby each line of text is examined for what it reveals about the phenomenon under investigation. The holistic reading generated insights into the way in which interviewees approached the interview and how they chose to frame their experience. For example, some participants presented in-the-moment reflections which touched on some very painful (and often unresolved) thoughts and feelings, whilst others made it clear that they had arrived at a narrative which served them well and which they did not wish to unsettle through further reflection. The selective reading focused on specific features such as repetitions of certain phrases and formulations (e.g. 'I can't understand'; 'I don't understand'; 'I just don't understand') or moments in the interviewee's account that they identified as a significant turning point in their experience (e.g. 'And then all hell broke loose'). The detailed reading identified the underlying concerns which informed the various aspects of experience that were being described. For instance, an interviewee's reflections on their relationship with the future constitute an example of an underlying concern. In the final phase of the analysis, I compared the results from the individual analyses and contrasted them with one another to generate tentative conclusions about how people experience and make sense of living with advanced cancer. These can be grouped under two theme headings, as follows:

Theme 1: The Challenge of Having to Engage with Death Awareness as Something That Cannot Be Sidestepped

Despite there being great variability in the meanings interviewees gave to their experience as well as the ways in which they spoke about these, all of them acknowledged that being diagnosed with advanced cancer was something that presented them with the challenge of how to manage a new death awareness. They all shared a sense of being confronted with something of enormous significance that could not be ignored and that required their attention in order to be managed in some way. One of the participant's observations: 'It's like in my face all the time and the only way is to turn your head to the other side but it doesn't last long, you know' captures this experience well, as does another participant's comment: 'Yes, you're in it and yes, you can't get out of it'. But perhaps the most powerful expression of the experiential quality of being confronted with the facticity of one's own mortality is contained in the following quotation:

> You have these strong feelings. And I have to live with that I suppose. I mean as I said I've been very depressed and now I feel like I'm getting out of it but the situation is such that some days I feel very alone and sad and unable to do anything because the only thing I can think of is that I'm going to die. And that's the only certainty that I have. I know we do all have that and I know people say (…) you could cross the street and be run over by a bus. But you live your life not thinking about it. I have to deal with it. My bus is here. All the time.

Theme 2: A Changed Relationship with Time

Being confronted with the prospect of their own death occurring in the not-too-distant future unsettled participants' relationship with the dimension of temporality. They described how both past and future took on a different meaning as time was running out. With the loss of a previously presumed future came the need to find meaning in a present which is not dependent upon long-term plans and assumptions about the 'normal' life-course. As one participant noted: 'What is so difficult to grasp when you get a diagnosis like this is that the progression of your life isn't going to happen in the way that you naturally expect'. The lost connection with an anticipated future can make it very difficult to find meaning in the present, leading some to describe how this can 'take the point out of things':

> One difficulty I have (…) is that a lot of things are pointless because there isn't a future (…) I'm not doing things for a future so that can take the point out of things, and an interest in a way.

At the same time, however, the loss of future prospects enabled an intensification of experiences of the present moment. Several participants drew attention to the sensual pleasure of drinking coffee, the joy of being with nature or listening to music, and they described how sharing experiences with friends and family had become more meaningful and rewarding since they had received their diagnosis.

The experience of one's past, too, can be changed by the loss of the future, and past events acquire a new significance because they will not be followed by more of the same. One participant's reflections on two intimate relationships she has had in the past illustrate this process very well:

> If I think about two men that I loved in my life, my relationship with them (…) is different because I'm not going to be able to go on and have another man. So somehow they have a weight (…) in my life, so it's the weight that changes, you're not actually changing events but the weight is changed because there isn't going to be a future.

Participants described how a changed relationship with the past can generate both positive and negative experiences. For some the past became a source of regret (e.g. 'I look at the past with horror') whilst others took the opportunity to revisit and celebrate their life story by producing a record of it (e.g. in the form of a photo album or a book).

In conclusion, the existentially informed hermeneutic phenomenological analysis of ten participants' reflections on living with advanced cancer suggests that living with advanced cancer constitutes a traumatic interruption of one's familiar way of being in the world and is experienced as an existential challenge which requires the individual to find a way of re-configuring their relationship with time and to find a way of living meaningfully without a presumed future. The results from this study indicate that the challenge of living with a terminal cancer diagnosis opened up an experiential space with qualities that were quite different from those that the research participants had been used to previously and that had characterised their lived experience of life without advanced cancer. The next question that arose for me was whether the phenomenon of finding oneself in a different experiential space was one that was commonly encountered by people with a terminal cancer diagnosis, rather than perhaps being specific to the group of ten participants we had spoken to.

Integrating the Results from Qualitative Studies of Patients' Experience of Living with Terminal Cancer: A Metasynthesis

Due to its commitment to a detailed exploration of meanings, qualitative research tends to use data from relatively small numbers of participants. This means that it can be difficult to draw wider conclusions from an individual piece of research. Meta-synthesis is a methodology that provides us with an opportunity to integrate findings from several qualitative studies to produce a conceptually more robust account of the meaning and significance of an experiential phenomenon than would have been possible on the basis of a single qualitative study alone. This is why I opted for this approach for the next stage in the study of the lived experience of cancer.

Metasynthesis

According to Ludvigsen et al. (2016), metasynthesis offers a methodology for systematically aggregating, integrating and interpreting findings from a collection of qualitative research reports.

There are a number of different approaches to conducting metasyntheses and researchers have different views regarding issues such as the ideal number of studies that should be included in a metasynthesis and the nature of the inclusion/exclusion criteria for the selection of eligible studies. There are also differences in approach regarding the extent to which primary findings from individual studies should be re-interpreted, for example by re-labelling and/or re-grouping themes. The aim of a metasynthesis can be theory development or it can be to simply bring together research findings that are pertinent to a particular research question in order to build a cumulative body of knowledge. Depending on the aim, the researcher's approach to the findings reported by the primary studies may differ quite significantly. However, as Thorne (2015, p. 1348) argues, any metasynthesis should constitute 'a distinct piece of scholarly research and not merely an option for organising and displaying available literature in the field'.

The present metasynthesis was conducted with the help of a research assistant, Luisa Wirth, who is also co-author on publications reporting the study (Willig & Wirth, 2017, 2019). The aim of our metasynthesis was to produce a synthesis of phenomenological studies of the experience of living with terminal cancer so as to gain a more complete understanding of the parameters of this experience and to provide a deeper insight into the lived experience of terminally ill cancer patients. The approach to metasynthesis taken in this research was informed by guidance provided by Bondas and Hall (2007) and Ludvigsen et al. (2016). The present metasynthesis aspired to offer novel interpretations of existing findings through their integration and to facilitate theory development rather than to simply aggregate the results of existing studies.

We started by selecting 23 qualitative studies of the experience of living with terminal cancer published between 2011 and 2016 in peer-reviewed English-language journals. To be selected, a study had to be phenomenological in orientation, based on semi-structured interviews as a method of data collection, with participants who were over 18 years of age and aware of their terminal cancer diagnosis. In total, just over 300 participants' accounts of their experiences were included in the metasynthesis, providing us with a much larger body of data than we could have generated ourselves in the time we had available. Participants were between 26 and 92 years old, and they were living with a wide range of types of cancer (27 in total).

Our analytic procedure started with the production of a summary table of the results of the primary studies in the form of themes. They were derived by extracting themes which the authors of the 23 studies themselves had identified in their results sections as well as by creating our own themes in cases where the authors had presented their findings in narrative form. The theme labels we ourselves created sought to capture the experiences described in the narratives. Once completed, our summary table contained a total of 151 themes. The next stage involved a process of integration and interpretation of the themes which was done by allocating each theme to a theme cluster. Theme clusters were based on shared meanings and were given labels which captured the shared meanings. This process generated 19 theme clusters in total.

The final step in the analysis involved a process of 'clustering the clusters' so that overarching experiential concerns could be identified. This was done through a process of joint reflection and discussion whereby both researchers examined the thematic content of the 19 theme clusters together, looking for meaningful connections and relationships between them. This led to the construction of four higher-order themes: *Trauma, Liminality, Holding on to Life* and *Living with Cancer*, thus capturing the parameters of the experience of living with terminal cancer, as follows:

Trauma captures the catastrophic interruption that a terminal cancer diagnosis constitutes as it impacts upon all aspects of the patient's life. This involves an intense sense of vulnerability and lack of physical and emotional safety and constitutes a major challenge to a person's trust in the world, and to its (relative) predictability and safety.

Liminality captures the experience of inhabiting an experiential space that is inbetween what was and what will be, a kind of twilight zone on the threshold of death which separates the person from the everyday world where being alive is taken for granted. It is characterised by an altered relationship with time, and it is not always experienced as negative as it can also generate new and precious experiences.

Holding on to Life captures the person's efforts to stay connected to life and to the living, and to resist being torn away from all that made life meaningful and worthwhile in the past. Such efforts include fighting the cancer and not giving up on treatments, focusing on little pleasures in daily life and maintaining a sense of the future; all these are important ways in which patients hold on to life in the face of the existential threat that their cancer poses.

Living with Cancer captures the impact of terminal cancer on the patient's day-to-day life, including often intensely unpleasant routines and their side effects as well as the challenges of being a cancer patient in the social world. This can involve a range of losses including a loss of dignity, a loss of energy, a loss of independence and a loss of control, but at the same time opens up opportunities for experiencing a sense of companionship and connection with other cancer patients.

The results from the metasynthesis confirmed that being diagnosed with advanced cancer opens up distinct experiential spaces which the person needs to learn to inhabit and find meaning in. To navigate this challenging terrain requires effort and commitment, demonstrating that patients are active and agentic as they search for ways in which they can rise to the psychological challenge of living in the face of death. This shows that suffering is not a passive state but a project in which the person is actively engaged.

Conclusion

In this chapter, I have described how my own experience of the distress generated by a cancer diagnosis provided the motivation to embark upon a research programme of qualitative research into the experience of living with cancer. Pursuing this research helped me process and make sense of my own experience, and at the same time, it offered me an opportunity to explore methodological possibilities for gaining a deeper understanding of the lived experience of cancer and how this experience might be brought into being within a particular social context. My choice of methods was shaped by the evolving questions that emerged, initially from the autoethnography and then from each of the consecutive studies. Different methods help the researcher generate different types of insights by shedding light on the phenomenon of interest from different angles. A research programme that uses a range of qualitative methods can, arguably, produce a more rounded understanding of a phenomenon than a mono-method study alone would be able to achieve. This resonates with a pluralistic approach to qualitative research (e.g. see Frost, 2009) and chimes with its commitment to generating multi-layered understanding(s) which reflect the complex, multi-faceted nature of human experience. The combination of methods used in the present research programme facilitates insights into the ways in which subjective experience is, at least in part, mediated and shaped by available discursive resources, and at the same time, it draws attention to people's active engagement with these resources as they find their own way of finding meaning in their experience. Such a binocular perspective helps to deepen and broaden our understanding of the experience of living with cancer, and it addresses the limitations inherent in each of the methods used. The in-depth focus on one individual's subjective experience that characterises the autoethnography is complemented by the wider lens applied through the metasynthesis, whilst the discourse analytic focus on sociocultural situatedness of experience is complemented by phenomenology's concern with lived, embodied experience. Such an approach to research allows us to examine experience in the light of discourse whilst at the same time paying close attention to experience as it is lived by those who describe it. It goes some way to addressing ethical concerns about deconstructing accounts of suffering and the stripping away of the subjective experiential dimensions that a discursive analysis inevitably entails (see Willig, 2015b), and at the same time it speaks to the sociocultural situatedness of experience which does not always receive the attention it deserves in phenomenological research (see Todorova, 2011). It is an approach that can examine how constructions of meaning around cancer can have a detrimental effect on the quality of life of people who are living with cancer, and, hopefully, contribute to creating a sociocultural context within which cancer is talked about in a way that is mindful of the impact of discourse on experience.

References

Anderson, L. (2006). Analytic autoethnography. *Journal of Contemporary Ethnography, 35*(4), 373–395.

Ashworth, P. (2003). An approach to phenomenological psychology: The contingencies of the lifeworld. *Journal of Phenomenological Psychology, 34*(2), 145–156.

Bondas, T., & Hall, E. O. C. (2007). Challenges in approaching metasynthesis research. *Qualitative Health Research, 17,* 113–121.

Ehrenreich, B. (2009). *Smile or die: How positive thinking fooled America and the world.* London: Granta Publications.

Ellingson, L. L., & Ellis, C. (2008). Autoethnography as constructionist project. In J. A. Holstein & J. F. Gubrium (Eds.), *Handbook of constructionist research* (pp. 445–466). New York: Guilford Press.

Ellis, C., Adams, T. E., & Bochner, A. P. (2011, January). Autoethnography: An overview. *Forum: Qualitative Social Research, 12*(1), Art. 10. http://www.qualitative-research.net/index.php/fqs/article/view/1589/3095.

Finlay, L., & Gough, B. (Eds.). (2003). *Reflexivity: A practical guide for researchers in health and social sciences.* Oxford: Blackwell.

Frost, N. (2009). Pluralism in qualitative research: A report on the work of the PQR project. *Social Psychological Review, 11*(1), 32–38.

Giorgi, A., Giorgi, B., & Morley, J. (2017). The descriptive phenomenological psychological method. In C. Willig & W. Stainton Rogers (Eds.), *The SAGE handbook of qualitative research in psychology.* London: Sage.

Gough, B., & Madill, A. (2012). Subjectivity in psychological science: From problem to prospect. *Psychological Methods, 17*(3), 374–384.

Holman Jones, S., Adams, T., & Ellis, C. (2013). Introduction. In S. Holman Jones, T. Adams, & C. Ellis (Eds.), *Handbook of Autoethnography* (pp. 17–47). Walnut Creek, CA: Left Coast Press.

Lakoff, G., & Johnson, M. (1980). *Metaphors we live by.* Chicago: University of Chicago Press.

Langdridge, D. (2007). *Phenomenological psychology: Theory, research and method.* Harlow: Pearson Prentice Hall.

Lubbock, T. (2012). *Until further notice, I am alive.* London: Granta.

Ludvigsen, M. S., Hall, E. O. C., Meyer, G., Fegran, L., Aagaard, H., & Uhrenfeldt, L. (2016). Using Sandelowskiand Barroso's metasynthesis method in advancing qualitative evidence. *Qualitative Health Research, 26,* 320–329.

Martin, C. (2000). *Writing your way through cancer.* Prescott, AZ: Hohm Press.

Mosher, C. E., & Danoff-Burg, S. (2009). Cancer patients versus cancer survivors. *Journal of Language and Social Psychology, 28*(1), 72–84.

Parker, I. (1992). *Discourse dynamics: Critical analysis for social and individual psychology.* London: Routledge.

Parker, I. (1994). Reflexive research and the grounding of analysis: Social psychology and the psy-complex. *Journal of Community and Applied Social Psychology, 4*(4), 239–252.

Potter, J., & Wetherell, M. (1987). *Discourse and social psychology: Beyond attitudes and behaviour.* London: Sage.

Propper, M. (2007). *Gestalttherapie mit Krebspatienten. Eine Praxishilfe zur Traumabewaltigung.* Koln: Peter Hammer Verlag.

Roy-Byrne, P. P., Davidson, K. W., Kessler, R. C., Gordon, J. G., Asmundson, R. D., Renee, D., … Stein, M. B. (2008). Anxiety disorders and comorbid medical illness. *General Hospital Psychiatry, 30,* 208–225.

Sellick, S. M., & Crooks, D. L. (1999). Depression and cancer: An appraisal of the literature for prevalence, detection, and practice guideline development for psychological interventions. *Psycho-Oncology, 8*(4), 315–333.

Smith, J. A., Flowers, P., & Larkin, M. (2009). *Interpretative phenomenological analysis: Theory, method and research.* London: Sage.

Stacey, J. (1997). *Teratologies: A cultural study of cancer*. London: Routledge.

Thorne, S. E. (2015). Qualitative metasynthesis: A technical exercise or a source of new knowledge? *Psycho-Oncology, 24*, 1347–1348.

Todorova, I. (2011). Explorations with interpretative phenomenological analysis in different socio-cultural contexts. *Health Psychology Review, 5*(1), 34–38.

Van Manen, M. (1990). *Researching lived experience* (1st ed.). Ontario: The Althouse Press.

Van Manen, M. (1997). *Researching lived experience* (2nd ed.). Ontario: The Althouse Press.

Williams Camus, J. T. (2009). Metaphors of cancer in scientific popularization articles in the British press. *Discourse Studies, 11*(4), 465–495.

Willig, C. (2009). "Unlike a rock, a tree, a horse or an angel...": Reflections on the struggle for meaning through writing during the process of cancer diagnosis. *Journal of Health Psychology, 14*(2), 181–189.

Willig, C. (2011). Cancer diagnosis as discursive capture: Phenomenological repercussions of being positioned within dominant constructions of cancer. *Social Science and Medicine, 73*(6), 897–903.

Willig, C. (2013). *Introducing qualitative research in psychology* (3rd ed.). Open University Press (McGraw-Hill Companies).

Willig, C. (2015a). "My bus is here": A phenomenological exploration of 'living with dying'. *Health Psychology, 34*(4), 417–425.

Willig, C. (2015b). Discourse analysis and health psychology. In M. Murray (Ed.), *Critical health psychology* (2nd ed.). Basingstoke: Palgrave Macmillan.

Willig, C. (2017). Reflections on the use of object elicitation. *Qualitative Psychology, 4*(3), 211–222.

Willig, C., & Billin, A. (2012). Existentialist-informed hermeneutic phenomenology. In D. Harper & A. R. Thompson (Eds.), *Qualitative research methods in mental health and psychotherapy: A guide for students and practitioners*. Chichester: Wiley-Blackwell.

Willig, C., & Wirth, L. (2017). A metasynthesis of studies of the experience of living with terminal cancer. *Health Psychology, 37*(3), 228–237.

Willig, C., & Wirth, L. (2019). Liminality as a dimension of the experience of living with terminal cancer. *Palliative & Supportive Care, 17*(3), 333–337.

Wray, N., Marcovic, M., & Manderson, L. (2007). Discourses of normality and difference: Responses to diagnosis and treatment of gynaecological cancer of Australian women. *Social Science and Medicine, 64*(1), 2260–2271.

Part II
Applying Qualitative Methods in Collaborative Research Projects

Chapter 6
Listening for What Is Not Being Said: Using Discourse Analytic Approaches in Mental Health Research

Julianna Challenor, Eugenie Georgaca, Rebecca Aloneftis, Nobuhle Dlodlo, and Helena Curran

Abstract This chapter explores the potential for discourse analytic research to address the topic of recovering the socially and discursively unsaid/unsayable through research in mental ill-health and distress. Psychological domains of distress, along with other affective and embodied experiences of the psychosocial subject, sometimes considered as extra-discursive phenomena or outside discourse, can be argued to create methodological challenges for discursive accounts. Drawing on research examples, the authors suggest ways in which different domains of unspoken distress can be discursively theorised. The chapter demonstrates how three different discourse analytic methods can illuminate which particular ways of knowing and speaking are left out or omitted from language, and once omissions are identified, investigate how this happens. This approach to discourse analytic research can suggest in whose interest it might be that certain discourses or discursive repertoires are not heard, in other words why it happens, and the effects of the absence for the individuals concerned. In the first study, Foucauldian Discourse Analysis is used to identify discourses of employability used by individuals tasked with aiding people back to work after unemployment. The near-complete absence of discourses of psychological distress in professionals' constructions of their roles and responsibilities towards their clients is notable and suggests that the possibility for psychosocial distress to be encountered through working/not working is excluded from current meaning systems. A second study draws on critical discursive psychology to examine rhetorical moves made by individuals who hear voices when constructing their identity. Voice hearers appear to have to make a discursive choice to fit with social norms and avoid stigma. The final example examines women's accounts of giving birth shared in groups and on social media, and draws attention to the absence of subjectively

J. Challenor (✉)
Metanoia Institute, 13 North Common Road, London W5 2QB, UK
e-mail: Julianna.challenor@metanoia.ac.uk

E. Georgaca
School of Psychology, Section of Social and Clinical Psychology, Aristotle University of Thessaloniki, Thessaloniki 54124, Greece
e-mail: georgaca@psy.auth.gr

R. Aloneftis · N. Dlodlo · H. Curran
Department of Psychology, City, University of London, London, UK

© Springer Nature Switzerland AG 2021
M. Borcsa and C. Willig (eds.), *Qualitative Research Methods in Mental Health*,
https://doi.org/10.1007/978-3-030-65331-6_6

female discourses elsewhere in the clinical and lay literature to make claims about a woman's power, positioning and sense of self in relation to giving birth.

Keywords Discourse analysis · Mental health · Extra-discursive · Foucauldian discourse analysis · Critical discursive psychology · Critical psychology · Visual discourse analysis · Voice hearing · Childbirth · Employability

Introduction

In this chapter, we argue that a discursive approach to research in mental health and mental distress is important for understanding not only what is being talked about and how, but also what is not spoken of, or not-said. We are interested in the ways that discourse analytic approaches can illuminate which particular ways of knowing and speaking are left out or omitted, and once identified, investigating how this happens. And finally, this method of research can suggest in whose interest it might be that certain discourses or discursive repertoires are not heard, in other words why it happens, and the effects of this absence for the individuals concerned.

Discourse analysis is a qualitative method that asks how a particular psychological or social construct comes to be through being spoken of, written about and enacted, in everyday interactions as well as in policy and institutional practices. Moreover, it examines the function of invoking and utilising particular discourses in terms of normalising types of experience and legitimising forms of knowledge and practice. It also investigates the effects this has for particular individuals and groups, whose experiences and practices are defined by these discourses. We would argue that the same interrogation can be made of what is *not* spoken of, thought, written about or enacted. Discourse analysis is suited to identify the gaps in discourse, that which is not addressed and talked about. Furthermore, it can be used to interrogate how something is left out of discourse, what processes are implicated, what function this omission serves and whose interests are being served by it. In other words, we contend that discourse analysis can be used to examine not only *what* is not said but, perhaps most importantly, *why* certain things are not said, and what function is served by the absence of alternative ways of speaking, thinking and doing. This effectively amounts to an investigation of the workings of power in defining reality and subjectivity. Highlighting the role of power opens up, in turn, possibilities for resistance, in terms of enabling more varied and empowering ways of defining experience and constructing subjectivities. In this chapter, we will illustrate what can be produced in taking this perspective, using three examples of research studies that use a range of discourse analytic methods to demonstrate how the not-said can be accounted for.

Accounting for the Not-Said

In arguing for this dual focus on both what is and what is not said, a question arises about the status of the not-said. Is the not-said to be considered to be 'outside' discourse or perhaps pre-discursive? The status of the not-said is intimately linked to the ways we theorise the relationship between experience, meaning-making and discourse. Willig (2017) argues that there are two poles in the theorisation of this relationship. On the one hand, there are approaches which view experience as primary, as having an embodied affective basis that pre-exists discourse. From this perspective, discourse may shape experience through determining how certain experiences can be talked about and understood, through covering up and constraining, or reversely foregrounding and amplifying, aspects of lived experience, but does not determine a phenomenon as it is experienced in its primary affective aspects.

An example of this might be an embodied experience, such as giving birth, or the emotional experience of psychological distress. This argument proposes that there are aspects of embodied and affective experience or material realities that cannot or ought not to be reduced to discourse. Critical realism has been offered as one way to give an account of an individual's experience while remaining within a constructionist framework. From this perspective, distress and other subjective experiences are conceptualised both as product of discourse and a pre-condition of existence. Critical realism attempts to account for the ways in which we are both constituted by discourse and simultaneously exist partly outside it. Drawing on Bhaskar's (1989, 2014) work, Sims-Schouten, Riley, and Willig (2007) describe critical realism's concept of "a relationship between deep material and social structures that are not object-like and concrete and that are, therefore, not directly accessible to the researcher. They can only be known through the phenomena that they generate, that is to say, their presence can only be deduced from the processes and experiences which they have made possible" (p. 105). Sims-Schouten and Riley (2018) have developed a method called Critical Realist Discourse Analysis (CRDA) with the aim of examining how individuals understand and experience their own mental health problems, founded in this view of a "…stratified model of reality" (p. 2). In theorising this approach Sims-Schouten and Riley also draw on Wetherell's (2013) proposal for a discursive focus on affect.

From this perspective, that which is not talked about may point to some aspect of embodied experience which is difficult to speak of, perhaps because of the nature of the experience or because of the limits of language. The not-said may be related to experiences that are beyond discourse and in this sense point to the pre-discursive or extra-discursive, that which lies outside discourse. In some cases, this can be seen to indicate experiences that are so primary they are inaccessible to discourse. In these cases the not-said can border on the unsayable, pointing to experiences that by their nature cannot enter discourse. What is left unaddressed in talk may represent experiences that, for various reasons, have not been put into words.

The other pole, according to Willig (2017), is occupied by a more traditional social constructionist perspective that sees discourse as primary and as constituting all experience. In this conceptualisation, there is no pre-discursive or extra-discursive experience; experience itself is produced by the action of discourses, which necessarily entail subject positions and thus constitute subjectivities. More generally, from a social constructionist perspective, material processes and structures, be it bodily, social or institutional, are always already inextricably interwoven with systems of meaning, knowledge and practice. From this perspective, that which is not talked about does not refer to some pre-discursive experience which has not been, or even cannot be, put into words, but to something that has been silenced and excluded in and by discourse. In other words, the not-said is that which is not-permitted, and in this sense it represents subjugated meanings and knowledges that are actively excluded from entering discourse and therefore shaping experience. From this perspective, then, what is left unaddressed in talk may indicate aspects of experience that, for various reasons, are not allowed to be put into words, and thus to become part of individuals' experience.

Subjugated forms of knowledge are linked to the operation of power in relationships between individuals, between individuals and organisations, as well as between organisations. This approach is founded on Foucault's (1982) claim that discourse constitutes experience, or what can be talked about, thought, felt and done. Through the constraining effects of discourse, power is enacted. When no discourses are available to talk about an experience, this experience cannot be had and therefore remains unaddressed. In the field of mental health, social constructionist approaches have argued that mental distress is to a large extent due to the operation of dominant discourses, mainly deriving from the biomedical model, which conceptualises distress as an illness, an effect of bodily dysfunction, and in this way precludes other, potentially more meaningful and empowering understandings of distress that individuals can draw upon to make sense of and manage their experiences (see, e.g., Cromby & Harper, 2009). Taking this stance further, postmodern, systemic, narrative and other social constructionist inspired therapy approaches have argued that the direction of therapy is towards deconstructing the dominance of the biomedical discourse and facilitating the development and utilisation by the therapy clients of other discourses that can render distressing experiences meaningful and manageable (Smoliak & Strong, 2018).

Regardless of whether they posit the existence of pre- or extra-discursive experience, both theoretical perspectives on the relation between experience and discourse view discourse as crucial in shaping experience. According to both, experiences that are considered to be psychological are filtered through a discursive lens in order to have meaning. Even if an experience exists on some level that is pre-discursive, the *forms* that the experience can take are discursively constructed. In mental distress, a raw sense of suffering is channelled and takes different forms through socially available systems of meaning. Discourse transforms a raw embodied state into a fully experienced phenomenon, and with this transformation power can be exercised to actively shape human experience through the dominant discourses available. Foucault's (1980) concept of power/knowledge underpins this account of subjectivity. An individual's account of themselves, their 'truth', is historically constituted, and accordingly constituted through power relations. From this perspective, discourse is a system for representing knowledge at particular historical, social and cultural points. Accordingly, identifying where and how individuals are subjected to power in the form of knowledge and the way they respond to it is central to discourse analytic methods. The process becomes one of uncovering how through discourses individuals can be positioned by language and knowledge regimes in ways that shape, constrain, and in some cases, exclude something central to the individual's subjective experience that, if acknowledged, would present opportunities for resistance.

We contend that attending to what is not said, what is left unspoken, is important in this attempt to highlight the effects of power and the way in which the mental health of individuals is constructed, as it points to aspects of experience that cannot be talked about, made sense of and ultimately fully experienced. The not-said refers directly to the constraining operation of power, to the aspects of meaning-making and experience that are inaccessible to speaking beings and unavailable to them to use in order to understand and manage their experiences. In this sense, attending to the gaps in talk, identifying what is not addressed, can be argued to be a more direct route into discursively investigating the operation of power than analysing the discursive constitution of subjectivity through dominant discourses. We certainly want to suggest that identifying what is not talked about and interrogating its functions and effects is a valuable part of discursive analysis, especially for those adopting more critical approaches that seek to address issues of power and resistance.

In what follows, we provide three examples of such discursive work, discuss the ways in which in each case the exploration of the not-said enhances our understanding of power, and in this way showcase the usefulness of this approach. Each study uses different versions of discourse analysis, and in doing so illustrates the flexibility of the method. The versions are Foucauldian Discourse Analysis (Willig, 2013), critical discursive analysis (Edley, 2001; Wetherell, 1998) and Machin and van Leeuwen's (2016) approach to analysing different modes of discourse, in this case, images on social media. A university ethics committee approved all of the studies.

In the first, which examines the discourse of professionals, we will show how what is left out of the construction of clients serves the interests of creating a legitimate professional identity, and in the course of doing so closes down, or neglects, important discourses and subject positions that clients can draw on. In the other two studies, with voice hearers and women after giving birth, we examine the effects of dominant discourses on experience. In these, what is not said reflects aspects of experience that are excluded by dominant discourses of voice hearing and giving birth, respectively.

Study One: Silencing Aspects of Experience in the Service of Constructing Professional Identity

In keeping with a focus on action orientation and context, an important part of analysing that which is not-said is examining its function. A first step is interrogating who articulates the text and in what interactional, institutional and socio-cultural context it is produced. An example of this is research by Dlodlo (2018). She interviewed five leaders of British social enterprises who were participating in programmes designed to enhance employability of clients at risk of social exclusion. A semi-structured interview schedule focused on how they constructed employability for their clients, who were unemployed individuals belonging to various vulnerable social groups. Of the five participants that took part in the study, four were white men, and one was a white female. Their unemployed clients had experienced issues with mental health or had physical and learning disabilities. One organisation worked with young homeless people. All but one had direct links with governmental organisations such as the Job Centre and IAPT (an NHS mental health provider; Improving Access to Psychological Therapies). The participants' organisations worked with clients on employment-related tasks such as Curriculum Vitae (CV) writing, interview preparation, coaching, job searches and placements.

Analytic Procedure

The transcripts of five interviews were analysed using Foucauldian Discourse Analysis. Willig's (2015) 6-step method was used, as it permits an exploration of what is considered pertinent to understanding the issues that are key to a Foucauldian approach to discourse analysis. Willig (2015) offers a detailed description of what each of the 6 steps asks of the data, and a simplified description is presented here to reflect the questions asked at each stage of analysis:

1. Discursive constructions: *Identifying the different ways the discursive object of employability is constructed using language, including references to its determinants and effects.*
2. Discourses: *What are the wider discourses within which the various discursive constructions of employability can be situated?*
3. Action Orientation: *When is the discourse being used and to what purpose? What function is being fulfilled, or what may be gained through constructing the employability in a particular way?*
4. Subject positioning: *What rights and duties are ascribed to different subjects through the use of the discourse? Taking up a subject position within discourse offers a position from which to speak and act, and positioning others in discourse has implications for what these others are expected to do and say. Positioning also determines whether and how subjects can exercise power in relationships with each other.*

5. Practice: *What can be said and done from those positions? How do the discursive constructions allow or disallow opportunities to act and make particular practices possible?*
6. Subjectivity: *What can be thought, felt and experienced from the subject positions that have been identified in the earlier stage? This final stage of the analysis can only make tentative claims.*

Results

We will describe the discourses with which participants construct employability for their clients, and consider what is left out of these constructions, together with the implications.

Neo-Liberalism as a Meta-Discourse

A neo-liberal discourse was identified as the dominant framework for constructing employability. Neo-liberalism interacted with all the other discourses and was considered to be a meta-discourse or a larger discursive framework, within which the participants' use of various discourses could be contextualised. Within this larger discursive framework of neo-liberalism, discourses were divided into two categories. The first constructed employability as an internal state attributable to the aspirational neo-liberal citizen. According to these constructions, intrinsic employability can be optimised within particular contexts. However, the barriers faced by clients challenged assumptions of the "citizen", or employable individual, and the participants' talk illustrated some resistance to these assumptions.

Yet, even as these assumptions were resisted, neo-liberalism remained relevant as a meta-discourse. It informed participants' use of the second discursive category, of paternalism, which was a way for them to resist some punitive aspects of neo-liberal citizenship discourses. Neo-liberal paternalistic discourses offered participants a way to accommodate their clients' vulnerabilities, whereas neo-liberal discourses of citizenship failed to do so (Fig. 6.1).

Neo-Liberal Discourses of Citizenship

Kock and Villadsen (2015) argue that citizenship is both a discourse and a mechanism by which discourse is enacted and in this study it interacted with all the discourses presented in the first category to shore up certain assumptions of the employable individual. According to Woolford and Nelund (2013), the neo-liberal citizen is active, and typically that is taken to mean employed. They are able to manage risks as an actuarial subject and are capable of self-management and privatised responsibility. Importantly, given the client group that the participants support,

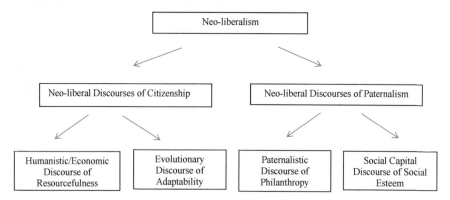

Fig. 6.1 Relationships between discourses

neo-liberal citizens are not reliant on government or social services for survival but are instead autonomous, self-reliant and empowered. Finally, the neo-liberal citizen is entrepreneurial in their ability to maximise personal interests (Woolford & Nelund, 2013). Participants constructed fostering these capacities as their main objective, suggesting that the main requirement for the employable individual is to be able to draw out some internalised sense of their own abilities. Participants talk about their role as helping clients to position themselves within society among other self-esteeming citizens, which will lead to the actualisation of the clients' own employability.

> *I wrote an article for the History of Employability professionals last year that really said you can only really do one thing with an unemployed person, increase their levels of self-efficacy around job searching and the job they want to do. Because if you don't address self-efficacy, you are forever pushing a person up a hill and the moment you let go, they are gonna roll back down again. (Christopher)*

Humanistic/Economic Discourse of Resourcefulness

Within this discourse of neo-liberal citizenship, employability is also constructed to include an individual's intrinsic capacity to be economically productive, and this is combined with an assumption that growth is ultimately fulfilling for the individual. The discourse of self-actualisation comes from humanistic theory in psychology, and claims that all human beings possess an innate drive towards growth. Constructions of employability here suggest an innate propensity in individuals towards employment. Any challenges that emerge around an individual's capacity to work are constructed as functions of inefficient, ill-suited, non-optimising working environments or barriers that can be overcome. Overcoming these challenges is described as a function of economically rational perspective taking.

> *All the evidence shows that clearly people are better off whilst at work than being out of work and that the majority of barriers to support people to go back to work can be overcome. (Adrian)*

Many times, they will consider something an obstacle, "I'm just a victim, a passive victim to it." When actually, when we talk to them about it, we can get them to see that it's actually a barrier and if we do something about it, we can get rid of it forever. (Christopher)

Here is an assumption that the employable individual or citizen is able to optimise their humanistic and economic 'resourcefulness' to eliminate employment barriers altogether. However, the sociopolitical factors, which exist outside of the individual, are not acknowledged as potentially complicating employment outcomes. Actual employment outcomes are of limited interest when the individual's employability is emphasised in this way.

Evolutionary Discourse of Adaptability

The discourse of 'adaptability' implies that a challenging environment can be valuable, because it stimulates an individual's ability to adapt their employability and to develop, in the form of gaining employment and career progression.

First and foremost, we look at the circumstantial side and say "Let's see if we can help this person have a lifestyle that is compatible with work". [...] This is my 20th year of being in the employment sector. I fell into the sector through having a nervous breakdown. Saw a psychiatrist for some months and ended up staring at the walls 20 hours a day at home. Started claiming employment benefits... (Christopher)

Participants position statutory settings like mental health hospitals and Job Centres as insufficiently stimulating or even stifling. Adaptability, and therefore employability, is constructed to facilitate economically rational choices about what one feels and does in a given environment. This use of language suggests that adaptability involves the 'rational' management of emotions according to the demands of the environment.

So what our guys do is a lot of work on challenging attitudes and behaviours, modelling the attitudes and behaviours [...]. To be able to switch an attitude on in an appropriate environment and go back to normal self when out of that environment...that's really vital for me [...] being able to help choose the attitude they show in a work environment. (Christopher)

Neo-Liberal Discourses of Paternalism

The neo-liberal meta-discourse permitted participants to uphold the expectations of neo-liberal citizenship, while using neo-liberal paternalistic discourses to accommodate their clients' dependence. Kettl (2006) demonstrates the ways in which neo-liberal paternalism is enacted through social entrepreneurs, such as the participants of this research study. The aim of neo-liberal paternalism, as Suvarierol (2015) writes, is to create citizen-workers through civic integration via mechanisms insistent upon the internalisation of moral codes that favour one's participation as an employed, active agent in a redefined community.

A Paternalistic Discourse of Philanthropy

This is arguably one of the seminal discourses available to social enterprises positioned as responding to social problems. Dean (2007) states, "…the essential nature of philanthropy is paternalism" (p. 4). Within this discourse, the philanthropist is a judge, mediator and pastoral carer for the poor. They take on responsibility for the poor individual's morality, in the service of larger societal goals of ensuring the individual's capacity for self-policing.

> *Often it takes me to be in a meeting with him and either talk for him or say "Look, he's not an angry guy. He gets really worked up, he is in a really difficult financial situation and he's fallen into a bit of bad luck et cetera". But if I wasn't there for that…dunno…he would probably get arrested, barred from places or whatever it might be, but no one knows why he is like that. I know why he is like that and there are reasons why he is like that. But no one else has that relationship, so they just see him as an angry guy. (James)*

Morality is key within this discourse, and participants take up a position of the moral, uniquely perceptive philanthropist. Without this benevolent oversight, their clients are positioned as unable to manage expected behaviour independently. The client's moral and social dependence is maintained by their persistent employment needs, which in this use of language is suggestive of moral needs. This permits a measure of social control for those who are yet to internalise the desired moral codes.

Social Capital Discourse of Social Esteem

Finally, employability is constructed as a product of socialisation to the surrounding society and to people. The client is encouraged to generate social capital by engaging in multiple, esteeming, socialising relationships. However, the paternalistic relationship that the client shares with the participant remains the most important. In it the client is intimately positioned to be seen and to see the world specifically through the provider's eyes. This is argued to be vital to triggering that initial generation of social capital.

> *Offering things like doing the football and doing other sports and the trapeze and the drama is a way of engaging with them and not actually putting employment straight away to them but actually about saying "Listen, try it and see how you feel", get that relationship going. So it's about starting to build a relationship so that eventually they feel better about themselves and feel that they can actually take on people…and take on…because it's quite a very…it's a very hard journey for anyone who's not worked for a number of years to suddenly feel like they can get a job again. (Richard)*

The participants contrasted their socially esteeming, paternalistic relationship with the distant, though similarly paternalistic, relationships they understand other 'blinded' expert professionals to share with the clients. They construct institutional practices, such as Psychiatry or Job Centres, as pathologising, isolating and censuring the individual, thus limiting their potential social capital. The 'expert's' insulated subjectivity does not allow them to demonstrate the degrees of engagement and encouragement that facilitate 'social esteem' or favourable socialisation. The expert does not build social capital. They cannot accommodate the informality, and therefore freedom, that neo-liberalism espouses.

There is, there is documented evidence that the average level of expectations of clinical workers, uh, not all, obviously, you can't generalize, but the more severe and enduring, um, diagnoses, category of illnesses, that they work with, typically the lower expectations are in terms of work and recovery...Why would a psychiatrist, who only ever sees people on a ward, have any idea of what they are capable of achieving at work...Whereas to have people who see it from the other side and are conscious of the work side of managing mental health, as opposed to the clinical and the, um, incarceration, and the in-patient aspect of it. (Adrian)

Discussion

Drawing upon neo-liberal discourses, study participants constructed employability for their clients via the culturally dominant image of the 'homo economicus', excluding any psychological and mental health concerns that the clients might have. They constructed the process of helping their clients through notions of disadvantage or deficit rather than vulnerability or distress. In the broader sociocultural imaginary employability is treated as an individual characteristic, and unemployment is linked to individual psychological vulnerabilities. This view is reinforced by the appointment of counsellors in UK government Job Centres. The question of why these study participants systematically exclude psychological, emotional and mental health issues from their depiction of employability therefore becomes particularly pertinent.

From a discursive perspective, we would focus on the function that this omission has for participants and their clients, and we would start by examining who articulated this discourse and what subject position they construct for themselves. If we take into account that the research participants are social entrepreneurs, leaders of social enterprises, it is no surprise that they foreground a neo-liberal ideal of people as individual entrepreneurs seeking self-improvement through calculated actions, and portray the obstacles to employability in terms of social disadvantage that hinders the process of self-improvement and socioeconomic ascent. In this way, the study participants construct their clients as in need of enhancing their entrepreneurial skills and thus legitimise their own professional identity. It may be hypothesised that if the research participants were employment *counsellors*, they would foreground psychological and mental health discourses and instead silence entrepreneurial and socioeconomic aspects, when discussing the employability of their clients.

Most discourse analytic research of mental health professional perspectives has focused on the discursive strategies through which professionals account for their practices of assessment, diagnosis and treatment. These studies have shown that, when professionals are called upon to account for their practice in a research study, they actively develop strategies of legitimation of their actions, through evoking expertise and mobilising dominant discourses in order to pathologise their clients and naturalise their actions (Liebert & Gavey, 2009; Stevens & Harper, 2007). In other words, mental health professionals actively construct their identity through legitimising their knowledges and practices (Georgaca, 2013). Systematically silencing understandings of their clients that do not fit in with their professional role seems to be one more of the strategies that professionals have at their disposal. We would argue, in conclusion, that when studying professional discourse, investigating what is left out can shed light on the construction and legitimation of professional identities. Excluding aspects of client experience and identity, apart from shaping professional identities, has repercussions for clients. We will address this more directly below.

Study Two: Dominant Discourses and the Construction of a Mentally Disordered Identity

While discourse analytic studies examining the talk of mental health professionals tend to focus on the discursive strategies of accounting for professional practices and legitimising a professional identity, studies examining client perspectives tend to investigate the discursive resources that clients draw upon to understand their distress and the effects of these discourses on their experience and identity (Georgaca, 2014). In this second example, Aloneftis (2017) examined the ways in which individuals who hear voices make sense of the voice hearing experience and the effects of this experience on their identity. The eight participants were all members of the UK Hearing Voices Network (HVN), an organisation that takes a pluralistic approach to understanding the phenomenon of voice hearing. Seven females and one male, aged between 19 and 20 years, and who identified as voice hearers were interviewed.

The study illustrates how individuals who hear voices get caught up in a dilemma in which they must denounce or disavow important aspects of their experience in order to claim a socially acceptable and valued identity. The subjective experience of distress is explicitly linked here with identity constructions and power relationships in every day and institutional settings.

Analytic Procedure

The discursive approach in this study operates on the assumption that language has a performative function. It is where identity work occurs and due to this an analysis of discourse is a useful method for investigating identity construction (Benwell & Stokoe, 2006). Moreover, adopting a discursive perspective enables researchers to critically examine the power implications of particular identity constructions and the ways in which these are reinforced by institutions and practices (Parker, 2002).

This study draws upon Davies and Harré's (1990) theory of positioning, which is helpful for the examination of the active role the individual plays in choosing between the discourses available to them. Positioning theory was used in the analysis to identify how participants positioned themselves within available discourses of voice hearing and with what consequence for identity construction. However, this is a cyclical process, because discourses have an impact on individuals and practices, and conversely the way that participants position themselves serves to reinforce or undermine discourses (Sims-Schouten et al., 2007). Critical discursive psychology is therefore both agentic and deterministic (Burr, 2015). Despite individuals being determined by discourse, they are also considered to be creative actors in the way they deploy language and construct accounts to accomplish a purpose (Edley, 2001). It is in this positioning within available discourses that identity work occurs (Davies & Harré, 1990).

The study sought to address the following research questions: How do people who hear voices talk about their experiences? What resources in the social domain do they draw upon to negotiate this identity? What are the consequences for the way in which this identity is negotiated? The critical discursive method used here entails a dual analytic focus, combining conversation analysis and post-structuralism (Billig et al., 1988; Edley, 2001; Wetherell, 1998). A micro-level analysis of the action orientation of participants' talk looked at what participants tried to accomplish in interaction. This stage of the analysis examined the discursive strategies that participants utilised, the rhetorical devices they drew upon to support their discursive strategies, the interpretative repertoires (common ways of talking about things formed by shared social consensus) employed, the ideological dilemmas (deliberations, contradictions and inconsistencies in talk) posed and the subject positions (how participants positioned themselves in discourse) used to do identity work.

The macro-level of analysis looked at the wider discourses that participants drew upon to construct the experience of hearing voices, attempting to locate the discursive constructions without losing the action orientation of talk. This level of analysis seeks to address power implications and address questions such as: What possibilities of action do the identified discourses enable? Whose interests are being served by the prevailing definitions of voice hearing? What is the relationship between discourse and practice? And how are these discourses and practices maintained, resisted or transformed? (Willig, 2013).

Results

Participants used two types of interpretative repertoires to construct the experience of hearing voices. Each of them was pursued through different discursive strategies (Fig. 6.2).

Of interest is the polarity of these constructions, which was observed both between interviews and within the same interview. We take these polarities to reflect the dilemmatic nature of talk, illustrating that what participants are trying to accomplish with their talk is dependent on both the immediate interactional and the broader sociocultural context. In this study, it was useful to explore the differential identity

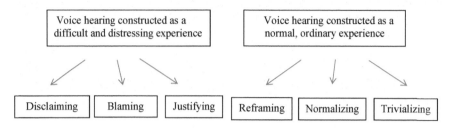

Fig. 6.2 Interpretative repertoires and discursive strategies of voice hearers

constructions found in the material through the concept of negative and positive identity construction (Bucholtz, 2009), as well as by examining the orientation of identity construction in relation to the in-group or the out-group (Wetherell & Edley, 2009). Negative identity practices are employed where individuals want to distance themselves from a rejected identity and emphasise identity as an intergroup phenomenon, whereas positive identity practices actively construct a chosen socially valued identity and thus emphasise the intragroup aspects of social identity (Bucholtz, 2009).

By drawing on the interpretative repertoire of voice hearing as a difficult and distressing experience, participants created a division between themselves and non-voice hearing populations through maximising difference in terms of their distressing experience. The construction of voice hearing as a distressing experience exemplifies negative identity practices, because participants seek to define what voice hearers *are not* by rejecting pathological notions of voice hearing and distancing themselves from negative constructions in the social domain. This repertoire is associated with discourses of pathology and is why, when using it, participants oriented towards avoiding being positioned by others as 'mental patients' within biomedical discourses of psychopathology.

With the second repertoire of voice hearing as a 'normal' experience, participants used rhetorical devices to normalise the experience of hearing voices and in doing so attempted to achieve a greater level of proximity with the rest of the population. With this interpretative repertoire, participants minimised difference by constructing their experience as ordinary. This was an example of positive identity construction, whereby participants attempted to disclaim any relation to the dominant discourses of pathology that might be ascribed to them through building up their credentials as 'normal' people.

Voice Hearing Constructed as a Difficult and Distressing Experience

Disclaiming

Participants adopted this strategy to disclaim pathological constructions of voice hearing in the social domain, when they perceived their identity to be under threat, for example when voice hearing was associated with pathological labels and notions of dangerousness. In this strategy, participants overtly rejected pathologising assumptions linked to voice hearing. Thus, through minimising the pathological associations to voice hearing, they tried to recover a valued identity as voice hearers.

The three areas that they look upon is, one is just general prejudice, you're mad, you're crazy, you're bad. The other area is basically in some respects it's your fault that you've suffered it and the other respect is in some warped sense, you must be weak in some respect or suffered a breakdown. And that's absolute rubbish on all three fronts. (Jack)

Through using a three-part list (*"you're mad, you're crazy, you're bad"*) and extreme case formulation (*"absolute rubbish"*), Jack initially articulates and then strongly rejects the negative, pathologising attributions that he sees as socially ascribed to voice hearers.

Blaming

This strategy apportions blame to others—the media, institutions, health professionals, pharmaceutical companies—for negative constructions of voice hearing in the social domain. This is not simply an attempt to reject pathological notions of voice hearing, as with the previous strategy. This strategy goes further in seeking responsibility for these presumably unfounded negative attributions. Apart from implicitly reinforcing the claim to the falsity of these attributions, this strategy serves to construct voice hearers as honourable moral agents, who are wronged by the misguided representations of others. Here, participants construct their identity in relation to what they are not and in direct comparison with others, who are positioned as not understanding and not knowing.

Society in general and the media. I think the media more than anything. The media, maybe psychiatry a little, drug companies. I usually blame drug companies for most things. But actually more than psychiatry or the pharmaceutical industry is the media, and you know it's the media for so many things, but it is, you know, this kind of need to print shocking scary things because that's what people want to read. And then print them in a really ill-informed way and report them in an ill-informed way, like every time something awful happens, there's like a query about whether the person who did it had mental health problems. (Neve)

I don't think they would have people cycling in and out of hospital if they would stop putting this as a "Oh it's a pathology", "oh you're nuts" that kind of thing. Ah, "I really must keep you away from society, because you're a bit of an embarrassment". (Zoe)

Neve uses repetition (*"you know"*), generalisation (*"every time something awful happens"*) and extreme case formulation (*"shocking scary things"*, *"really ill-informed"*) to maximise the impact of her claims that, more than *"psychiatry"*, *"the pharmaceutical industry"* and *"society in general"*, *"the media"* is responsible for the disastrous circulation of negative stereotypes regarding individuals in mental distress. Zoe voices in direct speech the exaggerated and misguided claims that people in general (*"they"*) make when talking to people with mental health difficulties.

Justifying

Participants also repeatedly justify the mental state and actions of themselves or others, when confronted with pathological constructions of voice hearing. In this way, they distance themselves from negative constructions of voice hearing though explaining how they have come about and why they do not conform to available constructions.

> *My brother said "Yea well everything you say when you're unwell is all gobbledygook". And that really, really hurt. Because it was like, you know, "I'm maybe unbalanced and not, and confused and not remember things, but it's still, I'm still me?" And to scrub out everything I'm about when I was showing those symptoms is very hurtful. (Angie)*

> *I have been abusive myself and people have kept out of the way from me. But the thing is I'm more frightened of them, than they are of me really. That's what we want to get the voice across, because all you hear about in the papers is "Paranoid schizophrenic, stabbed somebody", and so on and so forth and been arrested and they're usually down on the ground or something being manhandled by the police. And it's probably the voices telling them to do it. And they're more frightened of the police than anybody needs to be frightened of them. Cause I've been known to carry a knife but I didn't know that I was doing it. Do you know what I mean? Afterwards someone's told me and I couldn't believe it was me. It's like you're a different person, but you're very frightened. Cause hearing voices is frightening. (Anna)*

Angie recounts an episode in which, faced with her brother's accusation that in periods of crisis she does not make sense, she reformulated her mental state as being *"unbalanced"*, *"confused"* and *"not remembering things"* and argued that it is a state of mind that expresses aspects of her being (*"what I am about"*) that should be understood and respected. Anna attributes both her and other voice hearers' *"abusive"* behaviour to the experience of hearing voices, which affects their state of mind. Moreover, she indirectly attributes some extreme reactions of voice hearers to their fear, caused by the voices and by other people overreacting to their altered state of mind and aggressive conduct.

Voice Hearing Constructed as a Normal, Ordinary Experience

The discursive strategies employed to construct voice hearing as a normal and ordinary experience resulted in normalised accounts that minimised and reframed pathological notions of this experience. These are positive identity practices, because they seek to delineate what voice hearers are like, through asserting their proximity with the rest of the population, and thus ascribing to them the socially valuable identity of a 'normal' person.

Reframing

Reframing involves restating a situation so that it may be perceived in a new light. Wherever possible, participants attempt to reframe their experiences in ways that allows for a less problematic identity, for example, by constructing themselves as atypical members of pathological categories relating to the experience of hearing voices. The discursive strategy of reframing allowed participants to distance themselves from a position that is potentially problematic and particularly one that does not enable possibilities for action.

> *My voices have been more compassionate and reasoning and helpful as such on occasions, but I tend to be the exception to the case there, whereas most of the group their voices can be at times distressing, dark, aggressive, and cause them quite some distress. (Jack)*

> *Well, a psychiatrist explained to me years ago, that because I could recognise my hallucinations as hallucinations they weren't true psychosis. Now I get delusions, which I believe are true. I don't see them as delusions, so if somebody, psychiatrists, wants to argue they are delusions, I would debate that with him or her. So, they could say I'm psychotic on that. But the hallucinations, I can see as hallucinations, so they're called a pseudo psychosis, not a total psychosis. (Lauren)*

In the extracts above participants stress the difference of their experience from what is constructed as a 'typical' experience of hearing voices. They thus construct themselves as atypical members of the mental health diagnosis of schizophrenia or psychosis, repudiating the implied category entitlement.

Normalising

Participants used this discursive strategy to construct the experience of hearing voices as an ordinary experience. This strategy reduces perception of difference and otherness by establishing a degree of proximity with the rest of the population.

> *Well, it is normal but it's not seen that way, I don't think, by other people. [R: How do you think it is seen by others?] …Either it's scary cause you might be dangerous or it's scary cause it's completely weird and people just can't understand what I'd be like, so they're just kinda like "I can't relate the inside of my head to the inside of your head", which is really bizarre, cause the inside of my head works in a similar way to well everyone, the inside of everyone's head is pretty weird. And whenever you find out something about somebody's ways of thinking or beliefs and things, you're like "What? It doesn't make any sense!" So, everyone's different and weird and I don't think it, you know, I relate it quite often to my voices, are quite often troublesome to me in the night? That, you know, If I'm stressed they'll wake me up at like 3 in the morning, and kind of make lots of noise, but I know from other people that don't hear voices, that when they're stressed they wake up at 3 o'clock in the morning with their thoughts racing round in their heads. And that's completely normal. And I'm like "Well it's not so different from that! It's just like my body and my brain reacting to the fact that I'm stressed and disrupting my sleep. And for you it's your thoughts, for me it's the voices". (Neve)*

Neve uses extreme case formulation ("*completely weird*"), direct speech quotes and generalisation ("*everyone's different and weird*") to construct an argument that her voice hearing experiences are more similar to other 'normal' experiences than others would be willing to acknowledge. She also uses personal footing, presenting her own experience and comparing it to that of others around her, in order to ground her claims to personal knowledge and experience.

Trivialising

Participants use this discursive strategy to minimise the distress they experience. These constructions allow participants to remain in control, save face and reassure others. One of the strategies adopted is to use humour to cope with difficulty (Gelkopf, 2011). The alternative would mean participants having to acknowledge the sometimes very distressing and severe consequences that the experience entails for themselves and others.

> *One of my ways of kinda coping with things that have happened that have been really difficult, and this is my family's way of coping with everything, is with humour. So I've got like a collection of kind of hilarious stories about things that have happened when I've been in hospital, because hospital's been horrendously traumatic...but usually a few things happened that are quite funny, and they're particularly funny if it's something silly that I've done, cause I like making fun of myself so I'll maybe say to somebody "Oh like that time when I was in hospital and dadadadada happened" and then they'll laugh and someone might be like "Oh! what hospital were you in?" or something, and then I'll like make light of it. (Neve)*

Here, Neve uses direct quotes, extreme case formulation (*"horrendously traumatic"*), repetition and vague expressions (*"kind of"*, *"like a"*) to describe her deliberate use of humour to trivialise distressing situations and experiences.

Discussion

This study examines the effect of dominant discourses of voice hearing and psychosis, both lay and professional, on the identity construction of people who hear voices. It demonstrates that voice hearers are very aware of these discourses and are active in managing their positioning with respect to them. This is in line with other discourse analytic studies of mental health service users diagnosed with psychosis (Benson et al., 2003; Harper, 1995). Faced with the position of being severely mentally disturbed and potentially dangerous to themselves and others implicated in the diagnosis of a severe mental disorder, they can either accept it, with all the repercussions this has for their identity, or reject it and adopt a 'normal' subject position (Georgaca, 2004). The polarity between pathology and normality constructed by the dominant biomedical discourse of mental illness leaves no room for any position other than being 'mentally ill' or 'being normal'. The price of adopting the 'being normal' position is to deny the strangeness of voice hearing and to silence the distressing and disturbing aspects of this experience, as well as other psychotic experiences. There is no possibility of acknowledging, making sense of, and attempting to manage bizarre and disturbing experiences without adopting an unwanted pathological identity. Safe-guarding a positive 'normal' identity implies rejecting the disturbing aspects of one's experience, leaving no possibility to acknowledge and deal with them. We see here the operation of power in the form of dominant discourses forcing individuals caught up within them into particular binaries of subject positions, which end up silencing, excluding and leaving unaccounted for significant aspects of their experience. Here, paying attention to what is left out, what is not talked about, is important in order to identify the discourses at play and their effects in terms of shaping individual experiences of distress.

Analysing, through the gaps, the operation of power of dominant discourses, also points towards strategies of resistance. In this case, resistance to the power of the biomedical discourse necessitates deconstructing the polarity between normality and pathology. This would involve a simultaneous process of normalising distress and de-sanitising normality, in other words acknowledging both the continuity between the two and the deeply disturbing and distressing aspects of 'normal' experiences (Parker, Georgaca, Harper, McLaughlin, & Stowell-Smith, 1995). This is the direction that many self-help organisations in the field of mental health have taken (Campbell, 2013), and with regard to hearing voices the international hearing voices movement in particular (Longden & Dillon, 2013; Romme, Escher, Dillon, Corstens, & Morris, 2009).

Study Three: Sanitising Bodily Processes

A biomedical discourse shapes human experience through defining, ordering and constraining what can be felt, also with regard to bodily processes. An example of the simultaneously productive and constraining role of the biomedical model is given in the work of Curran (2019) around childbirth, specifically women's accounts of giving birth, as they share them in groups and in social media. This study is rooted in a premise, born of an emerging social narrative (McNish, 2017) that childbirth is constructed in non-'woman-oriented terms' (Grosz, 1989), within dominant biomed-ical and maternity discourses, and in turn the social contexts of naturally occurring talk between women. This study seeks to make sense of this absence of a subjectively female discourse in relation to what it says about a woman's power, positioning and sense of self in relation to giving birth. Twelve participants took part in three focus groups of 4. They were white or Asian women from the UK, Europe or the USA, and all the women had given birth more than 12 months previously. All were currently living in the UK, in London. Some of the women had more than one child, and some were pregnant at the time of the focus groups. The emancipatory aim of this research prompted three research questions: What dominant discourses around childbirth are available? How do women take up or resist those discourses in their own construc-tion of childbirth? What might that mean for both childbirth practice and a postnatal woman's subjective experience?

Analytic Procedure

Childbirth is both a practice and a process that is embedded within social, historical and institutional contexts. Explicit themes of gender, power, sexuality and medicine meant that a Foucauldian Discourse Analytic framework was deemed an appropriate research method. Willig's (2015) six-step method (described above) was applied to texts produced from three focus groups, each comprising four postnatal women talking to each other about childbirth. The participants were recruited through mother-and-toddler playgroups, personal contacts and social media sites. Focus groups took place in hired private spaces in three different locations and facilitated with the aim of eliciting something as close as possible to naturally occurring talk. Helena, the researcher, offered participants her own stake in the research, through disclosing her own experience of childbirth, as Potter and Hepburn (2005) suggest.

A second analysis of visual images of childbirth posted on Instagram was also carried out; this will be summarised later.

Results

What follows are three examples of discourses elicited from the focus groups. They all serve to limit a woman-oriented discourse and the consequent subjective experiences of childbirth. Instead, a 'natural' maternity discourse, a biomedical discourse, and a masculine discourse are drawn on to construct childbirth as a perfect, natural process, and/or one in which women are the vessels for a healthy baby, and/or governed by a strikingly male lens.

'Natural' Maternity Discourses

In the naturally occurring talk of the focus groups, childbirth was intensely, and quite fearfully, constructed as part of the participants' sense of self. Participants talked of being justified or judged in relation to their capacity as a woman and a mother. Hannah described what the leader of an antenatal group had told her:

> *"She said, 'Well you know what, I would just like to say that the ultimate childbirth experience and what you could all see as kind of a success story would be if you ended up having a home birth, because if you end up having a home birth, that just means you are awesome at childbirth'". (Hannah)*

When asked to talk about their experience of giving birth, the participants positioned themselves quickly into split camps of 'natural' (vaginal) birth or Caesarean Section. The explanation around having a C-Section, particularly a planned one, was much more extensive and justifying. The ideal birth, as prescribed by Hannah's antenatal maternity group leader, was *"home birth"*. *"Home birth"* is presented as the epitome of natural, which means you are "*awesome at childbirth*". This feeds into both a maternity discourse of natural as best, in which you are "more likely to feel satisfied with your labour" and "less likely to experience psychological problems like depression" (NCT, 2019), incorporating criticism of hospitals and medical intervention as overly controlling and therefore bad. By prizing the female 'naturalness' of birth this maternity discourse conversely constructs those who have navigated birth with anything other than natural ease as un-natural and a failure. The birthing woman is positioned as one to be observed and judged, as Sally experienced:

> *And I even overheard... and I shouldn't be critical, but it's something that happened and it sticks with me. I heard... someone came into start their shift, and the lady said, "Oh, how is she getting on?", and she said, "Well [inhales] [pause], she is doing alright, when she does it properly".*

To acknowledge childbirth as something emotionally and physically messy is made difficult by the 'natural' discourse of birth and the women described a need to tidy up their talk in their everyday lives when they talked about their experience of giving birth, into neat, clean, external and medicalised narratives of birth type, timings, location and pain relief used. Implicit in the 'natural' discourse was an expectation that women give birth independently, and without any (internal or external) fuss or mess. It was this absence of mess, chaos, gore—the 'not-said-ness' of childbirth—which was paramount; out of all the focus groups comprising over 5 h of talk about childbirth, the word 'blood' was said six times, 'vomit' five, and 'vagina' just twice.

Through the not-said, and not-seen, and within a scrutinising maternity discourse constructing childbirth as natural, women are positioned in a conflicting, eradicating and shameful way, where 'natural' is best but simultaneously unacceptable.

Biomedical discourses: the mother as vessel for a healthy baby

> *This other poor lady, um... she was quite adamant, like, you know, "The baby is coming." And then the midwife who, like... you know, they, whatever, examined her, and they were like, "No, it's not." You know, "You're a first-time mum. It's not coming." And, um [...], I think, like, somebody had told her to have a shower or... anyway, so she was in the shower. And she was like, "Can you get the midwife? The baby is really coming". And, um..., the midwife came, luckily, and it, kind of... it fell [laughter] out as she got out of the shower. (Renata)*

Another way in which women's subjectivity seems to be eradicated in childbirth links to the discourse that constructs the woman as a vessel for a healthy baby. All at once the birthing woman is constructed as a risky, threatening object and a passive, disposable entity. Renata recalls the story of the baby merely "*falling out*", and a 'lucky' one at that, as the vessel achieves its purpose and the baby survives.

That a woman is "supposed to efface her own subjectivity" (Bordo, 1993, p. 79) in childbirth evokes Foucault's (1998) thinking on discourses around women, their sexuality, their reproductive function and on the body as a site of disciplinary power. Taking up this discourse, Beatrice questions whether her subjective experience is even a valid consideration, given the baby was born healthy:

> *But it was those little things along the way that I hadn't really expected it and it, it did really take away from the kind of, the experience of childbirth. But then part of me sits here now*

and thinks, "Do I really care?" She came into the world, she's happy and healthy, um, does it, does it, any of these really matter, because it wasn't life and death at any point and it was quite controlled and, and carefully done.

There was frequent talk about actual and feared loss or death of the baby through numerous miscarriages and ectopic pregnancies throughout all focus groups. Nothing was said, however, about the loss a woman may experience in the moment of birth, as if both ideas cannot exist together. The birthing woman is constructed as a vessel through participants' accounts of being monitored, restrained, told to lie down on their backs, get in the (birthing) pool or get out of the pool. Dominant medical discourses construct this control as necessary for the safety of the baby. This medicalisation of birth, in which women are constructed as a vessel for a healthy baby, might be considered to represent the operation of a technology of power (Foucault, 1988), a means to control and prevent obstetric negligence claims, which in 2018 represented a significant 48% of the total value of all medical negligence claims in the UK (NHS, 2018).

'Masculine' Discourses of Birth

When distress *was* talked about in relation to childbirth during the focus groups, it was often introduced through a third, absent person or through a male lens. Masculine metaphors of war or murder scenes were recruited into the women's talk. It was thinking about how her husband saw and constructed their child's birth that allowed Sophia to re-construct what had previously been her "*great, really good birth*" to something that she definitely did not like and did not want to do again. The masculine lens was drawn on to allow her to construct a messier, more difficult birth in the absence of the not-said female-subjective one.

The masculine discourse was also constraining, as women describe its inability to accommodate either the physical or emotional chaos of childbirth. Sally described her husband's limiting, silencing reaction both to her being cervically examined; "*...my husband's reaction was to go to the toilet and throw up, you know*", and of her wanting to talk about the birth afterwards: "*Like, "Move on", basically, in not so many words*". The male lens constructs childbirth as intolerable and disgusting, needing to be curtailed and ended at the moment of birth. This suggests, as King (2004) argues, that "even in this supposedly equal, liberated society, femaleness is still disturbing enough to require supervision and containment by forms of discipline that men are not subjected to" (p. 36).

That discipline also manifests in repeated requests for pain relief to a male other, be it the husband, partner or clinician. This has something of a protective yet withholding function, as if women need to be both sheltered from yet bravely endure childbirth, the most threatening of all bodily experiences in its otherness to the male standard.

So it was awful, the whole... I had my playlist, I had the candles, I had all these things that my husband laughed about and said, "You're just going to be begging for that epidural". "No, I'll be fine". I tried the gas and air, threw up, as in similar to you. It didn't work and there was no anaesthetist around, which didn't help. (Anya)

My husband was very proud that I didn't have any pain intervention. (Sophia)

And I remember [laughter] saying straight afterwards to my husband… I was like, "Don't ever let me not have an epidural again". (Renata)

The notion of pain that is constructed as controllable by a male gatekeeper highlights something glaringly not-said in the women's talk about childbirth: the original sexual pleasure which creates the potential for childbirth, including any mention of sex, female sexuality and sexual organs. This can be contrasted with an image posted by the Empowered Birth Project on Instagram, with over 15,000 'likes', which shows a woman touching her clitoris for pain relief whilst the baby is crowning, accompanied by a caption, "Mammas, please don't be shy about touching yourselves!" (Empowered Birth Project, 2018a). This potential for the woman to relieve her own pain can be argued to be an example of an aspect of birth that a male discourse prevents, and which as Sophia says; "*…could quite easily be told to you and like…what is the myth about that that they can't say that to you?*" When birth is constructed as an event to be controlled by a male gatekeeper, woman's agency and sexuality is diminished at the moment of becoming a mother, kept as a shameful secret.

Visual Discourse Analysis: Birth as 'Real' or 'Unsee-Able'

In addition to the textual discourse analysis, a second form of analysis was employed using images posted by postnatal women about childbirth on Instagram, aiming to pursue the emancipatory rationale of this study as well as consideration of the not-said. For the purpose of the study, Instagram is considered to be a space where women can communicate and construct birth in a way that has the potential to exist outside the dominant discursive framework. Machin and van Leeuwen's (2016) discourse analysis framework for multimodal data was employed cyclically, to focus on meanings in relation to the signifier, signified and wider significance of the images selected. The first of the three stages of analysis focuses on the signifier, the visual evidence that is depicted, in terms of colour, objects or people within the image. The second stage focuses on the signified, the range of meanings that can be contained within the signifier, and arguments for how potential for meaning is realised in the context in which the image is presented. For example, whiteness in an image depicting childbirth may be interpreted as indicating cleanliness, calm or purity, and when contextualised as an image used by a hospital promoting its birth facilities, interpreting it as both clean and calm is plausible. The third stage of the analysis focuses on the wider significance of the image, particularly in relation to social theories, in which legitimisation or medicalisation, for example, can be argued to constitute, or disallow, particular identities, activities and values.

The disappearance of a woman's needs at the moment of birth found in the discourse analysis of focus group talk was also reflected in the visual discourses. A direct representation of what a vaginal birth actually looks like was in early 2018 actively censored by being removed from prominent visual social media platforms

Facebook and Instagram along with "pornography, graphic violence, profanity and other subject matter deemed too offensive for the public eye" (Vigos, 2018). In contrast, posting an image of a dead foetus was permitted, because it was posted (to 1.6 m followers) by a pathologist interested in the object as a medical curiosity (Hernandez, 2015).

Another image removed from social media in 2017 is worth considering (Empowered Birth Project, 2018b). The image in question does not show a vagina, a crowning baby, or a naked woman. It features centrally a woman, her breasts covered with her dark purple lace bra, her chest smeared with a little blood, holding her just-born baby over her bare, stretch-marked stomach, with the purple umbilical cord linking the not-yet-birthed placenta to her baby. In the image, there is an uncensored representation of the woman's intense emotional experience, which communicates horror and relief, agency and involvement in birth; unquestionably, this woman is more than a mere vessel. The setting is not within a medically controlled and mediated environment; indeed it's a messy, cluttered darkly lit domestic bedroom, with a sexually dark red bedspread in the background, far from a clean, white, sterile hospital context. The removed image shows physical and emotional mess, together with female distress, alongside the birth of a baby, all actively communicated by the woman in the photo.

Discussion

In these accounts, like those of voice hearers discussed above, we see clearly the way women are trapped in the dominant discourses of childbirth, both as a natural process and as a medical procedure. Both discourses normalise and sanitise the experience of giving birth, excluding any non-linear, contradictory feelings and understandings that women may have. They also efface the woman-subject, turning her to a carrier, a vehicle for the safe delivery of a baby, making her subjective experience of the process secondary and irrelevant. The combined effect of these is that women have no way of expressing, acknowledging and ultimately fully experiencing the messiness, the physical brutality, the pain and the intense ambivalence of the birthing process. This is another example of the way in which discourses define reality and experience, silencing and making inaccessible to the people who are caught up within them aspects of physical, psychological and emotional experience. In this example, noticing and interrogating what is left out, in this case the sheer physicality, messiness and ambivalence of the birthing process, allows us to examine the operation of power in terms of dominant discourses shaping individual experience.

Uncovering the operation of power can point towards strategies of resistance. In this case, encouraging women to voice their experience, ideally in mutually supportive groups and environments, might open up possibilities of more varied and complex accounts of the birthing experience. At the end of each of the three focus groups, the women taking part all independently agreed that a debrief with medical professionals about the birth would have been helpful in processing their experience. Consistent experiences of nobody asking, nobody wanting to hear about the birth within a medical context were reported. The women talked about wanting to voice their experience, have their distress validated, heard and held. This somewhat simple act might bridge the gap between the personal/female and the professional/male discourses, and be a way of disrupting the existing constructions of childbirth, so that a female-subjective discourse may be heard. Foucault (1998) claimed resistance is possible wherever normalisation and domination exists, as power is always shifting and unstable.

The Empowered Birth Project's goal of normalising the act of birth through showing it visually is one way that this resistance is contesting dominant power on what Foucault termed a 'micro level' (Foucault, 1998). The personal and female space of social media, showing actual childbirth, and with it a female-subjective discourse, which allows for a more mixed and messy, yet agentic expression and therefore experience of birth, is a way to do this. To this we might add the micro-levels of resistance shown by the women taking part in the research; two of whom, it should be noted, specifically requested their own name to be used in the study, with five declaring feeling comfortable with either their own name or a pseudonym being chosen. This can be considered, perhaps, a micro-act of resistance, which demands that they, and a woman-oriented discourse of childbirth, are both seen and heard in social, academic and ultimately clinical spaces. Thus, encouraging women's voices and the physical impact of circulating visual representations might operate as acts of resistance to the medicalisation, normalisation, sanitising and silencing of the disturbing aspects of women's experience of giving birth.

Conclusion: Power, Resistance and Potential for Action

The three studies presented here demonstrate how attending to the not-said and, most importantly, questioning the function of the not-said and its effects on the individuals affected by it, foregrounds the issue of power. Examining the operations of power can, in turn, open up possibilities for resistance. This, we contend, is one of the strengths of discourse analysis, and what provides it with its critical edge.

Attending to power is essential to the field of mental health research. Parts of experience that have been actively excluded through the operation of dominant discourses, such as a biomedical discourse in psychology, can be brought into the discursive framework and be thought about or spoken about in different, more empowering ways. The different purposes or reasons for the exclusion can be examined, limiting professional procedures can be questioned and strategies of resistance identified. These three studies all suggest different ways of uncovering the operations of power in what is currently dominant, deconstructing it and opening up gaps for other discourses and practices to emerge and gain ground. Discourse analysis seeks to "amplify the subjugated voices" (Miller, 2008, p. 258). It aims to identify and bring forth ways of talking and discourses that go against the grain of the dominant ones, and thus allow previously unacknowledged aspects of experience to be heard and felt.

At the beginning of this chapter, we briefly outlined some arguments that have been made about the place, or status, of the subjective experience of what it is that is not-said in discursive approaches. The limitations and criticisms of the methods described above depend on this status. If the not-said is considered to be outside discourse, discursive methods are limited to providing findings that must remain provisional. There is no way of either confirming or disconfirming what is being claimed when situated within a framework that suggests some experience will remain inaccessible to language. Participants themselves may not recognise the claims that are being made on their behalf and for a research method that aims to draw out the workings of power, researchers must remain acutely reflexive and alive to the potential for the abuse of power that lies with their own role. If, on the other hand, all experience is considered to be the product of discourse, then the argument can be made that the method neglects the possibility that individuals do possess and exercise agency, even if this remains limited. It is difficult to give an account of the choices that are actively made by participants in their talk, and this too may seem to participants to be counter to their own subjective experience.

Moreover, as it has been rightly noted (Willig, 1999), discourse analysis is reluctant to move beyond deconstruction to make recommendations for improved social and psychological practice. Through deconstructing harmful professional views and practices and opening up alternative spaces and positions discourse analysis does not directly lead to possible interventions, but can inform them (Harper, 1999). It has been argued that, if discourse analysis is to move beyond deconstruction towards a more direct impact in the field of mental health, it would need to take some important steps, which would include placing emphasis on the links between research, implementation and interventions, forging alliances between discourse researchers, mental health service users and critical professionals, and making tactical use of research findings through utilising multiple forms of dissemination and consultation (Harper, 1999, 2006).

We argued above that investigating the not-said can be a valuable part of a critical agenda in mental health research and practice. Moreover, we would argue that attending to the not-said, alongside to that which is said, can be pursued regardless of the status one gives to the not-said, be it as pre-discursive or as excluded from discourse. We contend that epistemological questions regarding the relationship between reality, experience and discourse, however important they might be, cannot detract discursive researchers from pursuing a critical agenda of problematising constraining knowledges and practices, which are sustained by dominant discourses, and opening up spaces for more empowering modes of experiencing, understanding and acting. We hope we have demonstrated in this chapter that attending to the not-said can be a poignant strategy for pursuing this critical agenda, which is much needed in mental health research and practice.

References

Aloneftis, R. (2017). *Discursive strategies in negotiating the voice hearing identity: A critical discursive approach* (Unpublished Doctoral thesis, City, University of London).

Benson, A., Secker, J., Balfe, E., Lipsedge, M., Robinson, S., & Walker, J. (2003). Discourses of blame: Accounting for aggression and violence on an acute mental health inpatient ward. *Social Science and Medicine, 57,* 917–926.

Benwell, B., & Stokoe, E. (2006). *Discourse and identity.* Edinburgh: Edinburgh University Press.

Bhaskar, R. (1989). *Reclaiming reality.* London: Verso.

Bhaskar, R. (2014). Foreword. In P. O. Edwards, J. Mahoney & S. Vincent (Eds.), *Studying organisations using critical realism: A practical guide* (pp. V–XV). Oxford: Oxford University Press.

Billig, M., Condor, S., Edwards, D., Gane, M., Middleton, D., & Radley, A. (1988). *Ideological dilemmas: A social psychology of everyday thinking.* London: Sage.

Bordo, S. (1993). *Unbearable weight: Feminism, western culture, and the body.* Berkeley: University of California Press.

Bucholtz, M. (2009). 'Why be normal?' Language and identity practices in a community of nerd girls. In N. Coupland & A. Jaworski (Eds.), *The new sociolinguistic reader* (pp. 215–229). Basingstoke: Palgrave Macmillan.

Burr, V. (2015). *Social constructionism* (3rd ed.). London: Routledge.

Campbell, P. (2013). Servicer users/ survivors and mental health services. In J. Cromby, D. Harper, & P. Reavey (Eds.), *Psychology, mental health and distress* (pp. 139–151). London: Palgrave.

Cromby, J., & Harper, D. J. (2009). Paranoia: A social account. *Theory & Psychology, 19,* 335–361.

Curran, H. (2019). *"Nobody told me": An integration of discourse analysis on constructions of childbirth* (Doctoral thesis in progress, City, University of London).

Davies, B., & Harré, R. (1990). Positioning: The discursive production of selves. *Journal of the Theory of Social Behaviour, 20,* 43–65.

Dean, H. (2007). The ethics of welfare-to-work. *Policy and Politics, 35*(4), 573–589.

Dlodlo, N. (2018). *Employability as a treatment goal? A Foucauldian discourse analysis* (Unpublished Doctoral thesis, City, University of London).

Edley, N. (2001). Analysing masculinity: Interpretative repertoires, subject positions and ideological dilemmas. In M. Wetherell, S. Taylor, & S. Yates (Eds.), *Discourse as data: A guide for analysis* (pp. 189–229). London: Sage.

Empowered Birth Project. (2018a, December 11). *Instagram.* Retrieved from Instagram: https://www.instagram.com/p/BrO9mB0jYio/.

Empowered Birth Project. (2018b, May 12). *Instagram.* Retrieved from Instagram.com: https://www.instagram.com/p/BiqV6EfBKMU/.

Foucault, M. (1980). *Power/Knowledge: Selected interviews and other writings, 1972–1977.* New York: Pantheon books.

Foucault. (1982). 'The subject and power': An afterword. In H. Dreyfus & P. Rabinow (Eds.), *Michel Foucault: Beyond structuralism and hermeneutics.* Chicago, IL: University of Chicago Press.

Foucault, M. (1988). Technologies of the self. In L. H. Martin, H. Gutman, & P. H. Hutton (Eds.), *Technologies of the self* (pp. 16–49). London: Tavistock.

Foucault, M. (1998). *The history of sexuality Volume 1: The will to knowledge.* Harmondsworth: Penguin.

Gelkopf, M. (2011). The use of humor in serious mental illness: A review. *Evidence-Based Complementary and Alternative Medicine ECAM,* 1–8.

Georgaca, E. (2004). Factualisation and plausibility in 'delusional' discourse. *Philosophy, Psychiatry and Psychology, 11*(1), 13–23.

Georgaca, E. (2013). Social constructionist contributions to critiques of psychiatric diagnosis and classification. *Feminism & Psychology, 23*(1), 56–62.

Georgaca, E. (2014). Discourse analytic research on mental distress: A critical overview. *Journal of Mental Health, 23*(2), 55–61.

Grosz, E. (1989). *Sexual subversions: Three French feminists.* Sydney: Allen & Unwin.

Harper, D. J. (1995). Discourse analysis and 'mental health'. *Journal of Mental Health, 4,* 347–357.

Harper, D. J. (1999). Tablet talk and depot discourse: Discourse analysis and psychiatric medication. In C. Willig (Ed.), *Applied discourse analysis: Social and psychological interventions* (pp. 125–144). Buckingham: Open University Press.

Harper, D. J. (2006). Discourse analysis. In M. Slade & S. Priebe (Eds.), *Choosing methods in mental health research* (pp. 47–67). London: Routledge.

Hernandez, D. (2015, October 31). *Splinter.* Retrieved from Splinternews. https://splinternews.com/meet-the-people-who-run-instagrams-most-horrifying-acco-1793852492.

Kettl, D. F. (2006). *The global public management revolution.* Brookings Institution Press.

King, A. (2004). The prisoner of gender: Foucault and the disciplining of the female body. *Journal of International Women's Studies,* 29–39.

Kock, C. E. J., & Villadsen, L. S. (2015). Citizenship discourse. *The International Encyclopedia of Language and Social Interaction* (Bind 1, s. pp. 115–121). Chichester: Wiley.

Liebert, R., & Gavey, N. (2009). "There are always two sides to these things": Managing the dilemma of serious adverse effects from SSRIs. *Social Science and Medicine, 68,* 1882–1891.

Longden, E., & Dillon, J. (2013). The hearing voices network. In J. Cromby, D. Harper, & P. Reavey (Eds.), *Psychology, mental health and distress* (pp. 151–156). London: Palgrave.

Machin, D., & van Leeuwen, T. (2016). Multimodality, politics and ideology. *Journal of Language and Politics, 15*(3), 243–258.

McNish, H. (2017). *Nobody told me: Poetry and parenthood.* London: Blackfriars.

Miller, L. (2008). Foucauldian constructionism. In J. A. Holstein & J. F. Gubrium (Eds.), *Handbook of constructionist research* (pp. 251–274). New York: Guilford Press.

NCT. (2019, January 11). *National Childbirth Trust.* Retrieved from www.nct.org.uk, https://www.nct.org.uk/labour-birth/different-types-birth/other-types-birth/what-straightforward-birth.

NHS. (2018). *Annual report and accounts 2017/18.* London: NHS Resolution.

Parker, I. (2002). *Critical discursive psychology.* Basingstoke: Macmillan.

Parker, I., Georgaca, E., Harper, D., McLaughlin, T., & Stowell-Smith, M. (1995). *Deconstructing psychopathology.* London: Sage.

Potter, J., & Hepburn, A. (2005). Qualitative interviews in psychology: problems and possibilities. *Qualitative Research in Psychology, 2*(4), 281–307.

Romme, P., Escher, S., Dillon, J., Corstens, D., & Morris, M. (2009). *Living with voices: 50 stories of recovery.* Ross-on-Rye: PCCS Books.

Sims-Schouten, W., Riley, S., & Willig, C. (2007). Critical realism in discourse analysis: Presentation of a systematic method of analysis using women's talk of motherhood, childcare and female employment as an example. *Theory & Psychology, 17*(1), 101–124.

Sims-Schouten, W., & Riley, S. (2018). Presenting critical realist discourse analysis as a tool for making sense of service users' accounts of their mental health problems. *Qualitative Health Research.* https://doi.org/10.1177/1049732318818824.

Smoliak, O., & Strong, T. (Eds.). (2018). *Therapy as discourse: Practice and research.* Palgrave/Macmillan: Basingstoke.

Stevens, P., & Harper, D. J. (2007). Professional accounts of electroconvulsive therapy: A discourse analysis. *Social Science and Medicine, 64,* 1475–1486.

Suvarierol, S. (2015). Creating citizen-workers through civic integration. *Journal of Social Policy, 44*(4), 707–727.

Vigos, K. (2018). *Allow uncensored birth on Instagram.* Retrieved from Change.org, https://www.change.org/p/nicole-jackson-colaco-allow-uncensored-birth-images-on-instagram.

Wetherell, M. (1998). Positioning and interpretative repertoires: Conversation analysis and post-structuralism in dialogue. *Discourse & Society, 9*(3), 387–412.

Wetherell, M. (2013). Affect and discourse—What's the problem? From affect as excess to affective/discursive practice. *Subjectivity, 6,* 349–368.

Wetherell, M., & Edley, N. (2009). Masculinity manoeuvers: Critical discursive psychology and the analysis of identity strategies. In N. Coupland & A. Jaworski (Eds.), *The new sociolinguistic reader* (pp. 201–215). Basingstoke: Palgrave Macmillan.

Willig, C. (1999). Introduction: Making a difference. In C. Willig (Ed.), *Applied discourse analysis: Social and psychological interventions* (pp. 1–21). Buckingham: Open University Press.

Willig, C. (2013). *Introducing qualitative research in psychology*. Maidenhead: Open University Press.

Willig, C. (2015). Discourse analysis. In J. A. Smith (Ed.), *Qualitative psychology: A practical guide to research methods* (pp. 143–167). London: Sage.

Willig, C. (2017). Interpretation in qualitative research. In C. Willig & W. Stainton Rogers (Eds.), *The SAGE Handbook of Qualitative Research in Psychology*. London: Sage.

Woolford, A., & Nelund, A. (2013). The responsibilities of the poor: Performing neo-liberal citizenship within the bureaucratic field. *Social Service Review, 87*(2), 292–318.

Chapter 7
Re-claiming the Power of Definition—The Value of Reflexivity in Research on Mental Health at Risk

Mariya Lorke, Carolin Schwegler, and Saskia Jünger

Abstract Being confronted with health risks implies challenges to mental health and well-being, requiring persons to find a balance between threat and confidence. The 'power of definition' with respect to health risks predominantly lies with professionals, implying that there is one appropriate way of understanding and interpreting risk-related information. This chapter will invite for a reflection on the potential of qualitative research in re-claiming the power of definition, offering the opportunity for a co-construction of concepts such as risk, vulnerability, and mental health. The aim is to highlight the particular value of different methodological approaches for opening up definitional spaces between scientists and research participants. It is grounded in the assumption that persons faced with a health risk construct their personal narratives to find a meaningful way to manage their situation, embedded in their biographical and social context. Narrative interviews with persons faced with a mental health risk were analysed in a circular process using complementing methodological perspectives from two disciplines: ethnology and linguistics. The findings were situated within a sociology of knowledge framework, focusing on the power of definition concerning a person's health and health risks. Herein, particular attention was drawn to ethical and methodological issues of assessing concepts such as 'risk' or 'vulnerability'; and the importance of (self-)reflexivity in conducting research in this field. Methodological reflection on these issues may contribute to constructively dealing with the tension between a standardised biomedical conception and an open, bottom-up approach to health knowledge in a medically oriented scientific environment.

Keywords Mental health risk · Risk perception · Dementia · Psychosis · Narrative approach · Semantics · Linguistic analysis · Ethnological approach · Sociology of knowledge · Meaning-making

M. Lorke · C. Schwegler
Cologne Center for Ethics, Rights, Economics, and Social Sciences of Health, University of Cologne, Cologne, Germany

S. Jünger (✉)
Department of Community Health, University of Applied Health Sciences, Bochum, Germany
e-mail: saskia.juenger@hs-gesundheit.de

© Springer Nature Switzerland AG 2021
M. Borcsa and C. Willig (eds.), *Qualitative Research Methods in Mental Health*,
https://doi.org/10.1007/978-3-030-65331-6_7

Introduction: Mental Health 'at Risk'—Challenging Definitions and Methodologies

From a sociology of knowledge perspective, knowledge is thought to be created through a process of discursive construction (Berger & Luckmann, 1966). Scientific knowledge—including medical 'facts'—is conceived of as socially, culturally, and historically contingent (Fleck, 1979). Of central interest is the process of the social production, transformation, and circulation of knowledge (Keller, 2011). This includes the roles, the positions, and the level of (non-)authority assigned to different stakeholders within the whole research undertaking.

While there are promising approaches such as user involvement or participatory, user-led research (e.g. Byrne & Morrison, 2010), the field of mental health research is still shaped by the predominant Western[1] paradigm of biomedical research. This has implications for the entire research process, including the definition of research questions (who defines them and which questions are considered relevant), theoretical foundations, the choice of methodologies and methods of data collection and analysis, the interpretation of findings and the conclusions drawn from these, as well as the publication and implementation of outcomes. As a consequence, the way of doing research shapes the reality of 'mental health'.

This chapter will invite a reflection on the potential of qualitative research in re-claiming the power of definition concerning mental health. Focusing on the experiences of persons 'at risk' for a mental health problem, it aims at offering the opportunity for a co-construction of concepts such as risk, vulnerability, and mental and (neuro)cognitive health. The aim is to highlight the particular value of the merger of different methodological approaches for opening up definitional spaces between scientists and research participants. It is grounded in the assumption that persons faced with a health risk construct their personal narratives in order to find a meaningful way to manage their situation and to (re-)gain a sense of agency, embedded in their biographical and social context. Drawing on the technique of (self-)reflexivity,[2] the potential and the challenges of qualitative research with regard to mental health risk will be discussed.

---

[1] The term 'Western'—despite not being undisputed—is used in this chapter in order to describe a "*mind-set, a worldview that is a product of the development of European culture and diffused into other nations like North-America*" (Ermine, Sinclair, & Jeffery, 2004, p. 5). 'Western' comprises an archive of knowledge and systems, rules and values, as well as intellectual, political, economic, cultural, and social constructs extracted from and characteristic of Europe and the Western hemisphere (Pellegrino, 1992; Smith, 2012). It includes fundamental attitudes to nature, reality, and knowledge (Sachs-Jeannet, Sagasti, & Salomon, 1994), hereby shaping the institutionalised social system within which knowledge production is embedded.

[2] We use the term (self-)reflexivity in the sense of a self-critique concerning the process of conducting research and producing knowledge. This self-critique demands examining our role as researchers, reflecting on how our particular background (such as our disciplinary and institutional socialisation, biography, values and attitudes, bodily constitution, or relationship to the interviewees) may interact with the research process, and on the power of presentation when publishing this research (Breuer, Muckel, & Dieris, 2019).

Being 'at Risk' in the Context of Dementia and Psychosis

Techno-scientific progress in biomedicine implies increasing opportunities for the early detection of disease risks (Aronowitz, 2009; Clarke, Shim, Mamo, Fosket, & Fishman, 2003). Advances in the field of predictive and preventive medicine can be considered a blessing, since ever earlier prediction is associated with the promise of better chances to prevent and treat disease and suffering. However, being confronted with health risks also implies challenges to mental health and well-being, requiring persons to find a balance between threat and confidence (Gillespie, 2012).

Both for psychosis and for dementia due to Alzheimer's disease (AD), efforts during the past decades were—and still are—directed at as precise and as early as possible diagnosis of prodromal stages of the conditions long before the full clinical picture can be observed.

In the case of AD, research aims to clinically identify early symptomatic stages such as mild cognitive impairment (MCI) or the even preceding subjective cognitive decline (SCD) (Albert et al., 2011; Jessen et al., 2014). MCI is associated with a risk for the development of dementia which is increasing in combination with a biomarker-positive testing (cerebral amyloid deposition and aggregation of tau protein; Jack et al., 2018).[3] In the case of psychosis, symptom assessment checklists and criteria for a 'high-risk' state were developed to identify the impending risk for transition to psychosis. Terms such as the clinical-high-risk state for psychosis (CHR), at-risk mental state (ARMS), or ultra-high-risk state (UHR) are used to describe the condition of individuals assumed to be in a pre-psychotic phase and to identify the impending risk for transition to psychosis (Fusar-Poli, 2017).

While there is agreement that early intervention is beneficial in terms of a person's long-term development, there is currently no unequivocal evidence concerning the most effective and efficient preventive interventions for either conditions. Concerning treatment options, in case of AD no cure exists to date. Meanwhile, the combination and probabilistic form of medical risk factors leaves the individual unclear concerning their relative effect, and without certainty about the future. Notwithstanding this, the 'power of definition' with respect to health risks predominantly lies with professionals, i.e., scientists or health professionals, implying that there is one appropriate way of understanding and interpreting risk-related information, and transforming it into health-promoting behaviour.

---

[3]MCI is connected with a 33% risk for developing dementia (Mitchell & Shiri-Feshki, 2009). MCI in combination with biomarker-based AD is associated with an increased risk of up to 59% for the development of dementia in the next three years (Vos et al., 2015). If the biomarkers remain inconspicuous or partially inconspicuous, risk probabilities of 5 and 23% apply. This means, so-called persons at risk do not only have to deal with the designation 'persons at risk' or 'MCI-patients' but also with the medically determined probabilistic understanding of risk (cf. Jack et al., 2018).

Making Sense of Risk—Risk Literacy and Meaning-Making in Mental Health

People confronted with a health risk need to make sense of the information communicated to them, such as probabilities, percentages, prognoses, as well as recommendations regarding prevention and treatment. Meaning-making can be considered as crucial in the process of coping with a challenging situation in life (Park & Folkman, 1997). Risk literacy is defined in terms of mathematical and logical transfer skills such as understanding percentages, estimating an individual risk based on a population risk, and deriving appropriate decisions and actions from the 'correct' risk appraisal (Gigerenzer, Gaissmaier, Kurz-Milcke, Schwartz, & Woloshin, 2007). However, critical health literacy as the capacity to critically appraise information against the background of one's personal lifeworld, values, and preferences, is much less in the focus of research and public debates (Sykes, Wills, Rowlands, & Popple, 2013). Hence, it can be argued that the capacity to make sense of one's own health risk and to translate this meaning into some form of coping is predominantly defined from a scientists' and health professionals' perspective, and is associated with patients' virtues of listening to and adhering to medical advice. In relation to risk literacy, Samerski (2013) describes the phenomenon of 'epistemic confusion' since a person needs to conflate a statistical risk profile with his or her personal situation in order to be considered as 'risk literate'.

Scientific Knowledge Production and Power Relations in Mental Health

Definitions of at-risk states in mental health require discussions about the transition between 'order' and 'disorder'. Psychiatric and neurocognitive diagnoses are used to categorise the emotional and behavioural traits to be considered as 'disordered', hereby setting standards for 'normality' (Albert et al., 2011; Timimi, 2014).[4] The conception of 'disorder' is highly debated in the field of mental health (Frances, 2014; Gronemeyer, 2013; Schaarschmidt, 2018; Wakefield, 2012). Psychiatry claims for itself the power of definition as to which behaviour or cognitive state is healthy and which is deviant, pathological, and in need of treatment. Discussions about the nature of a mental disorder, its aetiology, and the validity of risk factors are led among clinicians and scientists, while people experiencing the risk-related symptoms or syndromes are usually understood as the recipients of the resulting knowledge,

---

[4]All preliminary stages of dementia symptoms are defined as still being able to perform everyday tasks without larger limitation, even if now and then it may be necessary to overcome word finding disorders, forgetfulness and disorientation (as with MCI). Only in a second step biomedical markers of risk become relevant, but then with a strong classification and the label 'risk for AD', not only cognitive decline (of any category).

not as experts entitled to partake in the debate or in the planning of their thera-peutic process. Moreover, explanatory models tend to be increasingly dominated by biomedical perspectives (Bearden & Forsyth, 2018), while other approaches such as psycho-dynamic explanations or patients' self-experience are upstaged (Schultze-Lutter, Schmidt, & Theodoridou, 2018). At the same time, mental health problems and cognitive decline are seriously stigmatised, resulting in social labels based on arbitrary societal and medical norms. For example, medical, scientific and public discourses about dementia or schizophrenia tend to be catastrophising (e.g. Zeilig, 2014), shaping the political, social, and medical narratives around AD and psychosis. In this chapter, we aim at adopting a bottom-up approach to gain an in-depth under-standing of the individual constructions of meaning among persons whose mental health is considered being at risk: How do they make sense of this information? How do they describe their situation, either with or without referring to the term risk? What are the implications of the awareness of their risk for their everyday life?

Researching Mental Health 'at Risk': Methodology and Method

Narrative interviews with persons faced with a health risk in different clinical fields (psychosis and dementia due to AD) from two studies (RisKomp, hereinafter 'study on psychosis' and PreDADQoL (cf. Rostamzadeh et al., in press), hereinafter 'study on AD') will constitute the empirical base for the analyses in this chapter. The differences between the approaches in both studies are described in more detail in Box 1. Overall, narratives will be analysed in a circular process using comple-menting methodological perspectives from two disciplines: ethnology[5] and linguis-tics. Herein, particular attention will be drawn to methodological and ethical issues of assessing concepts such as 'risk' and 'vulnerability'; as well as the importance of (self-)reflexivity in conducting research in this field.

The two studies we refer to in this chapter both employ a qualitative design emphasising significant similarities in terms of the value of narratives. We aim at addressing the benefits and challenges of mental health research based on narrative knowledge, outlining the role of (self-)reflexivity in the research process by merging the findings from 20 interviews (10 from each study). In the following paragraphs, we will provide a short overview of the methodology used in both studies, focusing on sampling strategy, interviews, reflection, and analysis.

---

[5]For this contribution, we employed an *ethnological approach* to make use of a theoretical frame-work for comparative analysis with the aim to gain insight into both cultural phenomena and research processes concerning 'persons at risk' of psychosis or AD. While *ethnography* refers to a method-ological approach based on fieldwork for the in-depth study of a particular culture, *ethnology* allows for comparison and the identification of overarching structures, principles, and relationships (Flem-ming, 2010). *An ethnographer is constructing a theory that will make intelligible what goes on in a particular social universe. A comparativist (i.e., an ethnologist; author's note) is trying to find principles common to many different universes* (Goodenough, 1956, p. 37).

Sampling Strategy

Since there are hardly any evidence-based guidelines for the ideal size of the sample (Guest, Bunce, & Johnson, 2006), the decision on the sample size was taken based on the research question, the choice of methods, the sampling strategy and the availability of research resources. Also, we took the conventions in research literature and practice (Mason, 2010) into consideration. Our project partners[6] recruited the study participants according to collaboratively defined inclusion and exclusion research criteria, based on medical indications.

Data Collection

The qualitative data of 'persons at risk' were collected by means of narrative interviews (psychosis) and episodic interviews with a main narrative and a minor semantic part (AD) which both led to a significant proportion of uninterrupted narratives and free-flowing interactions (see methodological details below). As a central method of ethnographic as well as linguistic approaches (Deppermann, 2013; Groleau, Young, & Kirmayer, 2006), narrative and episodic interviews produce data that can give an insight into a person's individual perceptions, stratifications of experience, and entanglements of life-events (Schütze, 1983). A particular feature of our study on AD was the inclusion of one close other (e.g. spouse or close family member) with each patient. It is a common practice in memory clinics that a relative is closely involved in the diagnostic procedures and the counselling appointments. It was hence our aim to learn more about their individual perception of the (troubling) prospect to be a caregiver or even the present experience of being a 'pre-caregiver' (Largent & Karlawish, 2019). The dyads (of patients and close others) were interviewed separately but directly one after another.

Methodologically, we aimed at generating hypotheses on how persons confronted with the condition of being 'at risk' interpret this information and how they make sense of it in the context of their lifeworld. We therefore strived for a participatory perspective in defining our central concepts based on our interviewees' individual perceptions and experiences, in order to generate theories on the subjective meaning of risk grounded in these empirical findings, and to let them re-claim the power of definition.

With a view to such explorative outcomes, the methods of the guided narrative interview (Nohl, 2017) and the episodic interview (Flick, 1997) seemed to provide a fruitful ground for data collection (cf. Box 1). In both studies, a topic guide was used flexibly in the interview process in order to provide adequate space for the individual narrative construction. By asking further in-depth questions on aspects brought up

---

[6]In the case of psychosis, the FETZ (Cologne Early Recognition and Intervention Centre for mental crisis), and in the case of AD, the ZfG (Cologne Memory Clinic), both at the department of Psychiatry and Psychotherapy at the University Clinic of Cologne, Germany.

by the interviewee or questions on concrete situations of experiences the interviewer could stimulate the generation of additional complementing and/or more detailed accounts. This can provide not only information on the personal background and perceptions of risk, but also on how these are described in the interviewees' everyday language and embedded in social processes and cultural contexts.

Interview Procedures

In the study on psychosis, we used narrative interviews with the aim to put our interviewees' own perspective, interpretation, and subjective constructions of meaning at the centre of their accounts. A flexible topic guide was employed to allow for the unfolding of free narratives and the emergence of unexpected topics. We started the interview with an open question on a concrete situation in which individuals got confronted for the first time with the information of an increased risk. To elaborate more in depth on issues raised during the interviewees' initial open narrative, focused questions were used for explication, reflexion, or to invite for more detailed accounts (Groleau et al., 2006; Nohl, 2017). For in-depth exploration, the interview guide included topics based on existing research (family, identity, othering, health literacy) and additional questions formulated by the research team during the preparation phase. These were mobilised flexibly throughout the interview procedure (opening/formal phase, opening question, additional in-depth questions, closing phase), taking up the interviewees' preceding accounts and referring to their wording.

In the study on AD, we used episodic interviews as a useful approach to relevant experiences in life. The underlying idea is the differentiation of so-called world knowledge into two parts: Firstly, episodic knowledge which comprises knowledge that is linked to concrete circumstances (time, space, persons, events, situations), secondly, semantic knowledge which is more abstract, generalised, and decontextualised from specific situations and events (Flick, 1997). In the episodic part, which leads to narrations, the interviewer asks (chronologically) for specific situations from the life of the interviewee (before and after risk prediction and within those two times for situations of the everyday life, social environment, current situation, expectations, visions for the future, hopes and worries) in order to gain episodic knowledge. It is particularly important for the later linguistic analysis that central terms are not predetermined and that the questions are as 'innocuous' as possible from a lexical point of view. For example, "Can you describe to me how and why you got here?" (the interviews took place in the memory clinic). In-depth question: "Can you tell me a specific situation that explains to me how you felt about it?". With a reduction to deictics (here, it) the interviewees are invited to select and moreover name the central aspects themselves.

The last part of the episodic interview focuses on semantic knowledge which is achieved through semantic questions, i.e. questions for personal definitions, perceptions and understandings of certain terms which were used by the interviewee during the interview or are generally of interest for the study. The statements can be combined and contrasted with the narratives and also help to interpret certain statements of the interviewees (as well as the quantitative data of the study; cf. Rostamzadeh et al. (in press)).

Reflexivity

In order to make researcher's thoughts, feelings and subjective factors in the research process visible, we decided to employ different reflection methods in the two studies.

In the case of psychosis, we developed a reflection-tool integrated in the interview guide consisting of two subparts—notes (descriptions) and memos (interpretations and feelings). It enabled the researchers not only to analyse the 'subjectivity factor' in the overall analysis process, but also to reflect their own attitude and behaviour after each interview and so contribute to an increased richness of data.

In the case of our study on AD, we added metadata to each interview as material for the reflexive process. It includes additional aspects of the interview that cannot or was not recorded via audio taping, conversations and expression from the counselling physician, and impressions from the first meeting with both participants from one dyad (patient plus one close other). Concerning the analysed interview data, the linguistic approach of the interactional analysis (Deppermann, 2008) is not only focusing on expressions the interviewee utters but also the interviewer's assertions. In this way, the interviewer's statements also become objects of the (team) analysis and evaluation which encourages the reflection process. Since linguistic analysis is focusing on 'how' and not only 'what' was communicated, it is necessary for the interviewer to try to avoid certain key terms and predeterminations of vocabulary.

Analysis

In both studies, we focused on the multi-perspectivity of perception and strived to reveal various levels and modalities of the concepts concerned. The following paragraphs will demonstrate this by means of a detailed description of findings concerning the interviewees' perception and appraisal of their condition of being 'at risk', and by reflections on the methodological opportunities and challenges we encountered throughout the research process. The data used in the following discussion part originate from the interviews (psychosis and AD), the reflection-tools (psychosis), and single aspects of the metadata protocols (AD) (Box 1).

In the field of health sciences, interviewees' statements are often analysed from a thematic point of view, considering the interview as textual access to the social or psychological reality of interviewees, hence representing a more realist approach to data analysis (Willig, 2012). By contrast, in our analysis we strived for a more relativist perspective, understanding the interview narratives as situated co-constructions between interviewee and researcher.

Our *ethnological approach* was embedded in the **Reflexive Grounded Theory** methodology (Breuer et al., 2019). To enrich and complete our core data set of narrative interviews, we worked with additional data in the form of field notes, memos, and "thick descriptions" (Geertz, 1973) based on our self-reflection tools. Furthermore, we integrated reflexivity in the process of data analysis as a tool to make the researchers' subjectivity visible (Reichertz, 2015). Apart from this methodological triangulation (Denzin, 1970), we also strived for a researcher and theory triangulation which can be considered as crucial for an ethnological approach to our research field. The involvement of different disciplines within the research team allowed for a complex range of perspectives on the data, approaching it from different angles in terms of concepts and theoretical frameworks. The ultimate goals of our analysis were (1) to get as close as possible to the actors and let them speak for themselves, in their images and narratives; and (2) to generate preliminary theoretical explanations based on the empirical data.

The *linguistic approach* of interactional analysis (Deppermann, 2008) understands interviews as situated practice in which social structures of meaning are jointly created. Both the interviewees' and the interviewers' assertions are focused upon equitably during the process of analysis (even though the research questions and overall results might focus the interviewees' perspective only). As Deppermann (2013) points out, this approach prevents the analysis of the interviewee's statements without the reflection and analysis of what the interviewer emits or adds to the conversation—and most importantly 'how' he or she communicates. For this reason, it is essential that the audio-data is transcribed into the linguistic GAT2 system (Selting et al., 2009) which is close to the "Jefferson transcription system" and implies that overlaps of conversation elements, interruptions, and pauses are accurately represented. Furthermore, it appears to be a fruitful approach to consider the questions 'what', 'how', and 'why' successively and iteratively during the analytical process to shed light on relevant spoken elements, linguistic practices, forms, and semantic aspects as well as functions of those (Birkner, 2006).

For an *integration of both the linguistic and ethnographic approach*, we employed a comparative meta-analysis of the existing data in both projects in order to explore in-depth the findings and the methodological lessons learned from doing research on risk in the context of mental health. After data from the two projects had been analysed separately to answer the respective research questions, we discussed our findings and observations across both projects within the research team; and we compared our category systems in terms of intersections and differences. In this way, we identified our central categories with regard to the condition of being at risk (cf. section 'Insights from the Interviews: Naming, Explaining, and Coping'): naming, explaining, and coping; and we discovered overarching issues in terms of reflecting on our methodology and the research process (cf. section 'Methodological Reflection: Negotiating Vulnerability and Normality' and Box 2).

Box 1: Overview of the two studies presented in this chapter

	Study on AD	Study on psychosis
Name	Ethical and Legal Framework for Predictive Diagnosis of Alzheimer's Disease: Quality of Life of Individuals at Risk and their Close Others (PreDADQoL)	Health Literacy in Persons at Risk—From Information to Action (RisKomp)
Project leaders	Ceres, the Cologne Center for Ethics, Rights, Economics, and Social Sciences of Health, University of Cologne University Hospital Cologne Fundació ACE Barcelona	Ceres, the Cologne Center for Ethics, Rights, Economics, and Social Sciences of Health, University of Cologne University Hospital Cologne
Study design	Binational longitudinal mixed methods study including an ethical and legal framework (cf. Rostamzadeh et al., in press)	Multi-method study including systematic reviews and qualitative interviews
Aims of the study	(1) to determine attitudes and expectations towards the AD-risk prediction and elucidate the effect on the participants' QoL in order to provide a guideline for information and counselling; (2) to discover semantic content and multiperspectivity of concepts such as risk, QoL, satisfaction and well-being	(1) to better understand health literacy of 'persons at risk' in four different clinical fields, (2) to underpin it conceptually and (3) to make it fruitful for health care
Participants	Persons at risk for dementia due to AD, namely patients with MCI, who can optionally undergo a risk prediction, and one close other (family member; as an individual, not as a proxy informant) each (person at risk + close other = dyads)	Persons with an increased risk of developing a certain disease or an unfavourable course of the disease in four clinical fields: familial breast and ovarian cancer, coronary heart disease, psychosis and AD
Data of the project	Quantitative data from 50 dyads at 3 visits (in Cologne and Barcelona), qualitative data from 15 dyads at 2 visits from the German side only	Qualitative data from 40 narrative interviews (10 in each clinical field), 40 body-maps and 40 field notes data sets
Data used for this chapter	10 episodic interviews with narrative parts of around 30 min each, 5 from baseline (before predictive testing), 5 from the 3-month follow-up	10 narrative interviews with an average duration of 61 min, 10 field notes data sets
Data type	Audio-data, transcripts (GAT 2, basic)	Audio-data, transcripts, field notes data sets
Collection of metadata	Demographic data, medical records/explanations, interview metadata (interviewers' impressions and crucial non-verbal aspects on the background, the atmosphere or information the physicians shared with us in advance/after the interview) → used only additionally	Socio-demographic data (age, sex, marital status, cultural, educational and professional/occupational background) and field notes

(continued)

(continued)

	Study on AD	Study on psychosis
Method	Episodic interviews with a main narrative and a minor semantic part (Flick, 1997)	Narrative interviews (Nohl, 2017)
Interview topics	Everyday life, social environment, current situation, expectations, visions for the future, hopes and worries	Perceptions and experiences of risk, health and sickness, identity, family, everyday life, current situation, coping strategies, otherness and health literacy
Procedure	Chronological according to the participants' experiences, beginning with the first impression or feeling of impairment (at baseline), impressions and feelings since the risk disclosure (at 3-month follow-up), both thematically open	(1) Open question ("Tell me about the first time when you were confronted with the topic of being at risk of developing psychosis?"), (2) free part and (3) body-mapping exercise ("How would you depict the feeling of being at risk of developing a psychosis?") with comment on the drawing
Significant aspect	Questions and in-depth questions on concrete situations and experiences, semantic questions	Narrative interviews combined with memos (to make the researcher subjectivity visible)
Method of analysis	Linguistic interaction analysis with a focus on lexical and semantical aspects; metadata protocols as an analytical support, but focused on the aspects of perception that are revealed trough individual linguistic expressions (Birkner, 2006; Deppermann, 2008, 2013)	The process of data analysis was embedded in the Reflexive Grounded Theory (Breuer et al., 2019) based on three pools of data—the interviews (as audio and transcription), the body maps (incl. the verbal comments on them) and the field notes data sets (in the form of self-reflexion tools)

Results and Discussion

The following section consists of two subparts, which draw a common line of methodological reflection across both projects, hereby emphasising the opportunities and challenges that our teams faced doing qualitative research on mental health within the context of risk and medical prediction. It encompasses *content-led* results in negotiating vulnerability and normality from a bottom-up perspective ('Insights from the Interviews: Naming, Explaining, and Coping'), and *process-led* reflexivity discussing the interview as a method of data generation, the negotiation of roles and responsibilities, as well as ethical reflections throughout the research processes ('Methodological Reflection: Negotiating Vulnerability and Normality'). The sub-sections mirror methodological opportunities and challenges in the field of tension between biomedical understandings of risk and a person-oriented bottom-up approach.

Insights from the Interviews: Naming, Explaining, and Coping

The notions of vulnerability and normality play a central role in all steps of the research process and in all levels of content generation. Defining the persons at risk as a vulnerable group in the beginning of the research process challenged the idea of mental resilience, the explanatory models of risk, and raised questions about the factors that trigger and/or regulate this vulnerable condition. We will present findings from both studies along three categories that we identified in the interviews with regard to the condition of 'being at risk': naming, explaining and coping. These categories are selected because they thematically summarise essential stages of the process that occurs within the scope of 'being at risk' or 'learning to be at risk'.

Naming

The naming of risk can have diverse implications in the context of different conditions, as the following comparison of our interviews will illustrate. During the interviews with persons at risk of psychosis, it became clear that the naming of this condition in the context of the diagnostic process had been perceived as a relief rather than a threat. One reason was the affirmation of one's own perceptions, and an 'acquittal' of being suspected of working oneself up into the perception of strange sensations, and all symptoms being just an imagination:

PSYP03 (Interviewee; study on psychosis)[7]

```
436   When you talk to some friends or so about it, who don't really know anything about
437   it […] I've already heard it once or twice: Yes, I think you're exaggerating a bit,
438   or something. That is of course […] hurtful. But if someone who's studied that and
439   says that, uh, so… says: Yes […] You're right, you have that… and you actually
440   have a problem, that's very affirmative… in, so, for me […]. Well, it didn't
441   scare me now either, but I thought by myself: Now I know […], I can do something
442   about it. That's the first step.
```

The hard-to-communicate experience of ambiguous symptoms was replaced by a tangible and nameable condition of being at risk of developing psychosis. The latter might be perceived as more favourable, presumably because it can be explained by biomedical knowledge and is more strongly connected to body processes.

The impact of risk on people's lives and the notion of naming and vulnerability also became obvious in terms of the role as a "patient", which reveals the close relation between the phase of naming and explaining the 'at risk' condition. This role could be seen pragmatically, willingly engaging oneself with it, as reflected in the first quotation; or as an enigma, to a certain extent associated with a loss of definitional control, as emerging from the second quotation:

---

[7]The interviews were conducted in German language. Quotations were literally translated by the research team; for better readability, language and grammar were smoothened (e.g. omission of repetitions).

PSYP01 (Study on psychosis; P: interviewee; I: interviewer)

```
1098 P:  (laughs) Has now rented a, uh, practice or so, a room and I am now one of the
1099      first patients, so.
1100 I:  Oh so, ok. Because
1101 P:  =Is it called 'patients'?
1102 I:  Yes, there are always discussions about it. Some say clients, others say
1103      patients=
1104 P:  =Bähh, clients. Like somehow it's a … as if I give her money (laughs)=
1105 I:  =Yes, I, uh, I always find that difficult, because I actually also don't want to
1106      say 'patient' either, because you are now my interview partner, for example. But
1107      when you're so medically minded, you automatically say 'patient'.
1108 P:  =Yes, so I don't find anything reprehensible about the term, so, it, I'm just de
1109      facto one.
```

PSYP04 (Interviewee; study on psychosis)

```
1015  And yet the feeling afterwards was as follows: Now somehow for one and a half or two
1016  hours we have spoken to each other and described the problem as it were and that from
1017  this comes a diagnosis, yes, a diagnosis, or that somebody somehow can get an idea of
1018  something, uh, … and just then with such standardised questionnaires somehow, uh,
1019  therefore, hard to imagine… for me, or… yes, if you are perhaps not a specialist,
1020  uh, that you then have a clear picture of what is happening with these diagnostic
1021  instruments.
```

In our interviews with persons at risk for AD, the 'possibility to give a name' to the situation after the predictive biomarker testing sometimes is not experienced as a relief but as a reason for their behaviour and a confirmation of their perceived cognitive problems or the distrust towards their own mind. One participant (AD04, MCI patient) pointed out that with a conspicuous test result she "had something to say" when someone wonders why she "behaves so strangely". Her husband (AD04, close other), who was interviewed as part of her dyad, supported the positive effect in his narrations. He mentioned that with a conspicuous test result he knew that his wife "did not deliberately ignore him" but "acted in her disease". In this case, a medical label in the form of a risk status helps especially (close) others to classify the perceived 'abnormal behaviour' and to find explanations for it—even if those aren't entirely certain.

In the baseline interview—before the predictive testing—most of the participants showed a strong reaction to the terms 'dementia' or 'Alzheimer's disease dementia', even if the interviewer did not use the word in her own expression, but only referred to the associated documents or situations in the interviewee's life. This reveals a different attitude to 'naming' at baseline compared to the follow-up interview after the predictive testing. In the baseline-interviews from our study on AD, some participants started to tell a story about a specific situation in which the idea of 'being at risk for dementia' simply became 'dementia' and led to a different treatment or even discriminating actions as in the interview segment below (AD01). For the linguistic analysis, it is crucial that the naming is performed by the participants themselves to be able to analyse 'how' and 'why' something is communicated.

AD01 (Study on AD, baseline interview segment with an MCI patient)

```
204 P:  on the referral he wrote dementia (.) he knows ehm he doesn't KNOW what that
205     I have dementia -
206 I:  the family doctor?
207     no that is true (-) he doesn't [know;]
208 P:                                 [ yes ]
209 I:  assumed maybe [non that ] was his assOMPtion.
210 P:               [yes yes- ]
211     he assumed that I have dementia;
212 I:  hmhm.
213 P:  that's why the reception the receptionists are eh were suddenly different (.)
214     different to me;
215 I:  oh okay I understand
216     but this is they don't mean it (.) do you think they mean is in a harmful way?
217 P:  no no ((laughs))they a shout over as if I were deaf or so and MRS SCHMI::::D
218     ((anonymized)) as if I was not normal -
219     they are they don't know how to talk those to those with dementia ((laughs)),
220 I:  you are more experienced there right you gathered experience with your mother how
221     to handle this did you say before;
222 P:  yesyes -
223 I:  and the receptionists maybe learn when there is written dementia on the sheet of
    paper
224     learn to talk slower or something like that don't you think,
225 P:  yesyes ((laughs)) that is what they learn but he they don't KNOW that I have
    dementia
226     and talk like that to me because of a sheet of paper (.) yesyes.
```

At the beginning of the segment (204/205), the interviewee emphasises that although "dementia" was on her referral from the family doctor, the latter does not know whether she really has dementia. She emphasises the word "know" (204) and agrees with the interviewer that it's an assumption (211) but explains the consequences immediately (213/214). From the emphasis on "know" (depicted in capital letters) one can derive that the contrast between 'knowing' and 'not knowing' is very important to the interviewee ('assuming' is introduced by the interviewer). The doctor's actions are perceived as irritating within this attitude. Later, after she had shared her experience about the receptionists who suddenly behaved quite differently (and visibly inexperienced) towards her due to the label "dementia" (217ff.), she returns again to the aspect that the doctor did 'not know' anything concrete about her health status (225) and that it is not okay to talk to her like this (she emphasises "so/like this") only because of a piece of paper (226) which underlines her distinction between knowing and not knowing/assuming again. Asking the question 'why' she points out consequences (actions of receptionists) and a responsible party (sheet of paper), one can consider that she describes the deterministic aspect of the situation she was put in.

In both studies, we found that the label 'at risk of developing psychosis/AD' plays an important role in the process of negotiating the entanglement between symptoms and personality, as well as the interrelation between labels for (naming), potential causes of (explaining), and ways of dealing with (coping) the condition of being 'at risk'. While the naming of risk can be experienced as a relief and a source of agency, it can also entail a perceived loss of control and feelings of being trapped in deterministic attributions.

Explaining

Current studies on physician-patient conversations in oncology show that physicians strongly concentrate on treatment, while pushing questions about the cause of disease into the background—even if patients repeatedly want to discuss the origin (Bentz et al., 2016; Imo, 2017). In our studies, the situation is different, because on the one hand there is no treatment and healing (AD) and on the other hand therapies are protracted and assumed to accompany persons for a lifetime (psychosis). The question of origin or source is therefore one of the most pressing concerns here. In the case of psychosis, our study shows that individuals' explanatory models of origin of the (risk of) disease consist of internal (undeserved—genetic; deserved—behavioural) and external (undeserved—family, social environment and life events) factors. Drug use can serve as a good example for these closely intertwined factors. On the one hand, drugs are seen as a risk factor for getting mentally ill and the experienced symptoms as a side effect of a certain lifestyle:

PSYP01 (Interviewee; study on psychosis)

```
266   And of course, especially when you start smoking grass, you get to grips with
267   the story, where it actually comes from and how it works and what THC actually is
268   and, um, then, in the course of that, you naturally also come across studies that …
269   talk about the increased risk of psychosis from long-term consumption and … (?)
270   Yes, and almost … (laughs) I smoked that for almost six years. Um … therefore …
271   Well, I knew the risks, but I didn't care about them.
```

On the other hand, drug use is perceived as a 'defence mechanism' and a way to regulate stress: Drugs play the role of 'a catalyst' that brings problems up to the surface early enough to make them obvious for oneself and the others, hereby accelerating the process of searching for help. This unavoidably raises questions of responsibility: "I have the feeling that I have ruined an area in my whole life!" (PSYP08). This feeling of guilt and responsibility has been an object of research in other clinical fields (e.g. the notion of 'genetic responsibility' in familial breast- and ovarian cancer—Etchegary et al., 2009, Hallowell, 1999). Here again, the tension between biomedical versus individual biographical explanations (Holmberg, Waters, Whitehouse, Daly, & McCaskill-Stevens, 2015) becomes obvious. For the researcher, this may imply being confronted with an expectation to provide an 'objective' opinion in the context of a narrative interview, for example, concerning the question of whether or not one is responsible for the condition of being 'at risk'.

Parallel to this notion, individuals attempt to 'normalise' this 'at risk'-condition by labelling the "awkward moments" and "crazy thoughts" as "normal" for each human being. The border between disease and health in this case is not marked by the fact that these crazy thoughts emerge but by the way of handling them. Our findings demonstrate that persons 'at risk' perceive the concept of risk in a fluid dimension, with the impossibility of defining a starting and an ending point.

PSYP04 (Interviewee; study on psychosis)

```
796   But also a thing I didn't think about at all before, so… so the basic attitude,
797   someday, you know? You can get any type of illness at some point, come down with
798   something, or somehow suffer from something. But so that, uh, there could actually be
799   something that somehow comes from the head and so without external influences, or
800   not. To say: Ok, you have this and that disease concretely, but that it is somehow
801   something that is not tangible.
```

In our interviewees' narratives, we identified indications of how they construct meaning concerning their situation; for example, they described their risk as an inherent part of their biography. This reasoning was based on three sources of information: (1) risk prediction is based on symptoms which are perceived as an inherent part of the personality ("dreamy person" (PSYP03), "class clown" (PSYP01), "I grew up with it" (PSYP06), "I usually fantasize" (PSYP09), "I was always the weirdo" (PSYP10)) and thus a part of their 'normal' everyday condition; (2) prior experience with other therapies; and (3) intuition.

In our study on AD, the question of origin or source was not one of responsibility, even though behavioural risk factors have been described as well.[8] The risk is depicted much more deterministically ('the disease hits you') regardless whether the factors are internal or external. The essential way of dealing with the question of the origin culminates in considerations about heredity and detailed stories about family members with dementia. Some participants are quite sure that this will be their or their partner's "fate" (99), others hang on the hope "that the cup will pass them by" as the participant in AD02 (091, 098).

AD02 (Study on AD, baseline interview segment with an MCI patient)

```
87 P:   yes MAYbe I am er (.) I am OLDer than my brothers and they are quite er demented;
88      one of them Max ((anonymised)) we always- with him I always went outside for a walk
89      but this is difficult now;
90 I:   why,
91 P:   yes he is quite er er: demented now and I hope that this cup will pass me by (--)
92      but you never er know -
93 I:   could you describe this feeling to me in a more detailed way?
94 P:   I REALLY have poor preconditions with our parents it was like that with my father
95      first and with my mother later but she wasn't so (.) so aggressive then-
96      but I am the third er the first but now the least ((laughs)) it doesn't always
97      hit everyone.
98      I hope like I said that the cup will pass me by but my wife says that it is the
99      family's fate (--) so far.
100     she also called ((the clinic)) and made the appointment.
```

The process of 'explaining' in the case of risk for dementia due to AD sometimes even starts before the (new) 'naming' and may change in the course of the prediction procedures. Perceptions and explanations are different before and after predictive testing:

Before the predictive examination, two types of participants' perceptions were observed. Some pointed out that they are suffering from dementia, others that

---

[8] Biomedical factors for dementia due to AD are also combined with modifiable risk factors, such as lifestyle-related factors (unhealthy diet, alcohol consumption, smoking, cognitive inactivity, physical inactivity and low education), cardiovascular risk diseases (diabetes, hypertension, obesity) and psychosocial factors (depression, social inactivity) (Livingston et al., 2017).

they are only 'cognitively impaired' and there is a strong possibility of remaining or improving beside the option of dementia (cf. Schwegler, Rostamzadeh, Jessen, Boada, & Woopen, 2017). Simultaneously, the latter explain duties or aspects from their everyday life to demonstrate how they are integrated, needed, and still perform well. For example, the interviewee (AD01) in a later segment points out that she could no longer take care of her mother if she had dementia herself. After the predictive examination, participants with two suspicious biomarkers (biomedical interpretation: 59% likelihood to develop dementia due to AD within the next three years) did not mention the possibility of remaining or improving anymore, but still narrate stories around their good performance to explain aspects of their capabilities to their interview partner.

In summary, our findings show that different attribution patterns are involved in the process of explaining one's situation of being 'at risk'. Relevant dimensions concerning the origin or source of one's risk are related to questions of fate and guilt, internal or external causes, changes in explanatory models before and after risk testing and disclosure, as well as the endeavour to normalise one's experiences and integrate them into one's personal narratives. These different layers of interpretation are strongly intertwined with the individual's perceived and enacted opportunities to cope with their condition.

Coping

The analysis of our interviewees' accounts showed that the process of meaning-making (Park & Folkman, 1997) with respect to the at-risk state is closely related to individual coping mechanisms. The narratives reveal differences between persons at risk of psychosis and AD in terms of their coping strategies and also with regard to their experienced sense of agency and quality of life (QoL).

Coping in the context of risk for psychosis implies the notion of vulnerability in terms of keeping-up with everyday life on the one hand and reflecting on one's individual illness prevention on the other hand. The notion of risk, the process of meaning-making and coping appear to be tightly entangled. The risk symptoms are perceived as a particularly strong and sophisticated warning and defence system enabling individuals to get control over the condition of imbalance. Risk is seen not as the enemy that should be controlled, but much more as a team player who can help to control the symptoms, and as a protective mechanism for mental health of each human being. As the quotations below exemplify, our interviewees' narratives show the potential of meaning-making as a resource for (re-)constructing order instead of surrendering to disorder; for "achieving congruence between an individual's global meaning and the appraised meaning of a particular event" (Park & Folkman, 1997, p. 116). Discussing risk with others is described as a strategy to understand and deal with it. At the same time, it should not be given "too much space" in order to keep the balance:

PSYP08 (Interviewee; study on psychosis)

```
361  As I've just explained, with me it's stress that causes the symptom to get
362  worse. Well, I think it makes sense to know what's there, but it shouldn't
363  be over-, uh, over-dramatized.
```

In contrast to the medical understanding of risk as a threat, our interviewees' accounts suggest that they also associate an idea of agency with risk, as the following quotation illustrates.

PSYP10 (Interviewee; study on psychosis)

```
28   That is, there is a very high risk of, um, getting schizophrenia or
29   psychosis. Um. I know that in most cases it is determined by stress and
30   diet, thus determined by life. If one lives a healthy life and avoids
31   stress, then risk will in any case be lower.
```

The individuals in our study on AD are considered vulnerable because of their experienced and medically ascertained cognitive impairments (MCI diagnosed). Although they are still fully capable of shaping their everyday lives, they and their relatives noticed that they display cognitive difficulties. In addition to the risk, these individuals have to live with 'first symptoms' which they have to understand and evaluate for themselves. One understanding of risk (in combination with minor symptoms) is to implicitly go through and review the family history. Risk is strongly linked to heritability, and in a next step to subjective certainty of suffering from AD, combined with fear towards this condition. 'Being at risk for AD' basically does not trigger thoughts of consequentialist agency, but traps some persons in deterministic attributions and the search for explanations.

Overall, coping appears to be a process starting long before a risk disclosure following predictive testing. Due to interviews at two points in time (before/after predictive testing), our study on AD can shed light on different phases, variations and manifestations of this coping process in individuals with MCI symptoms and a risk for dementia due to AD:

Before the predictive testing some patients showed verbal self-distancing from the possible disease or diseased persons: From a linguistic point of view, it is very interesting that the interviewee in AD01 in her story (213–219) uses descriptive elements and deictic expression to distance herself both in terms of time and space from "those with dementia"/"them". This is in line with the attitude that dementia is just an assumption.

Directly following predictive testing, conspicuous test results can be shocking and unexpected as described in AD03 as "a punch back" (039) which led to a "breakdown" (042) and needed "time to digest" (045).

In the segment AD03, one can see from the progress of the conversational sequence that *normality can be restored within the narration*: The interviewee begins at a normality, which he summarises by himself as "everything was fine" (043). This normality was disturbed by the conspicuous test result. Afterwards, he establishes a 'new normality' by comparing himself with a 'truly diseased' person on the one and (average) persons at the same age on the other hand: "my father had it really badly, but with me, it is something totally different. What I have is normal for my age, but just, er, conspicious" (051–053).

After the predictive testing, in the light of first symptoms, some individuals developed a more 'conscious experiencing' of future actions regardless of a result with two, one or none suspicious biomarkers.

AD03 (Study on AD, 3-month follow-up interview segment with an MCI patient)

```
032 I:   and then you came back in agAIn for the risk disclosure [right],
033 P:                  [yes ].
034 I:   when the results were [THERE]-
035 P:                        [yes ]
036      er yes then the situation was a LITtle different.
037 I:   mhm;
038 P:   the professor was with us (.) huh,
039      and er this and that (-) and this and that was (.) of course a punch back (-)
040      er (---) but told me again YES oKAY but within a small er rANge
041      that one can do something or something IS to do if something happens -
042      an there I was inside I won't say broke down this would be OVERstated.
043      but damn it, that CAN't be (-) so far they told me everything was fine and it gets
044      better and then they told me so to say unconcerned nevertheless we found something;
045      then I needed some amount of time to digest that;
046 I:   and now,
047 P:   yes er basically like always;
048      before some days were good some were bad,
049      that is so to say normal in my age if I may put it this way (-)
050      I am continuing normally now.
051      my father so to say had it badly (-) really badly,
052      but with me (-) it is something totally different.
053      what I have is normal for my age (-) but just er conspicuous.
```

As this section illustrates, the interview can be a space for the negotiation of questions about self-perception, self-awareness, agency and determinism, as well as for the narrative restoring of (a new) normality.[9]

Methodological Reflection: Negotiating Vulnerability and Normality

Throughout the research process, by means of reflexivity, we aimed at creating a space for re-defining the power of definition, including notions of vulnerability and normality, with regard to risk. In the following, we will discuss central methodological issues that emerged in the course of our studies. These include the planning and preparation of the study, the sampling strategy, the interview process, roles and responsibilities between researcher and interviewee, ethical considerations, as well as data analysis and interpretation. Our reflections aim at providing insights into

---

[9]Alongside to the role of meaning-making, the interrelation between coping with risk and QoL became visible in both projects during data analysis. For example, the episodic interviews in our study on AD provided us with the opportunity to capture differences between individual descriptions of QoL (in the narrative part), concrete specifications (from the semantic part), and a 'scientific' understanding used in common definitions of QoL (c.f. Rostamzadeh et al., in press; Woopen, 2014).

opportunities and challenges related to the practice of doing research on risk in mental health.

Ethical Considerations Concerning the Notion of 'Vulnerability'

In the process of designing the research, we classified the condition of being considered as a person 'at risk' as vulnerable. This had implications for our ideas of the appropriate way to encounter our study participants during the interview situation, and for our assumptions about the impact of risk on their lives.[10] But which impact does this vulnerable condition have on the research process and the interview topics, and how can the researcher handle it?

Although the narrative interviews were conducted based on a flexible topic guide and open dialogue, the potential distress caused by certain individual topics was a central concern in the research process. It is true that in an open research format, informants determine themselves, based on their own relevance criteria, which aspects of risk experience and understanding of health and disease are in focus. This however does not exclude the possibility that sensitive, stressful or traumatic experiences may be brought up in the course of the interview. For the interviewees, this could mean a danger of being confronted with these experiences again and of overemphasising their 'vulnerable condition at risk' or their 'patient role' through the narration. We therefore took precautionary measures to avoid additional stress for the research participants presumably caused by the narrative interview. At the outset of the study, thorough reflections on the balance between potential benefit and harm for study participants were made in the context of applying for ethics approval. During the interview, we made continuous careful considerations, weighing our curiosity as researchers and the wish to attain as much information as possible against the fear of undue confrontation and intrusion, and the wish to protect the interviewees from distress. At the end of the interview, we offered our participants the opportunity to give us a signal of stress or unpleasant feelings, using a feedback form they could return to us in a sealed envelope. In some cases, we made a follow-up telephone call or emailed participants when we had the impression that the interview may have left them behind too agitated. Overall, our participants described their experience of the interview situation as comfortable and caring; however, it could also be perceived as a distressing situation. Some of them described it as pleasant to talk to someone unknown who is not a family member or their physician, or they reported that it had been interesting and helpful for them to reflect on their situation during the narrative interview. This is in line with observations by other authors about the potential of the narrative interview as an 'identity-forming action or discursive production of the self' (Lucius-Hoene, 2002, p. 178) that may even have a healing effect (Rosenthal,

---

[10] After considering risks and benefits for the informants, as a first step, the research team developed a guideline for the conduct of the interviews, for the process of pseudonymisation and for the publication of the results according to the "principle of non-harm" (Hopf, 2005).

1995). Since there is no guarantee for this positive effect, we nevertheless directed our efforts at avoiding stress and possible harm.

In the course of the interviews for this study, it became obvious that the topic of family is one of the most sensitive when doing qualitative research in this clinical field. A major question was how to ask about family without aggravating this vulnerable condition?

In spite of various discussions and researcher self-reflection, we cannot offer a general solution. After analysing the data, we realised that each researcher's decision whether to ask further questions or not and when to change the topic was based on 'inner feeling'. The choice is based on an ethical judgement that researchers will need to make for themselves, and preferably discuss with colleagues in the team, or use other spaces for reflection such as intervision or research workshops.

Qualitative Research in a Medically Oriented Scientific Environment

In the process of research conceptualisation, our teams faced the challenge of two fundamentally different approaches in the way of designing the research process. In a medically oriented environment, operationalisation of research questions is expected to follow a standardised approach based on predetermined definitions of risk and QoL. This confronted us with conflicting ideas about the appropriate sampling strategy or the suitable ways of collecting data.

As a compromise, concerning the criteria for in- and exclusion of participants, we agreed on medically defined criteria of 'persons at risk' of developing psychosis or AD.[11] This decision requires a further methodological reflection on our sampling strategy. Defining biomedical inclusion and exclusion criteria is an attempt to objectify individuals' intuitive feeling of risk and automatically excludes persons who feel at risk without having a biomedical explanation of this feeling. This strategy should be critically reconsidered in future studies. A possible solution is to circumvent the strict—and temporary—medical criteria by including an additional criterion of 'feeling at risk'. The recruiting process could take place both in cooperation with the medical prediction centres and randomly with the help of adverts or announcements. Concerning the operationalisation of research questions, we encountered challenges in terms of the degree of openness and standardisation in approaching concepts of interest such as risk or quality of life (QoL). Our studies aimed at an open, discovery-oriented approach providing a bottom-up perspective in order to generate a definition grounded in empirical data. In our study on psychosis, the iterative process alternating between data collection and analysis (Palinkas, 2014) offered a fruitful ground for several transformations related to the research setting, methodology and research relationship between interviewer and interviewee. However, such an approach meets resistance and requires methodological negotiation in a primarily medically oriented research environment.

---

[11] The only individuals who can currently obtain a predictive test in clinical practice are patients (medically) as MCI.

We also realised how different methodologies can result in divergent findings on a seemingly consensual concept such as QoL. In our study on AD, the overall focus of the mixed methods approach (cf. Box 1) was on the effect of risk prediction on the QoL of persons at risk and their family members. We aimed at contrasting the findings of the common and established standardised questionnaires on QoL, satisfaction with/in life and well-being with the findings of the qualitative approach: Within the narrative parts of the episodic interviews—in which we explicitly avoided terms such as QoL, satisfaction or well-being—together with the semantic part of the interview—in which we explicitly asked for subjective specifications of those terms—we were able to shed light on the subjective descriptions of the semantic field of QoL and related concepts such as well-being and risk. This can lead to a reasonable appraisal of the individual meanings of QoL and may hence help to strengthen the appreciation of the qualitative approach in relation to the quantitative data. Interestingly, the analysis of the subjective definitions revealed that the concrete expression 'quality of life' is mostly understood in monetary terms ("to have enough money to life a good life"), while the expressions 'well-being'/'satisfaction' might be better terms in everyday language to represent the health-related understanding of 'having a good life'.

Hence, in a medically oriented scientific environment, researchers need to face the blurred borderline between objectivism and subjectivism, general and specific, fact and interpretation in the context of qualitative research in mental health.

Data Generation—Asking About Risk

Concerning the assumed impact of risk on people's lives, our strategy of mitigating harm and bias included a reserved attitude towards the label of 'being at risk' and avoiding the use of this wording in the beginning phase of the interview. In both of our studies, the medical understanding of risk is presented to our participants during their clinical diagnostics and treatment, but the understanding of risk in both instances differs. In order to bridge this definitional gap, we decided not to employ a single or fixed definition of risk, but "to elicit the perspective of those being studied" (Sofaer, 1999, p. 1105). We used conversation techniques that minimise the use of 'objective definitions' of risk, and the emphasis on 'medical knowledge'. Throughout the interviews, we regularly explored the background of the narratives ("How do you know about that?" and "Could you explain your feelings and thoughts (in this specific situation)?") in order to create a space for individual frameworks of meaning, including the verbalisation of somatic (bodily) knowledge (Samerski, 2019).

While conducting the interviews and analysing the data, we realised that even if we agreed on a short and clear opening question, it had been slightly modified in each interview depending on the pre-conversation and the conversation atmosphere. This reveals on the one hand the researchers' own personal attitude towards the label 'being at risk of developing psychosis/AD' and on the other hand the ethical concerns related to the interview situation; the danger of introducing a label or a meaning of 'risk' that may be not relevant for the individual's life.

The Interview as a Setting and Format for Data Generation on Mental Health Risk

Our data analysis allowed for a methodological reflection on the interview as an appropriate setting for generating meaningful information. In the context of mental health, especially within our study on psychosis, we often meet interview-partners who have experience with conversations that aim at generating narratives (in the context of previous therapies or psychological conversations with professionals). The high ability of self-reflection among the interview-partners enabled a highly differentiated approach to the self and the disease, offering expert knowledge on symptoms, risk and individuals' daily struggles. From a researcher point of view, this should be considered as an important factor which influences the type of the collected data and poses challenges to their interpretation.

A further important task was to discover the different voices narrating the story. Narrative interviews in the context of mental health 'at risk' contain a great share of self-interpretation, narratives on psychological interpretations and external definitions. Additional data sources such as field notes and memos can be fruitful to enrich and complete the verbal way of telling about perceptions. These additional means of data collection require an increased awareness of the researcher's role in conducting the interview as well as control over the dynamics of proximity and distance during the interview. A look into the data reveals some of the researcher's strategies to stay "open" (DeWalt & DeWalt, 1998) and curious, keeping their attention independent from medical background information or therapeutic experience: emphasising empathy ("I can imagine how difficult this situation was"), personal disclosure, appreciation ("that's exciting") and re-questioning one's own question ("this question may not be so relevant, but I am curious to know").[12]

Negotiating Roles and Responsibilities in the Research Process

Our findings and memos reveal that the process of role definition during the interview was an issue from the interviewees' point of view. This became visible through discussions on the research questions ("Do you follow a specific common thread while asking these questions?" (PSYP01)), evaluations on the notion of representativeness of the project results ("I am wondering if what I say could be representative for others?" (PSYP02)), thematising their own role as a research participant ("Am I a patient, or a client, or what is the right term here?" (PSYP01)).

---

[12]An additional aspect that invites further analysis and reflection is the gender dimension of the research. All researchers are female and of different ages. Both gender and age certainly have an impact on the interview dynamics but due to space limitation, these aspects will not be further discussed in this contribution.

This 'patient-role' became visible in different stages in the course of the interview. Research participants adopted medical language not only when describing different diagnoses and symptoms, but also when reflecting on their coping strategies, everyday feelings and experiences and interactions with others. Apart from this adoption of terminology, role definition in general was not a very obvious, but still a constantly present issue in the interview process. We noticed interviewees switching between the role of the patient (having experience with diagnoses and therapies), the self-reflected and aware person (emphasising one's own importance in the process of managing mental health) and the knowledgeable person, "cognisant of researchers and doctors" (highlighting one's own position as an experienced person in communication with doctors and researchers). This helped us as researchers to minimise the risk of reducing the interviewees to their traumatic experience, or to exclude areas or phases of their lives that may be relevant to the research question (Loch & Rosenthal, 2002). On our part, we as researchers also took measures to minimise these risks, such as the use of questioning techniques for in-depth exploration, in some instances self-disclosure, scheduling sufficient time and space, re-establishing contact after the interview (Küsters, 2009), and a process-accompanying self-reflection among the research team.

Summary: Methodological Reflection and Research Ethics

The following questions (Box 2) are intended as a source for reflection, rather than guidelines or rules, when planning and conducting a qualitative study on mental health risk. The leading idea is to encourage considering the methodological decisions at each stage throughout the research process in terms of their implications for the data that will be generated. Eventually, methodological reflection on these issues may contribute to constructively dealing with the tension between a standardised biomedical and an open, bottom-up approach in a medically oriented scientific environment.

Box 2: Questions for reflection

Ethical considerations concerning the notion of 'vulnerability'	
Sensitive topics /traumatic experiences	Are there issues of responsibility or feelings of guilt related to the condition of being at risk (e.g. in terms of the interviewee's behaviour, implications of his/her situation for close others, or heredity)? If yes, what may the methodology of qualitative enquiry imply in terms of a confrontation with these feelings guilt? How can the researcher prepare for situations surrounding potential feelings of guilt in conversations with the interviewee? For example, the researcher may need to be prepared for being asked about his or her opinion about appropriate ways of dealing with the risk or about questions of responsibility; or he/she may need to make a trade-off between curiosity and the wish to protect the interviewee from potential harm by overly intrusive questions

(continued)

(continued)

Qualitative research in a medically oriented environment	
Research design	In an interdisciplinary, medically oriented research environment, qualitative researchers will be challenged to make a trade-off between the demands of an open, circular research process guided by the premises of theoretical sampling and data saturation, and the expectations of an a priori elaborated, standardised, and linear research procedure usually expected in the medical field
Sampling	With regard to mental health risk, careful considerations are required concerning the operationalisation of the 'condition at risk'. How are risk factors defined according to the current state of knowledge? Do medical guidelines on risk detection differ from discourses in the media? What do people think about their own risk? Based on our experience, we recommend scheduling time during the study preparation for detailed discussion with clinicians, but also with participants, about risk factors, different risk constellations, and in- and exclusion criteria for study participation. Recruiting interviewees could take place both in collaboration with medical prediction centres and using adverts or announcements
Data generation—asking about risk	
Using the term 'risk'	'Risk' may have a variety of meanings and implications, not only with respect to different mental health conditions, but also for different people and in different socio-biographical contexts. We therefore encourage researchers to reflect on the implications of when and how to introduce the term risk in the research process, including the first contact with the interview partners and the opening question of the interview. The choices will also depend on the recruitment process and on the procedures of clinical prediction and risk communication (for example, whether disclosure of the clinical high risk has already occurred and if yes, in which way, and how long ago)
The interview as a method of data collection	Researchers are encouraged to reflect on the choice of an interview as a setting and format for data generation on mental health risk. This is of particular importance when talking to persons familiar with a high degree of self-reflection, for example when experienced in psychotherapy. With regard to research on mental health risk, different knowledge systems come into play; these will also be reflected in the interviewees' narratives. Different stocks of knowledge may inform their reflections, for example normative ideas about their condition, adopted medical language and expert knowledge, or concerns uttered by family and friends. We therefore encourage researchers to stay alert concerning the different voices 'speaking' in the interviewees' narratives. In addition, other methods of data collection may be considered, allowing for non-verbal data generation
Negotiating roles and responsibilities in the research process	

(continued)

(continued)

Between disorder and normality	The condition of being 'at risk' for a mental health problem introduces the negotiation between disorder and normality. We argue that both the interviewee and the researcher will locate themselves somewhere on the continuum between these two poles. As a researcher, one needs to engage in the reflection about how to deal with his/her own 'mental vulnerability', and will be required to reconsider this position in relation to different interview partners. This includes choices such as 'Will it be appropriate to employ self-disclosure in support of a trusting relationship with the interviewee?' or 'Which personal memories, threats or anxieties may the interview trigger in me as a researcher?'
Data analysis	
Tools and sources for reflection	When analysing data, it is important to keep in mind that narratives generated through qualitative enquiry are the result of a co-construction between researcher and interviewee. We therefore encourage researchers to employ diverse tools and sources for reflexivity, such as auto-ethnographic memos or thick descriptions following the interview, metadata-protocols, and discussions in the interdisciplinary research team. Herein, researchers can use questions such as 'What are my own thoughts, fears, and prejudice concerning the risk in question?'; 'Which implications do my assumptions have for the topics addressed in the interview, and for those neglected or hidden?'

Conclusion: Methodologies in Support of Reclaiming Power

Qualitative methodologies are a powerful way for people experiencing mental distress to speak for themselves. We argue that they can constitute a valid approach to understanding people's experiences and perspectives in mental health care as well as in mental health research (Powell, Single, & Lloyd, 1996). In the two studies presented in this chapter, we drew on approaches from linguistics and medical ethnology, and we used narrative methodology and reflexivity in order to open up definitional spaces between researchers and interviewees. A reflection on both the content and the process of the interviews conducted during both studies allows for some considerations concerning the power of definition. Constantly taking a step back and questioning our strategies and interpretations before, during and after the interviews provided the opportunity for re-defining concepts related to the notion of being 'at risk' for psychosis or dementia, such as vulnerability, QoL, and risk itself. The narrative and episodic interviews proved to be a fruitful source for the discursive generation of definitions, unfolding the multi-faceted understandings of health. It became evident that risk, beyond 'objective' scores and percentages, can have divergent meanings to different persons and in the context of different health conditions such as psychosis or Alzheimer's dementia. Risk is a mediator at the border between order and disorder; beyond being perceived as a threat, risk can also be a regulator in the process of negotiating normality. Persons being confronted with a health risk can (re)gain agency by either interpreting their risk as a source for self-awareness and self-care, or by trying to restore order and normality through their narrations.

Methodologically, our studies revealed particular opportunities but also challenges concerning the realisation of a qualitative approach in the context of a medically oriented environment. For example, our sampling strategies were shaped by the medically defined risk factors for psychosis and dementia, and methodological nego-tiations with our clinical partners were needed to convey the benefit of a discovery-oriented—rather than a standardised—approach to concepts such as risk or QoL. We also reflected on the interview as an appropriate format of generating meaningful knowledge, particularly among persons who are familiar with a high level of self-reflection, or with a view to different 'voices' speaking in the narratives, such as personal interpretations, but also knowledge and beliefs adopted from physicians, family, or the media. In the future, an even more open-ended and spirited approach to sampling and data collection may be worthwhile, for example, by including self-definitions of 'at-risk' states, or by employing pre-discursive forms of data collection such as in arts-based research.

In terms of disciplinary approaches, instead of being restricted even more by biomedical thinking, dementia and mental health research ought to refocus on a variety of disciplines such as sociology, anthropology, philosophy, or politics (Timimi, 2014) in order to accommodate a broader understanding of the person and their well-being. Biomedical, psychosocial, and cultural models of mental health should be appropriately balanced in order to do justice to a holistic perspective on mental health (Puras, 2017). In particular, user-lead research has the potential to overcome power asymmetries characteristic of biomedical study designs, and to be able to 'cut to the heart of issues that are important to service users themselves' (Pitt, Kilbride, Nothard, Welford, & Morrison, 2007, p. 60). Stories and storytelling can be considered as the heart of qualitative methodology, particularly in narrative, linguistic and ethnographic approaches. As a particular example, auto-ethnography can be a fruitful methodology, capable of generating dense accounts of a person's lived experiences by connecting these to cultural process and understanding (Liggins, Kearns, & Adams, 2013; see also Willig in this book).

In conclusion, when awarding people the opportunity to speak for themselves in the context of mental health research, their personal accounts and narratives can help challenge existing social constructions of their conditions. This can also allow for new perspectives on the experiences of people living with mental distress (Zeilig, 2014; Zimmermann, 2017). The narrative approach offers the potential to (re)arrange life events and experiences, and to attribute subjective meaning to their condition, which can be an important resource for coping with the at-risk state. Moreover, narratives allow for accommodating different forms and types of health knowledge, including intuition and somatic (bodily) knowledge. From a sociology of knowledge perspective, qualitative research can therefore offer the opportunity to contribute to new realities of mental health in terms of scientific knowledge production, diagnostics and treatment, as well as personal and public perception. Eventually, qualitative approaches to data collection, analysis, and interpretation open up spaces for reclaiming power concerning the experience, the definition, and the appraisal of mental health.

Acknowledgements The research described in this chapter received funding by the Robert Bosch Foundation ("Health literacy of persons at risk – from information to action (RisKomp)"; grant number 11.5.A402.0002.0) and by the Federal Ministry of Education and Research—BMBF as part of the Network of European Funding for Neuroscience Research—ERA-NET NEURON ("Ethical and Legal Framework for Predictive Diagnosis of Alzheimer's Disease: Quality of Life of Individuals at Risk and their Close Others (PreDADQoL); funding number: 01GP1624)". The sponsors did not have any influence on study initiation, conducting and reporting.

Both joint projects were conducted at the Cologne Center for Ethics, Rights, Economics, and Social Sciences of Health (ceres) under the leadership of Principal Investigator Prof. Dr. med. Christiane Woopen.

We are obliged to our interviewees for their time, their commitment and their openness in sharing their narratives with us. We would like to thank our clinical partners for the fruitful collaboration in the course of our empirical work; we are particularly grateful to Frank Jessen, Stephan Ruhrmann and Kai Vogeley for endorsing our project, and to Theresa Haidl, Mauro Seves, and Ayda Rostamzadeh for their relentless support in designing the study, defining in- and exclusion criteria, and recruiting our interview partners. Special thanks are due to Laura Harzheim who is part of the RisKomp project team; without her contribution, this book chapter would not have been possible. We would like to express our special gratitude to Maria Borcsa and Carla Willig for their careful editing; their constructive comments and wise suggestions greatly helped us to refine our manuscript.

Literature

Albert, M. S., DeKosky S. T., Dickson, D., Dubois, B., Feldman, H. H., Fox, N. C., … Phelps, C. H. (2011). The diagnosis of mild cognitive impairment due to Alzheimer's disease: Recommendations from the National Institute on Aging-Alzheimer's Association workgroups on diagnostic guidelines for Alzheimer's disease. *Alzheimers Dementia, 7*(3), 270–279. http://doi.org/10.1016/j.jalz.2011.03.008.

Aronowitz, R. A. (2009). The converged experience of risk and disease. *The Milbank Quarterly, 87*(2), 417–442. https://doi.org/10.1111/j.1468-0009.2009.00563.x.

Bearden, C. E., & Forsyth, J. K. (2018). The many roads to psychosis: Recent advances in understanding risk and mechanisms. *F1000Research, 7* (F1000 Faculty Rev), 1883. https://doi.org/10.12688/f1000research.16574.1.

Bentz, M. Binnenhei, M., Coussios, G., Gruden, J., Imo W., Korte, L., … Stier, S. (2016). Von der Pathologie zum Patienten: Optimierung von Wissenstransfer und Verstehenssicherung in der medizinischen Kommunikation. *Sprache und Interaktion, 72,* 1–43.

Berger, P. L., & Luckmann, T. (1966). *The social construction of reality: A treatise in the sociology of knowledge.* Doubleday: New York.

Birkner, K. (2006). Subjektive Krankheitstheorien im Gespräch. *Gesprächsforschung, 7,* 152–183.

Breuer, F., Muckel, P., & Dieris, B. (2019). *Reflexive grounded theory: Eine Einführung für die Forschungspraxis* (4th ed.). Wiesbaden: Springer VS.

Byrne, R., & Morrison, A. P. (2010). Young people at risk of psychosis: A user-led exploration of interpersonal relationships and communication of psychological difficulties. *Early Intervention in Psychiatry, 4*(2), 162–168. https://doi.org/10.1111/j.1751-7893.2010.00171.x.

Clarke, A. E., Shim, J. K., Mamo, L., Fosket, J. R., & Fishman, J. R. (2003). Biomedicalization: technoscientific transformations of health, illness, and U.S. biomedicine. *American Sociological Review, 68*(2), 161–194. https://doi.org/10.2307/1519765.

Denzin, N. (1970). *The research act in sociology.* London: Butterworth.

Deppermann, A. (2008). *Gespräche analysieren: Eine Einführung* (5th ed.). Wiesbaden: Springer VS.

Deppermann, A. (2013). Interview als text vs. interview als interaktion. *FQS Forum Qualitative Sozialforschung, 14*(3), 1–36.

DeWalt, K. M., & DeWalt, B. R. (1998). Participant observation. In B. H. Russell (Ed.), *Handbook of methods in cultural anthropology* (pp. 259–300). Walnut Creek: AltaMira Press.

Ermine, W., Sinclair, R., & Jeffery, B. (2004). *The ethics of research involving indigenous peoples: Report of the indigenous People's Health Research Centre to the Interagency Advisory Panel on Research Ethics.* Saskatoon (SK): Indigenous People's Health Research Centre.

Etchegary, H., Miller, F., deLaat, S., Wilson, B., Carroll, J., & Cappelli, M. (2009). Decision-making about inherited cancer risk: Exploring dimensions of genetic responsibility. *Journal of genetic counseling, 18*(3), 252–264. https://doi.org/10.1007/s10897-009-9218-z.

Fleck, L. (1979). *Genesis and development of a scientific fact.* Chicago: University of Chicago Press.

Flemming, I. M. (2010). Ethnography and ethnology. In H. J. Birx (Ed.), *21st century anthropology: A reference handbook.* Thousand Oaks: Sage.

Flick, U. (1997). *The episodic interview: Small scale narratives as approach to relevant experiences* (Discussion Papers—Qualitative Series). http://docshare01.docshare.tips/files/24191/241 911951.pdf.

Frances, A. (2014). *Normal. Gegen die Inflation psychiatrischer Diagnosen.* Köln: DuMont.

Fusar-Poli, P. (2017). The clinical high-risk state for psychosis (CHR-P), Version II. *Schizophrenia Bulletin, 43*(1), 44–47. https://doi.org/10.1093/schbul/sbw158.

Geertz, C. (1973). Thick description: Towards an interpretive theory of culture. In C. Geertz (Ed.), *The interpretation of cultures* (pp. 3–32). New York: Basic Books.

Gigerenzer, G., Gaissmaier, W., Kurz-Milcke, E., Schwartz, L. M., & Woloshin, S. (2007). Helping doctors and patients make sense of health statistics. *Psychological Science in the Public Interest, 8*(2), 53–96. https://doi.org/10.1111/j.1539-6053.2008.00033.x.

Gillespie, C. (2012). The experience of risk as 'measured vulnerability': Health screening and lay uses of numerical risk. *Sociology of Health and Illness, 34*(2), 194–207. https://doi.org/10.1111/j.1467-9566.2011.01381.x.

Goodenough, W. H. (1956). Residence rules. *Southwestern Journal of Anthropology, 12*(1), 22–37.

Groleau, D., Young, A., & Kirmayer, J. (2006). The McGill illness narrative interview (MINI): An interview schedule to elicit meanings and modes of reasoning related to illness experience. *Transcultural Psychiatry, 43*(4), 671–691. https://doi.org/10.1177/1363461506070796.

Gronemeyer, R. (2013). *Das 4. Lebensalter. Demenz ist keine Krankheit.* München: Pattloch.

Guest, G., Bunce, A., & Johnson, L. (2006). How many interviews are enough? *Field Methods, 18*(1), 59–82. https://doi.org/10.1177/1525822x05279903.

Hallowell, N. (1999). Doing the right thing: Genetic risk and responsibility. *Sociology of Health & Illness, 21*(5), 597–621.

Holmberg, C., Waters, E. A., Whitehouse, K., Daly, M., & McCaskill-Stevens, W. (2015). My lived experiences are more important than your probabilities: The role of individualized risk estimates for decision making about participation in the study of Tamoxifen and Raloxifene (STAR). *Medical Decision Making: An International Journal of the Society for Medical Decision Making, 35*(8), 1010–1022. https://doi.org/10.1177/0272989X15594382.

Hopf, C. (2005). Forschungsethik und qualitative Forschung. In U. Flick, E. von Kardorff, & I. Steinke (Eds.), *Qualitative Forschung. Ein Handbuch* (pp. 589–599). Reinbek bei Hamburg: Rowohlt.

Imo, W. (2017). Trösten: Eine sprachliche Praktik in der Medizin. *Muttersprache, 3*(17), 197–225.

Jack, C. R., Bennett, D. A., Blennkow, K., Carrillo, M. C., Dunn, B., Haeberlein, S. B., … Sperling, R. (2018). NIA-AA research framework: Toward a biological definition of Alzheimer's disease. *Alzheimer's Dementia, 14*(4), 535–562. http://doi.org/10.1016/j.jalz.2018.02.018.

Jessen, F., Amariglio, R. E., van Boxtel, M., Breteler, M., Ceccaldi, M., Chételat, G., … Wagner, M. (2014). A conceptual framework for research on subjective cognitive decline in preclinical Alzheimer's disease. *Alzheimer's Dementia, 10*(6), 844–852. http://doi.org/10.1016/j.jalz.2014.01.001.

Keller, R. (2011). The sociology of knowledge approach to discourse (SKAD). *Human Studies, 34,* 43–65.

Küsters, I. (2009). *Narrative Interviews: Grundlagen und Anwendungen* (2nd ed.). Wiesbaden: Springer VS.

Largent, E. A., & Karlawish, J. (2019). Preclinical Alzheimer disease and the dawn of the pre-caregiver. *JAMA Neurology, 76*(6), 631–632. https://doi.org/10.1001/jamaneurol.2019.0165.

Liggins, J., Kearns, R. A., & Adams, P. J. (2013). Using autoethnography to reclaim the 'place of healing' in mental health care. *Social Science and Medicine, 91,* 105–109. https://doi.org/10.1016/j.socscimed.2012.06.013.

Livingston, G., Sommerlad, A., Orgeta, V., Costafreda, S. G., Huntley, J., Ames, D., … Mukadam. N. (2017). Dementia prevention, intervention, and care. *Lancet, 390*(10113), 2673–2734. http://doi.org/10.1016/S0140-6736(17)31363-6.

Loch, U., & Rosenthal, G. (2002). Das narrative interview. In D. Schaeffer & G. Müller-Mundt (Eds.), *Qualitative Gesundheits- und Pflegeforschung* (pp. 221–232). Bern u. a.: Hans Huber.

Lucius-Hoene, G. (2002). Narrative Bewältigung von Krankheit und Coping-Forschung: Psychotherapie und Sozialwissenschaften. *Zeitschrift für qualitative Forschung, 4*(3), 166–203.

Mason, M. (2010). Sample size and saturation in PhD studies using qualitative interviews [63 paragraphs]. *Forum: Qualitative Social Research, 11*(3), Art. 8. https://doi.org/10.17169/fqs-11.3.1428.

Mitchell, A. J., & Shiri-Feshki, M. (2009). Rate of progression of mild cognitive impairment to dementia: Meta-analysis of 41 robust inception cohort studies. *Acta Psychiatrica Scandinavica, 119*(4), 252–265. https://doi.org/10.1111/j.1600-0447.2008.01326.x.

Nohl, A. (2017). *Interview und Dokumentarische Methode*, 3–13. https://doi.org/10.1007/978-3-658-16080-7_1.

Palinkas, L. A. (2014). Qualitative and mixed methods in mental health services and implementation research. *Journal of Clinical Child & Adolescent Psychology, 43*(6), 851–861. https://doi.org/10.1080/15374416.2014.910791.

Park, C. L., & Folkman, S. (1997). Meaning in the context of stress and coping. *Review of General Psychology, 30,* 115–144.

Pellegrino, E. D. (1992). Intersections of western biomedical ethics and world culture: Problematic and possibility. *Cambridge Quarterly of Healthcare Ethics, 1*(3), 191–196. https://doi.org/10.1017/s0963180100000360.

Pitt, L., Kilbride, M., Nothard, S., Welford, M., & Morrison, A. P. (2007). Researching recovery from psychosis: A user-led project. *Psychiatric Bulletin, 31*(2), 55–60. https://doi.org/10.1192/pb.bp.105.008532.

Powell, R. A., Single, H. M., & Lloyd, K. R. (1996). Focus groups in mental health research: Enhancing the validity of user and provider questionnaires. *International Journal of Social Psychiatry, 42*(3), 193–206.

Puras, P. (2017). Human rights and the practice of medicine. *Public Health Reviews, 38*(9). https://doi.org/10.1186/s40985-017-0054-7.

Reichertz, J. (2015). The meaning of researchers' subjectivity. *Forum Qualitative Sozialforschung/Forum: Qualitative Social Research, 16*(3). Article number 33. https://doi.org/10.17169/fqs-16.3.2461.

Rosenthal, G. (1995). *Erlebte und erzählte Lebensgeschichte. Gestalt und Struktur biographischer Selbstbeschreibungen.* Frankfurt/Main: Campus.

Rostamzadeh, A., Schwegler, C., Gil, S., Romotzky, V., Ortega, G., Canabate, P., … Woopen, C. (in press). Biomarker-based risk prediction of Alzheimer's dementia in MCI: Psychosocial, ethical and legal aspects—the PreDADQoL project. *JAD Journal of Alzheimer's Disease, 2021.*

Sachs-Jeantet, C., Sagasti, F. R., & Salomon, J. J. (1994). *The uncertain quest: Science, technology, and development.* Tokyo: United Nations University Press.

Samerski, S. (2013). Professioneller Entscheidungsunterricht: Vom Klienten zum mündigen Entscheider. *Leviathan, 41*(1), 144–163. https://doi.org/10.5771/0340-0425-2013-1-144.

Samerski, S. (2019). Health literacy as a social practice: Social and empirical dimensions of knowledge on health and healthcare. *Social Science and Medicine, 226,* 1–8. https://doi.org/10.1016/j.socscimed.2019.02.024.

Schaarschmidt, T. (2018, January 2). *Ich bin nicht verrückt, ich bin Revoluzzer* [online newspaper article]. Retrieved from https://www.zeit.de/wissen/gesundheit/2018-01/antipsychiatrie-psychiatrien-psychologie-patienten. Accessed 14 Apr 2019.

Schultze-Lutter, F., Schmidt, S. J., & Theodoridou, A. (2018). Psychopathology: A precision tool in need of re-sharpening. *Frontiers in Psychiatry, 9*(446). https://doi.org/10.3389/fpsyt.2018.00446.

Schütze, F. (1983). Biographieforschung und narratives Interview. *Neue Praxis, 3*(13), 283–293.

Schwegler, C., Rostamzadeh, A., Jessen, F., Boada, M., & Woopen, C. (2017). Expectations of patients with MCI and their caregivers towards predictive diagnosis of AD: A qualitative approach. *Alzheimer's and Dementia, 13*(7), 538. https://doi.org/10.1016/j.jalz.2017.06.641.

Selting, M., Auer, P., Barth-Weingarten, D., Bergmann, J. R., Bergmann, P., Birkner, K., … Hartung, M. (2009). Gesprächsanalytisches Transkriptionssystem 2 (GAT 2). *Ge-sprächsforschung –Online-Zeitschrift zur verbalen Interaktion, 10,* 353–402.

Smith, L. T. (2012). *Decolonizing methodologies: Research and indigenous peoples* (2nd ed.). London and New York: Zed Books.

Sofaer, S. (1999). Qualitative methods: What are they and why use them? *Health Services Research, 34*(52), 1101–1118.

Sykes, S., Wills, J., Rowlands, G., & Popple, K. (2013). Understanding critical health literacy: A concept analysis. *BMC Public Health, 13*(150). https://doi.org/10.1186/1471-2458-13-150.

Timimi, S. (2014). No more psychiatric labels: Why formal psychiatric diagnostic systems should be abolished. *International Journal of Clinical and Health Psychology, 14*(3), 208–215. https://doi.org/10.1016/j.ijchp.2014.03.004.

Vos, S. J. B., Verhey, F., Frölich, L., Kornhuber, J., Wiltfang, J., Maier, W., … Visser, P. J. (2015). Prevalence and prognosis of Alzheimer's disease at the mild cognitive impairment stage. *Brain, 138*(5), 1327–1338. http://doi.org/10.1093/brain/awv029.

Wakefield, J. C. (2012). Der Begriff der psychischen Störung: An der Grenze zwischen biologischen Tatsachen und gesellschaftlichen Werten. In T. Schramme (Ed.), *Krankheitstheorien.* Berlin: Suhrkamp.

Willig, C. (2012). Perspectives on the epistemological bases for qualitative research. In H. Cooper (Ed.), *The handbook of research methods in psychology.* Washington, DC: American Psychological Association.

Woopen, C. (2014). Die Bedeutung von Lebensqualität aus ethischer Perspektive [The significance of quality of life – an ethical approach]. *Zeitschrift für Evidenz, Fortbildung und Qualität im Gesundheitswesen, 108*(2–3), 140–145. https://doi.org/10.1016/j.zefq.2014.03.002.

Zeilig, H. (2014). Dementia as a cultural metaphor. *The Gerontologist, 54*(2), 258–267. https://doi.org/10.1093/geront/gns203.

Zimmermann, M. (2017). Alzheimer's disease metaphors as mirror and lens to the stigma of dementia. *Literature and Medicine, 35*(1), 71–97. https://doi.org/10.1353/lm.2017.0003.

Chapter 8
Interpersonal Process Recall in Systemic Research: Investigating Couple Therapists' Personal and Professional Selves

Maria Borcsa and **Bernadetta Janusz**

Abstract In this chapter, we discuss the Interpersonal Process Recall (IPR) or Stimulated Recall Interview (SRI) as a method and show its usage in investigating systemic couple therapy processes in two international research projects. IPR/SRI has been designed as a process-focused interview method for training and supervision, expanded into clinical, especially psychotherapy process research: patients and/or therapists watch video (segments) of the therapeutic situation and comment on their experiences during the session. The aim of the presented analysis is to study the mutual dynamic between the couple therapists' references to their professional practices and to their personal experiences during the interview. To achieve this aim, we employed two methodological approaches: dialogical analysis to investigate the distinction between the therapist's professional and personal selves, and the narrative storytelling approach in order to describe the therapist's positioning in terms of his or her discursive identities being displayed in the IPR/SR interview. We discuss the results in three aspects, describing (1) the therapists' discursive practices of presenting their professional and personal identities; (2) the shifting of their attention between the video episode from the session and displaying their mental state in relation to it; and (3) the thinking aloud phenomena as enhancing the insight into psychotherapeutic processes. We conclude with methodological reflections.

Keywords Interpersonal Process Recall · Stimulated Recall Interview · Self-Confrontation Interview · Psychotherapy research · Systemic couple therapy · Dialogical analysis · Positioning · Storytelling narrative analysis

M. Borcsa (✉)
Institute of Social Medicine, Rehabilitation Sciences and Healthcare Research, University of Applied Sciences Nordhausen, Nordhausen, Germany
e-mail: borcsa@hs-nordhausen.de

B. Janusz
Family Therapy and Psychosomatic Department, Jagiellonian University Medical College, Kraków, Poland
e-mail: bernadetta.janusz@uj.edu.pl

© Springer Nature Switzerland AG 2021
M. Borcsa and C. Willig (eds.), *Qualitative Research Methods in Mental Health*,
https://doi.org/10.1007/978-3-030-65331-6_8

Introduction

In this chapter, we discuss the Interpersonal Process Recall (IPR) or Stimulated Recall Interview (SRI) as a method and show its usage in investigating systemic couple therapy processes in two international research projects. The aim of the presented analysis is to study the mutual dynamic between the couple therapists' references to their professional practices and to their personal experiences during the interview. We discuss the results in three aspects, describing 1. the therapists' discursive practices of presenting their professional and personal identities; 2. the shifting of their attention between the video episode from the session and displaying their mental state in relation to it; and 3. the thinking aloud phenomena as enhancing the insight into psychotherapeutic processes. Methodological reflections conclude the chapter.

Interpersonal Process Recall (IPR) as a Qualitative Interview Approach

Interpersonal Process Recall (IPR; also Stimulated Recall Interviews,[1] see Vall et al. 2018 or Self-Confrontation Interviews, Breuer, 1991, 1995) was initially created as a qualitative research method to study students' thought processes during classroom discussions (Bloom, 1954). It was further developed as a process-focused interview method for training and supervision (Kagan, Krathwohl, & Farquhar, 1965; Kagan, 1980) and expanded into clinical research by Elliott (1984, 1986).

Since its beginnings, IPR/SRI has been used extensively in research on profes-sional know-how, competence and expertise in such fields as medical practice, pedagogy, athletics coaching, psychotherapy and psychotherapy training (Borchers, Seikkula, & Lehtinen, 2013; Cegala, McNeilis, & Socha McGee, 1995; Consuegra, Engels, & Willegems, 2016; Laitila & Oranen, 2013; Lyle, 2003; Rober et al., 2008; West & Clark, 2004).

IPR/SRI has been developed as a method of reviewing a video recording to recall thoughts and feelings that occurred during the time of the recording. Hence, with regard to psychotherapy research, IPR as an interview approach was designed to access a therapy participant's experiences as close as possible to the moment of the original interaction (Larsen, Flesaker, & Stege, 2008). One of the original methods introduced by Kagan et al. (1965) was to record a session and then immediately review the recording. Usually a trained member of staff interviewed the therapist and client separately. Obtained recordings of therapists' and clients' recalls would then be used in the therapists' training. They constitute the unique sources of information about what was happening in parallel in the session for the therapists and for their client

---

[1]In this chapter, we will use the terms Interpersonal Process Recall (IPR) and Stimulated Recall Interviews (SRI) in a synonymic way and often together as IPR/SRI. This reflects the two back-grounds of the authors: while research project 1 (see below) operates with the term IPR, research project 2 uses SRI.

(Kagan et al., 1965). An events paradigm model informed IPR as Elliott (1986) had clients listen to the entire session and rate specific 'significant events'. Later, Elliott (1986) and Elliott and Shapiro (1988, 1992) had clients select meaningful moments without watching the entire session followed by independent researchers who would then view these same moments to qualitatively develop models of change.

IPR/SRI as a particular interview format for data collection may be combined with different qualitative methodologies. The data obtained by IPR/SR interviews can be analysed through different methods, depending on the research question of the study, e.g. grounded theory (Henretty, Levitt, & Mathews, 2008; Rober et al., 2008) or dialogical analysis (Janusz, Jozefik, & Peräkylä, 2018; Macaskie, Lees, & Freshwater, 2015).

The Role of the Interviewer

IPR/SR interviews are communicative actions; they create their own interactional situation. Interviewer and interviewee as communicative partners influence each other during the interview situation. For this reason, and to meet the requirements of research quality criteria (Gass & Mackey, 2000; Lyle, 2003) researchers have formulated several guiding rules for the IPR/SR interview, such as: (1) minimizing the time delay between event and recall, (2) minimizing the possibility that research participants (interviewees) deliver explanations (their own a priori theories) about links between prompted actions and intentions, (3) designing procedures that create strong links between the interaction, which is the focus of the study, and the procedures for creating the recall, e.g. re-directing the interviewee into the past, maintaining the focus on the specific action during the investigated interaction. They also emphasized the need for constructing the questions and prompts in such a way that they do not alter the cognitive process being employed at the time of the investigated interaction (Gass & Mackey, 2000). Further, Lyle (2003) identified the need to reduce anxiety in interviewees by limiting the perception of judgemental probing, reducing the intrusion into the investigated action by minimalizing any discussion in the IPR/SRI which goes beyond the interaction under study (e.g. by talking about the view of the interviewer). Since the memory works rather through associations than through directive interventions, stimulating and employing an indirect route to the focus of the research seems to be important. What is more, the interviewee should be allowed to give relatively unstructured responses.

In psychotherapy research, the interviewer should help the interviewee to talk about his or her internal processes rather than about the content of the interaction during the therapy session (Elliott, 1986). Larsen et al. (2008) recommend accessing the recency and emotionality of the investigated session by helping the interview participants with such questions as: "What do you remember thinking at that point in the session?" (p. 27).

These guiding rules reflect the positivist epistemology, through which the interview is seen as an operationalization of accessing memories of the interviewee.

They try to minimize the fact that recalling is impacted by the here-and-now of the memorizing situation itself, i.e. the interview situation. Moreover, we think that the stimulus, i.e. watching the video, might create new emotional states overlaying with the past situation (sequence of the video shown), thus interfering with the memorizing process.

Taking these considerations into account, we agree with Breuer (1995) that we face two different action levels: Action 1: the action happening in the therapy session and Action 2: the IPR/SRI situation itself. With regard to this differentiation, the role of the interviewer has generally to be seen as significant and treated with a high level of methodological awareness. Furthermore, the interviewee is positioned on these two levels differently, which will be elaborated on in the next paragraph.

Two Positions of the Interviewee: The *Talking Subject* and the *Object of Talk*

As mentioned, IPR/SRI initially focused solely on past events to capture, interpret and clarify what happened in the recorded session. With regard to psychotherapy research settings, it was used merely for studying individual therapy. So far, little research has been conducted using IPR/SRI in multi-actor settings like couple and family therapy (Gale, 1992; Gale, Odell, & Nagireddy, 1995; Nyman-Salonen et al., 2020; Vall et al., 2018). This delay in systemic research studies might be due to the fact that classical IPR/SRI research and systemic therapy follow a different epistemological stance. While traditional IPR/SRIs are rooted in a positivistic epistemology, most systemic approaches refer to a constructionist (Gergen 2009) background. From a positivistic research framework, IPR/SR interviews are solely the operationalization of getting access to otherwise not accessible data (like motivations and intentions) or implicit aspects during a recorded conversation (like emotions), i.e. a means to an end. From a constructionist perspective, in the course of the interview the talk between interviewer and interviewee creates a new level of phenomena, where the interviewee is part of a new interaction (with the interviewer). In this conversation, created by the IPR/SRI, the interviewee refers to the past session always from a present perspective. This oscillating between two time frames generates two positions for the interviewee: the position of the interviewee here-and-now and the position of the interviewee in the recorded, past session. The positivistic epistemology conceptualizes these two positions by proposing that the interviewee remembers the past. However, content analysis of SRIs with therapists shows, that during the SR-talk we find at least nine categories of accounts: (1) memories related to the shown sequence, (2) further comments on the relevant situation and memories, (3) statements of the interviewee confirming or rejecting statements of the interviewer, (4) generalizing comments on one's own behaviour and experience or on the behaviour or experience of the clients with no direct reference to the presented sequence, (5) subsequent perception and interpretation of the sequence, (6) statements triggered by the thematization of specific aspects through the interviewer, (7) statements addressing the interview itself, (8) unclear, ambiguous statements and (9) other irrelevant statements not related to the subject of the interview (Breuer 1991).

We have to acknowledge that the interviewee in the present situation is the *talking subject*, whereas with reference to the past situation, the same person is the *object of the talk*. This difference refers to the two distinct narrative dimensions while talking about the sequence watched on video: the interviewee is at the same time the 'I as an author'—of his talk here and now—as well as the 'Me as an actor' in the story he or she is presenting (Hermans, 2001).

For these reasons, we will conceptualize IPR/SRI as a tool that is intended to evoke different self-positions; the IPR/SR interview can be seen as a particular social practice of storytelling. These assumptions will situate our analysis in narrative and conversation analysis research frameworks, and from this perspective, we will now refer to some aspects of the dialogical approach.

The Dialogical Approach as Conceptual Framework for Researching Systemic Therapy

Psychotherapy has been referred to as dialogical activity (Seikkula et al., 2011; Rober, 2005). Dialogue is an important concept in the philosophy of Mikhail Bakhtin (1984). We can distinguish the external dialogue between speakers (what we usually call conversation) from the internal dialogue of an individual. This concept refers to feelings, memories and other internal states that are evoked while participating in the conversation. In an external dialogue, the words of the speaker are met by the internal dialogue of the one who listens. Both, speaker and listener, speak and listen from certain positions of their selves, i.e. the internal dialogue contributes to the external in a reciprocal way. Internal dialogue brings into focus the inner conversation between different positions of self (Hermans, 2006), a condition which we can refer to as voices of the self. Thus, different positions of self are connected with internal voices, although the internal voices may of course contain the internalized perspectives of others. All in all, voices are usually defined as the internal, unspoken as well as spoken (and by that becoming external) manifestation of self-positions in the dialogical process.

During some moments of therapy, two selves of the therapist can emerge at the same time: the professional self, containing the professional voice, which is manifested by, e.g. planning further therapeutic procedures, and the personal self, containing the personal voice, which may be manifested by uncertainty or feelings of unease regarding these procedures.

The relation between the self and the others is seen as the starting point for dialogical analysis (Voloshinov, 1976), as the internal dialogue is mediated by what happens in the external conversation (and vice versa), e.g. the voice of uncertainty regarding performing the professional role can be prompted by what happened in the external, professional conversation. Generally, dialogical analysis focuses on the shifting of different positions of self, on internal dialogues and dialogical tensions between the positions and voices (Hermans & Dimaggio, 2007); in psychotherapy research external conversations are used to gain access to internal dialogues and through this, to understand the therapeutic conversation (Rober, 2014).

Dialogical Approach in Psychotherapy Research

Within the dialogical approach, the therapeutic relationship is seen as an active conversation of the internal and external voices of all participants in a therapeutic session. The content of the therapist's mind while conducting the session is the subject of particular interest of psychotherapy researchers. The inner conversation of the therapist (Bakhtin, 1986; Hermans, 2006) is connected to the idea of the polyphonic character of the therapist's internal dialogue (Rober 2005; Rober et al., 2008; Rober, Seikkula, & Latila, 2010). The distinction between the therapist's experiencing (personal) and professional self is central (Rober 2005, 2014), whereby different selves contain different voices. The experiential self involves voices related to personal beliefs, memories, experiences, etc., while professional self contains voices including professional knowledge and clinical experience (Rober, 2005, 2014). According to Rober (2014), the experiencing self contains "the observations of the therapist and the memories, images and fantasies that are activated by what the therapist observes" (ibid., p. 256).

As we mentioned above, the therapist's professional self derives from professional activities during the session, like hypothesizing and focusing on preparing responses (Rober, 2002); in this state of mind the therapist's role is largely one of an observer (Rober, 2005, 2014). In line with the idea of dialogical self (Bakhtin, 1986; Hermans, 2006), Rober (2005) describes the possible contribution of the therapist's internal dialogue to the therapeutic conversation: "the therapist can also reflect explicitly on his or her contribution to the dialogue [i.e., the therapeutic conversation; the authors]. He can create a mental space in his inner conversation in which he can reflect on what happens in the session, on the client's utterances and the invitations for a response that they imply" (Rober, 2005, p. 491). From this perspective, investigating the therapist's inner conversation after the session—e.g. by using IPR/SRI—is seen as a way of investigating the therapist's professional and personal selves and activities as one part of the therapeutic process.

Interpersonal Process Recall as a Storytelling Practice

The analysis presented below is based on the understanding of the IPR/SRI as a particular practice of storytelling. Storytelling is treated as the central way of sharing somebody's past experience with others, although it is not limited to it. Storytelling appears spontaneously or can be elicited in interviews (e.g. in IPR interviews). Conversation analytic studies of storytelling focus on the ways the telling is organized, carried out and delivered collaboratively.

Some researchers of storytelling practices (Labov, 1972, 1982; Labov & Waletzky, 1967) focus on the narrative structures the reportable event is conveyed through, such as: a chain of causal relations, the transformation of the narrative by the narrator's insertions of his or her subjective view on the described events, and the termination of the narrative by returning the time frame to the present. In our research design, we define and analyse the IPR/SRI as a conversational practice of storytelling: we are particularly interested in investigating the conversational ways of displaying different positions of the therapist's self while describing the investigated session.

Storytelling researchers define positioning as the discursive practice employed to accomplish and display different facets of identity that are relevant in different discursive contexts (Bamberg, 1997; Bamberg & Georgakopoulou, 2008; Davies & Harré, 1990; Lucius-Hoene & Deppermann, 2000, 2004a, 2004b). Davies and Harré (1990) describe positioning as the primary locus of the discursive production of selves, the basic mechanism by which a self and identities are acquired in social interaction. Bamberg (1997) distinguishes three levels of positioning: the level of the story, the level of the interaction and the level of displaying different facets of the narrator's identity. We will now discuss the three levels in more detail with reference to IPR/SR interview as a storytelling practice.

1. **Positioning on the level of the story involving the relations between the characters/actors of the story that is told.** This level of the positioning can be described by the question "How are the characters positioned in relation to one another within the reported events?" (Deppermann, 2015, p. 374). Harré, Moghaddam, Cairnie, Rothbart, and Sabat (2009) claim that the storyteller implicitly defines the actors by describing their way of relating to each other while the story develops. It means that characters in the story are positioned in relation to each other or vis-à-vis each other (Bamberg & Georgakopoulou 2008). This level of positioning is specific to narrative and other descriptive practices. Lucius-Hoene and Deppermann (2000) developed Bamberg's levels of positioning further. They point out that the described characters are designed by the narrator from his/her present point of view, they actively design the story by linguistic and narrative means. The IPR/SR interview can be seen as the specific narration that is designed to access and tell the story about the past interaction from the perspective of one actor who participated in the event under examination. The research design utilized in the research reported in this chapter pertains to investigating the reflections of therapists after couple therapy sessions. For this reason, positioning on the level of the story is particularly complex: it involves

three or four actors: both partners (i.e. the clients) and the therapist(s). Partners are intimately interconnected, the therapists act as professionals, and at the same time, during the examined interactional episode, they are actors in the same story.

2. **Positioning on the level of the interaction between the teller and the receiver of the story.** This interactional level refers to jointly organizing the turn-taking between the teller and the receiver of the story. This kind of turn-taking structure is seen as an accomplishment that needs to be negotiated in interaction. The storytelling can be categorized by different actions, e.g. complaining or explaining which are pursued in and through storytelling (Schegloff, 1997). While analysing the storytelling practices conversation analysis researchers put particular emphasis on the following interactional phenomena: the narrator adjusts his or her way of storytelling to the reception of the story, e.g. by providing corrections or redirections to pursue an intended reaction (Goodwin, 1986). For this reason, in spite of the authorship of the teller, what the story comes to be about is eventually arrived at through interaction (Goodwin, 1997). The reception of a story involves the interactants' alignment and affiliation (Stivers, 2008). Alignment refers to the recipients' support in the delivery of the story on the level of interaction, such as to accept the role of listener and make momentary evaluations of the story being told. Affiliation refers to the listener displaying support of and endorsing the teller's conveyed stance. It is also possible to resist the stance delivered, which is a sign of disaffiliation.

   Interviewer's positioning on the level of interaction involves: (1) endorsing or supporting the interviewee in order to facilitate him or her to get access to the interaction under study; (2) monitoring the production of the interviewee's story by interviewer's affiliations/disaffiliations and alignments/misalignments; and (3) creating a new interactional level of the IPR/SRI phenomenon by discussing the interaction under study with the interviewee here and now.

3. **Positioning of the narrators to themselves, through displaying particular aspects of self and identity.** This level of positioning is connected with the idea that selves exist as multiple, contradictory, contextual and distributed over time and place (Bamberg & Zielke, 2007).

   In this context, Deppermann (2015) refers to the description of category-bound actions, which are connected to attributes and ways of speaking. Category-bound activities are a form of actions that are conventionally associated with being a member of the relevant category (Sacks, 1992). In the research presented in this chapter, the couple therapists as interviewees (in the IPR/SRI) not only use certain therapeutic vocabulary but also their way of speaking, i.e. categorizing, expressing understanding can be associated with the style or register of this particular social group (Coupland, 2007) creating distinct discourse identities.

In the analysis presented below, we put emphasis on linguistic and narrative means by which the couple therapists display their professional selves and identities. We analyse their distinctive category-bound actions that are displayed, told and re-acted[2] in IPR/SRI dialogue. As the temporal organization of a storytelling involves the continuity between past action or event and the actual account, i.e. telling the story, the teller has the possibility of "*self-positioning by extra- and meta-narrative self-reflexive activities*" (Deppermann, 2015, p. 379). Through this particular conversational practice "tellers may explicitly take a stance toward past events and their past selves through meta-narrative retrospective comments, argumentations, and evaluations from the present point of view" (Deppermann, 2015, p. 379).

Using IPR/SRI to Analyse Couple Therapists' Perspectives on Their Professional Practices

In the following parts of the chapter, we will present two IPR/SRI segments that come from couple therapy research (see also Borcsa & Rober, 2016). We will analyse in what way couple therapists' professional practices and their personal experiences are commented upon in the IPR/SR interviews. To achieve this aim, we will refer to the distinction between the therapist's professional and personal self as described above, as well as to the conversational practices of storytelling, particularly to the therapist's positioning in terms of his or her discourse identities that are displayed in the IPR/SR interview. We will focus on the interplay between recalling the experiences from the session (positioning on the level of the story) and reflecting upon them in the IPR/SR interview (positioning on the level of the interview interaction).

The capacity to manage their professional talk is part of the training and professional experience of therapists. On the other hand, a considerable part of professional talk is neither predictable nor fully manualized, as it usually involves the complex, embodied interaction of two or more individuals. To some extent, the professionals control their conversational practices already during the talk. Some instances, however, might be reflected upon only thereafter, when the professional meeting is recalled and discussed. Such post hoc discussions create new dialogical space to rethink the investigated interaction.[3]

In the majority of cases the time dimension in the IPR/SR interview means sticking to the retrospective reports that represent access to direct, unordered accounts of previous thought processes (Lyle, 2003). We assume that the researcher can mainly recognize retrospection through the use of past tense, whereas the use of present tense mostly signals reflection. As mentioned, the main aim of the IPR/SRI talk has been to access the experiences of the participants as they emerged during the investigated interaction (thoughts, feelings and bodily sensations) (Elliott, 1986; Larsen et al., 2008). However, the intersubjective approach to IPR/SRI (Freshwater

---

[2]We use the term to *re-act* when the teller refers to himself as being an actor in the story he is telling. Re-enactment is used with a different meaning in systemic therapy as well as acting-out in psychoanalytic therapy.

[3]Traditionally, in psychotherapy the supervision is considered as the professional meeting where the earlier psychotherapeutic session(s) are discussed and reflected upon.

& Rolfe, 2001; Macaskie et al., 2015; Rubin & Rubin, 2005) is not limited to talking about experiences in the earlier interaction (recalling the past). Moreover, it also includes the co-analysis of the material, which means reflecting here and now in the conversation of interviewer and interviewee about the earlier interaction. We will be investigating the junction between recalling and reflection in the IPR/SRI data through the different dimensions of storytelling such as the past events told in the story, displacing of selves of the teller, and eventually the teller's meta-narrative comments in the IPR/SRI (Bamberg, 1997; Deppermann, 2015).

Procedure

In the section below, we present the analysis of two segments, coming from two different couple therapy research projects.

The first derives from a research project investigating the *Therapists Internal Conversation and Interactional Practices in the First Family and Couple Therapy Consultations*.[4] The research was conducted in the Department of Family Therapy at the Jagiellonian University Medical College in Cracow, Poland. The data presented in this chapter are part of a set of nine video-recorded first session consultations together with IPR/SR interviews with the therapists. The interviews with the therapists were conducted directly after the sessions. The therapists were asked to identify and comment on any moments in the video-recorded session which they found important or meaningful from the perspective of the therapeutic process or which caught their attention in any way. The researchers, who were also couple therapists, could also stop the session at any moment and ask the therapists to reflect upon it; what is more, the interviewers could comment by themselves and clarify the therapist's answers. Most importantly, the interviewers were instructed to steer the therapists' focus to the chosen moment of the session, irrespective of whether interviewers or therapists stopped the video in order to ask a question or comment upon.[5]

The second segment derives from the German cooperation in the *Relational Mind Project* (Seikkula, Karvonen, Kykyri, Kaartinen, & Penttonen, 2015; Vall et al. 2018; Nyman-Salonen et al. 2020).[6] The data presented is part of a set of 5 completed heterosexual couple therapies with a female and a male co-therapist in each case,

---

[4]The project was approved by the bioethics committee of the Jagiellonian University Medical College: KBET/273/B/2011.

[5]By now, results are published as follows: Janusz et al. (2018) show that gender assumptions held unchallenged by a therapist can create difficulty in introducing circular thinking, in terms of the therapist's inner conversation and the conversation during the session. Bryniarska, Tomasiewicz, Janusz, and Józefik (2019) illustrate that therapists' biographical experiential voices evoked in IPR tend to deepen reflection on the therapeutic process. Janusz, Matusiak, and Peräkylä (2021) show the emergence of the therapist's asymmetry of affiliation with both spouses.

[6]The research programme *The Relational Mind* is the first to look at dialogue in terms of both the outer and the inner dialogues of participants (clients and therapists), observed in parallel with Autonomic Nervous System (ANS) measurements. Funded by the Academy of Finland (Principal Investigator: Jaakko Seikkula) the project collaborates with Nordhausen University of Applied Sciences,

carried out at the Institute of Social Medicine, Rehabilitation Sciences and Health-care Research, UAS Nordhausen, Germany. The therapies had a total length of 2–7 sessions (each 90 min), autonomic nervous system (ANS) measurement took place during the second and sixth session,[7] the IPR/SRI followed within 24 h after these sessions, mostly directly after the session itself. IPR/SRIs were conducted with each participant of the therapeutic system individually, i.e. with the female client, the male client, the female therapist and the male therapist, and all interviews were video-recorded. A female clinician-researcher, sitting behind the one-way mirror during the therapy sessions, selected three situations during the consultation, which were later used for the IPR/SRIs. The selection process of the situation segments followed these rules: (i) visible emotional expression (weeping, laughing, etc.) of participants in the therapy session; (ii) a notable change in the interaction (e.g. vivid dialogue after a silence or a long monologue); (iii) visible synchrony in ANS measurements between two or more participants; (iv) a combination of these aspects; (v) one scene from the Reflecting Team intervention.[8] During the IPR/SRI, these selected three segments were shown to the interviewees; i.e. the segments to talk about in the IPR/SRI were chosen before the interview by the clinician-researcher and not by the participants in the interview situation itself.

In our analysis, we will be studying the therapists' comments on their professional practices in the systemic couple therapy consultations. We will follow the therapists' experiences identified by them as emerging in the course of the investigated sessions. We will discuss in what way the therapists achieved their recall and reflecting stance in the course of the IPR/SR interview.

Each extract will be introduced by a summary of the scene of the therapy session (as it is shown on the video), followed by the transcript of the IPR/SRI[9] and its analysis.

Germany; Aristotle University Thessaloniki, Greece and University Ramon Llull, Barcelona, Spain. The German part was approved by the bioethics committee of the Medical College of the University of Jena, Germany: 3953-12/13.

[7]We will not speak in this paper about the ANS measurement procedure or results; please refer to Seikkula et al. (2015), Karvonen, Kykyri, Kaartinen, Penttonen, and Seikkula (2016), Päivinen et al. (2016).

[8]During the Reflecting Team (Andersen 1991), the co-therapists turn to each other and reflect openly in front of the clients about the session.

[9]Extract 1 is translated from the Polish language, Extract 2 from the German language; transcription followed transcription rules; I = Interviewer, T = therapist; words in round brackets () signalize that the talk is hard to understand and an assumption; text in square brackets [] gives indication of meaning by the authors, > text in arrows < indicate non-verbal behaviour, (.) short pause, (2) length of pause in seconds.

Couple Therapy Research 1

The Scene from the Therapy Session: The Physical Arrangements in the Therapy Room

As the participants are entering the room, the husband immediately points to the fan heater (centred in the room) and asks whether it can be turned off. In response, the wife and the therapist express surprise, treating the husband's wish as unexpected. Both the therapist and the wife perceive the temperature of the room as too cold, while the husband experiences it as too hot, asking whether it can be switched off. Thereafter the therapist reorganizes the setting: he repositions the heater in such a way that it is more comfortable for both spouses.

IPR/SR interview. After the first minute of watching the session, the therapist stopped the video after the heater was repositioned and commented upon the sequence in the following way:

Extract 1: Transcript IPR/SRI with Male Therapist

```
01 T:  So here, I've (had) such a problem when he [the client] said this.
02 I:  I wanted to ask you exactly about his moment.
03 T:  OK.
04 I:  Shall we switch it on
       [in order to watch once more and they do watch it once more]
05 T:  Here, I was concerned about an alliance with her
06     that with her, we will be warming ourselves together and he
07     he will be over - heated and not acknowledged.
08 I:  And this was more or less the first minute of this meeting
09     so I understand that you were concerned
10     about being non-neutral, something like that?
11 T:  Yes.
12 I:  Mhm.
13 T:  At that moment when she said that
14     she is in the same climatic situation as I was.
15 I:  Mhm.
16 T:  And he in a different one.
17 I:  Because I remember that you-
18 T:  because he wanted to switch it off when I entered, being frozen
19 I:  I remember.
20 T:  Yes, completely frozen, it was diabolically cold there
21     but he says that he is too hot, and in the first moment
22     I wasn't sure whether he is serious or if something isn't ok with him
23     because it is diabolically cold, but he is too hot.
24     I understood this only in terms of his sensory faculties
25     of perception and sense of temperature, but not (.)
26     It is visible here that she is she can be reached but he is frozen.
27 I:  At this point?
```

```
28 T:  Yes, there is a clear difference between her degree of openness
29     and his. My idea here is indeed to take care of him
30     as she she has already bought [into the idea of therapy]
31 I:  Aha, 2nd minute [referring to the moment of the session]
```

In lines 05–07 the therapist indicates a risk of developing a stronger alliance with the wife than with the husband. By using the pronoun *here* (meaning here in the session as seen on the video) and then continuing in the past tense *I was concerned about an alliance with her*, he refers to his worries, indicating that they were evoked in him at the time of the session. Directly after that, by using the future continuous formulation *we will be warming ourselves together and he will be over-heated and not acknowledged* he indicates that already at the very beginning of the session he was troubled about developing an uneven alliance with both spouses in the further course of the session. The therapist demonstrates an awareness (professional voice) of the complex dimension of the therapeutic processes—the risk of developing a split alliance; the solution (as a kind of repair) is rooted in his physical action (repositioning the heater).

By using the psychotherapy related term *alliance* the therapist positions himself in the SRI as a professional who is able to reflect upon the session while conducting it. Besides expressing his concern, he situates himself also as one of the actors in the story (embodied experience of the temperature). Moreover, he constructs the position of an observer who is reflecting upon the course of the session.

In lines 18–23 he reveals his experiential, personal voice conveying his bodily sensations (*I entered being frozen*), which he felt at the beginning of the session (past tense: *I entered*). Continuing his utterance, the therapist shifts from his body related experiential voice of *being frozen* into another experiential voice conveying uncertainty and surprise related to the husband's perception of the temperature in the room (l.22–23), *I wasn't sure whether he is serious or if something isn't ok with him because it is diabolically cold, but he is too hot.* By maintaining his experiential voice, the therapist is presenting himself as an actor in the story. By recalling his experience during the therapeutic session (*I entered being frozen*) he positions himself in the embodied interaction with other participants: *it is diabolically cold, but he is too hot.* While remaining in the actor's position and evoking the personal voice, the therapist ends up expressing astonishment regarding the husband's embodied experience. Additionally, he introduces a normative statement: *something isn't ok with him,* as a possible explanation of the man's behaviour.

Continuing the topic, the interviewee shifts again into his professional voice by saying (l.24) *I understood this only in terms of his sensory faculties,* (past tense—referring to the investigated session), but at the same time indicating that now (after the therapy session, during the interview) he has attained additional understanding. This important shift between remaining an actor in the story (personal voice) and his self-positioning on the meta-narrative level enables him to realize the limitations of his earlier vision.

Thereafter, in line 26 he uses present tense *It is visible here* (in the video sequence) that *she is she can be reached but he is frozen.* He depicts the asymmetry in experiencing the temperature in the room as a metaphoric manifestation of the spouses' openness for the therapy (1.28): *Yes, there is a clear difference between her degree of openness and his.* The last part of his utterance is expressed from the position of professional self in the voice of explaining his behaviour: *My idea here is indeed to take care of him as she has already bought [into the idea of therapy],* giving to him the position of the director in the scene who is taking responsibility for integrating the husband into the therapeutic system. However, it isn't clear whether this complex understanding and planning of the therapeutic process was consciously available to him while he was acting or only ex post, i.e. after the session.

Next, we would like to present the second example (extract 2), which is taken from the Relational Mind Project. The investigated session with a heterosexual couple was conducted by two couple therapists (one male and one female); here we focus on the SRI with the male therapist.

Couple Therapy Research 2

The Scene from the Therapy Session: Making Comparisons Between Couples

The female client discusses an example where her friends, a couple, had brought off an agreement. She tells how the couple had tried to agree upon a floor covering. Every time they noticed that they did not find a way to see eye-to-eye, they put the topic aside and so were still able "to further look at each other". The female therapist asks her what her husband does not like about that. The woman says in response: "that I compare us with others". She would not want to do it exactly that way, but she would like to learn certain general principles by watching. She thinks it was a good way for the couple to reach an agreement; both moved towards each other, they were still close to each other and found a solution which would satisfy both. The female client wishes this also for her own relationship. In the scene played, the woman prevails as a speaker, the husband makes barely one utterance. The woman gesticulates with her hands during the entire speaking time, speaks in a loud voice and glances repeatedly over to her husband. The man displays few movements in this scene; he looks mainly at his wife, seemingly detached.

IPR/SR interview. After this sequence, the researcher stopped the video and started the interview:

Extract 2: Transcript IPR/SRI with Male Co-therapist

```
01 I:  Okay [name of the therapist], what did you think and feel at that
02     moment during the session?
```

```
03 T:  Um (.) I tried (struggle to be neutral) to keep an eye on both and
04      (.) um one immediately felt an impulse um (.) to stay more with the
05      man because I (1) otherwise I had the feeling oh that is now a topic
06      he does not like at all, so already when she started here, we have
07      among our relatives or friends or something a couple, well there I
08      noticed, comparing is not his thing, he thinks, it is silly now (.) and
09      I thought it was very interesting how he behaved just there - it
10      cannot be a coincidence > shakes his head from one side to the other<
11      but can also be such a thing, well I need a distance
12      i-it was not said n the therapy, the man did not say that
13      there to um (4) it is a little bit that I have a feeling
14      with Mrs [name], once she has constructed
15      such um a picture, she embellishes it, I called it
16      in my notes from the first session embellishment hang-up
17      while he has well the order hang-up(1) and um (3) well it took a
18      bit too long for me all the things she elaborated on, (.) yes (.) and
19      she always [name of the female therapist] and looked at me and um I
20      would have wished that she [female patient] looked (also) more
21      towards her husband, then she would have perhaps also realised that he
22      somehow well also, for me he had signalled it is enough now, I got it
23      by now, I have actually understood it by the second sentence (.) um
24      (1) I had the feeling she was explaining something to herself there,
25      it is all right, too, um hm (.) whether it is helpful for the process
26      one must simply see this is what crosses my mind (4)
27 I:  Mhm what did you feel at that moment?
28 T:  (2) well the feeling was, I know this feeling um, when someone
29      confronts you with comparisons, that I also rather go on the
30      defensive (1) so I was able to (.) um (.) empathise with Mr.
31      [1st letter of name]'s situation (1) and um at the same time um as
32      I like to tell stories, I could also empathise um with the woman,
33      who explains it so, um I am also quite fond of doing it [
34      incomprehensible 2-second sequence] so similar structures take place
35      also in my case sometimes, although I imagine that I keenly watch my
36      interlocutor with who I am talking in that moment
37      and wait for reactions (.) this is what I was emotionally going
38      through, so to speak
```

At the beginning of his utterance, in lines 03–06, the therapist uses past tense: *I tried, felt an impulse, I had the feeling,* thereby indicating that he is referring to his mental states that were invoked in him during the session, positioning himself as one of the characters of the story he is telling. He starts with his professional self, indicating that he was able to maintain a meta-perspective while conducting the session *I tried (struggle to be neutral) to keep an eye on both* (l.3). Immediately after this statement, he shifts into an impersonal experiential voice: *um one immediately felt an impulse um (.) to stay more with the man* (l.4). The emergence of the experiential voice seems to indicate an inner dialogue between voices: he was closer to the man in spite of his professional intention to *keep an eye on both.* It needs to be emphasized that both personal-experiential voices were told as a self-reflective observation: *one immediately felt an impulse um (.) to stay more with the man,* and *I had the feeling oh that is now a topic he does not like at all.* Thereafter, he shifts into the reflection on the patient's state of mind in the course of the session, using direct reported speech: *he thinks, it is silly now,* and again starts to describe his own mental processes in relation to the patient, positioning himself as an observer: *I thought it was very interesting how he behaved just there.* He maintains the position of the character in the story, but remaining in his professional role. He finishes his utterance by the meta-reflection: *it cannot be a coincidence.* Continuing, he comes again close to the husband by putting himself in the husband's shoes and thereby inferring his possible stance during the session: *but can also be such a thing, well I need a distance* (l.11). Through the dialogue between his experiential, personal voice (closeness to the husband) and his professional voice (the position of an observer), the therapist indicates the possibility to resonate with the patient's stance during the session. By saying, in the past tense, *I thought it was very interesting how he behaved just there,* the therapist seems to refer to his thoughts in the course of the therapeutic session. In the next statement by employing the present tense: *it cannot be a coincidence* and *but can also be such a thing, well I need a distance* he indicates the ongoing reflection at the time of the interview, which leads again to giving voice to the male client and his feelings: *well I need a distance.* The talk depicts thinking aloud phenomena (see also the pauses): *it cannot be a coincidence,* which at the same time can serve as auto-reinforcement, reassuring himself and the receiver of his talk about the validity of the statement.

Thereafter, starting in line 13 he presents the characteristics of both spouses from his point of view, commencing with the wife: *....in my notes from the first session embellishment hang-up, while he has well the order hang-up.* Introducing the symmetry in the description might indicate his efforts to regain the professional stance of neutrality,[10] after being closer to the husband's perspective (l.4–13). In this segment, the therapist positions himself entirely in the professional stance by referring to typical therapist's attributes: *in my notes.* In spite of not using therapeutic language semantically (see *alliance* in the example above), his way of speaking contains typical category-bound action related to diagnostic talk, in which the patients are classified. The presented segment does not indicate any new understanding or insight achieved, e.g. by recall of the past experience or putting into words something that was in his mind during the session. Rather, it can be treated as self-assurance by referring to the knowledge that was obtained and written down after the session. Anyway, he stays more distanced from the wife (l.17–18): *it took a bit too long for me all the things she elaborated on.*

In the next segments the therapist shifts again closer to the husband (without indicating his awareness of this move) by saying *I would have wished that she [female client] looked [also] more towards her husband, then she would have perhaps also realised that he* (l.19–21). The therapist positions himself as being inside the story by going back to his motivation in the moment of the session, while the account may

---

[10]Neutrality was initially understood as a particular attitude of the therapist manifested by temporal shifts of alliances between the therapist and each participant (Selvini-Palazzoli, Boscolo, Cecchin, & Prata, 1980), maintenance of neutrality in respect of the therapist's own belief and value systems (Tomm, 1984), and a particular therapeutic outcome (Brown, 2010). According to the Milan school (Selvini-Palazzoli et al., 1980), neutrality is one of the three central tenets of conducting family therapy sessions, the others being the *testing of hypotheses*, and *circularity*. In order to achieve the position of neutrality the therapist constantly forms hypotheses by which to understand the behaviour of a problematic client in a non-judgemental, relational way.

serve at the same time as a post hoc explanation for his *impulse* to stay more with the man. In lines 22–26 he elaborates on this in more detail: *then she would have perhaps also realised that he somehow well also, for me he had signalled it is enough now, I got it by now, I have actually understood it by the second sentence (.) um (1) I had the feeling she was explaining something to herself there, it is all right, too, um hm (.) whether it is helpful for the process one must simply see this is what crosses my mind (4).* The therapist explains his understanding of the non-verbal behaviour of the husband, once more giving him the direct speech: *I got it by now* on the level of the story plot. The interviewee positions himself in contrast to the female client, thereafter trying to give meaning to her behaviour, almost as a dialogue between an experiential voice and a professional position. Finally, the meaning-making is done in a psychologizing manner, validating it but immediately afterwards being questioned on the level of the therapeutic process by switching to the professional voice-stance.

In the next segment, after the interviewer's question (l.27), the therapist is able to accomplish his professional position (the symmetry in relation to each spouse). In lines 28–30 he uses the present tense while referring to the husband's potential internal stance during the session and his (therapist's) own characteristics: *I know this feeling, I also rather go on the defensive,* and by shifting into the past tense he finishes the sentence: *so I was able to empathise with Mr.* This also demonstrates a move towards reflecting upon a particular facet of his personal characteristics: *I know this feeling, I also rather go on the defensive.* Thereafter, by positioning himself on the level of the story, he shifts into the displaying of his therapeutic capacity in the session: *so I was able to empathise with Mr.* (l.30). The same shift of time perspectives and positions occurs in relation to the female client *I like to tell stories, I could also empathise um with the woman* (l.32). This segment shows that the personal, self-reflective voice regarding the therapist's general predispositions, interconnected with the personal voice on the level of the story, can lead to reflective insight into professional practices. In this moment of the interview, the therapist indicates his efforts to achieve his professional stance by maintaining symmetric empathy towards both spouses. The present segment can be seen as an example of employing a personal experiential voice—an awareness of one's personal characteristics—in order to accomplish a professional stance—an insight. Thereby the therapist shows in what way his personal resources may contribute to empathizing symmetrically with both spouses. Nevertheless, by the utterance *I imagine that I keenly watch my interlocutor with who I am talking at the moment* he introduces another difference between himself and the female client (l.35), indicating that he is still struggling with his neutrality.

Recapitulating extract 2, we observe that at the beginning of the SRI the therapist's experiential voice situates him closer to the husband: *um one immediately felt an impulse um (.) to stay more with the man.* Yet, he is not just re-acting this closeness but rather positions himself as reflecting upon this experience in the session. Recalling his internal states from the session together with employing a reflexive stance in the course of the IPR/SRI enables him to understand in what way he utilizes his personal resources in order to accomplish his professional identity, even if he is not regaining total neutrality.

Discussion

Understanding the IPR/SRI as a specific storytelling practice, and inspired by the distinction between personal and professional self, we described the complexity and the dynamics of recalling and getting reflective insight into therapists' professional practices in the course of IPR/SRI.

In comparing the similarities and differences of the two interviews, we realize that both therapists are discussing the aspect of possible asymmetries in the therapeutic system. Therapist 1 is referring to more closeness to the female client, therapist 2 to the male client. To overcome this felt asymmetry, therapist 1 intervenes directly in the scene, therapist 2, being more in the position of a listener and observer in the therapy situation itself, uses the IPR/SR interview to reflect upon the experienced situation.

From this perspective, therapist 1 (who himself stops the video) is explaining his intervention of repositioning the heater, therapist 2 (being confronted with a sequence chosen by the interviewer) is reflecting on the case and on his internal states being part of this therapeutic system; he presents resonances and reflections, almost in a self-supervisory manner. Through the differences in the therapy and research settings of the two projects, therapist 1 holds the sole responsibility for structuring the situation and the therapy process, in the second case we are dealing with a couple co-therapy, an other (female) therapist is taking part in the session.

In the following, we discuss the results on three levels: (1) therapists' discursive practices of positioning themselves through displaying their professional and personal identities; (2) the dynamics of interviewees' positioning in the IPR, i.e. shifting between the described episode and the interviewees' mental states: thinking by talking, recalling by thinking, feeling by acting out and (3) thinking aloud as the IPR related storytelling practice.

Displaying professional and personal identities. The interviewees' positioning—referring directly to the professional interaction or commenting on it retrospectively—seems to be particularly relevant while investigating professional practices. In extract 1, the therapist positions himself as the actor in the story by pointing out his bodily sensations and astonishment at the husband's perception of the temperature in the room. This specific reference to the level of the story (using past tense) evokes his experiential personal voice. Further on, by shifting into the present tense, and displaying such facets of his professional identity as interpretation, by attributing metaphoric meaning to the husband's bodily sensation (Davies and Harré, 1990; Bamberg, 1997; Bamberg & Georgakopoulou, 2008), he positions himself in the professional stance. Additionally, he uses a specific therapeutic code-choice (Sacks, 1992) by pointing at the husband's *openness* for the therapy.

The dynamic aspect of positioning appears in extract 2, where the therapist recognizes the felt proximity to the male client, which emerged in him in the course of the session (past tense). Although he talks from the position of experiential personal voice, he also displays his professional stance by situating himself in the position of an observer: *felt an impulse um (.) to stay more with the man.* From this position, he shifts into describing the relations between the other actors of the story (especially the husband and the wife), resonating with the male client's state in the session, expressing the voice of the husband: *he thinks, it is silly now; I got it by now* and *I need a distance.* He is continuing with the construction of personal similarities between the figures in the story and himself, and ending with a difference between himself and the female client.

In both presented cases of positioning, we need to acknowledge the specificities of IPR interviews that evoke situational identities (Bamberg & Georgakopoulou, 2008; Deppermann, 2015); the therapist is bound to recall his subjective mental states connected with his (actual) professional position: both, the IPR/SR interview situation as well as his professional identity, create a respective obligation. Both examples refer to the awareness towards keeping a neutral or a multipartial alliance with both spouses, which is a guiding principle of systemic couple therapy.

The analyses of the presented cases indicate that the inner conversation between the therapist's two positions of self (experiencing and professional) can be seen as a circular process, i.e. shifting from professional voice into experiential and vice versa. What is more, the circularity thereof is mediated by the therapist's observer stance, his shifting between the recall of the internal states in the session, making sense on the level of the story, and employing a reflective stance in the IPR/SRI situation.

When the process of shifting between the therapist's positions stops and only one type of voice (identity) is maintained within one topical segment of talk, this seems to create an obstacle for getting new insight or even recall. Extract 1 shows that maintaining the personal voice and the position of an actor in the story puts the therapist into the normative stance: *I wasn't sure whether he is serious or if something isn't ok with him because it is diabolically cold, but he is too hot.* Whereas in extract 2 enacting entirely the professional stance leads to categorization of the patients ….*in my notes from the first session, embellishment hang-up, while he has well the order hang-up, once she has constructed such um a picture, she embellishes it.*

Our analysis shows that shifting between different levels of the storytelling—being an actor in the story (personal voice) or displaying professional identity—leads to the activation of reflective insight into one's professional practices. While being stuck in one position, be it the personal or the professional, led to normative statements.

The dynamics of speakers' positioning in the IPR. The uniqueness of recalling social interaction, in this research a couple therapy session, lies in putting into words the embodied, mental experience that emerged in its course. Shifting between the personal and professional domain, being an actor in the story as well as an observer while commenting upon particular segments of the session seem to constitute the creative space produced by IPR, which is at the same time recalling, understanding and thereby using it as a source of insight.

Yet, it is also important to mention that during the IPR/SR interview the professional has the implicit or explicit understanding and memory of the entire investigated session; the interviewee uses knowledge which he did not have at the beginning (at the time of the episode that is brought to mind in the IPR). This was particularly evident in case 2, when the therapist mentions "the notes" he made after the session.

From this perspective, the calling to mind in the course of the IPR procedure is rooted (i) in the memory of the investigated moment, (ii) the memory of the whole session, (iii) the stimulus of the video playback of the session (the segment under investigation) and (iv) in the interaction with the interviewer (interviewer's questions or comments depending on the approach[11]).

Typically, the practice of storytelling is grounded in the reporting of the events that happened in the past. The teller either situates himself/herself in the position of an actor who actively took part in the described events or as an observer. His or her subjective comments are treated as insertions containing, e.g. his/her evaluation or reflection (see Labov, 1972, 1982; Labov & Waletzky, 1967). The storytelling in IPR focuses on sharing a therapist's professional or personal subjective experience while referring to the investigated event, the therapeutic session. The analysis shows that this kind of insertion - shifting between one's own mental states and referring to the investigated action (and vice versa) - creates a particular source of reflection and insight.

To sum up, IPR analyses show the appearance of new insight as a creative process of (re-) construction through the narrator's shifting between narrated story and his subjective states. We could say that shifting between the described episode and the interviewee's mental states creates such phenomena as: thinking by talking, recalling by thinking or feeling by re-acting the investigated interaction.

Thinking aloud as the IPR related storytelling practice. The present analysis of the conversational means of the storytelling indicated that in the IPR/SR interview the therapist shifts between the role of an actor engaged in the investigated moment, the observer of the session (Rober, 2005, 2014), and the interlocutor in the actual talk. Furthermore, we identified the practice of thinking aloud, which seems to be characteristic of the IPR related practice of storytelling.

Thinking aloud is displayed in a combination of recall, commenting on the video, shifting between time frames (in the session and in the interview situation) and eventually formulating insights in the here-and-now. The interviewees, being both actors and observers, bring both aspects together to make sense of what they see in the video. The very idea of thinking aloud involves actively looking for meanings and finding connections between different multimodal experiences during IPR/SR interview; the creative aspect of thinking aloud is depicted by a tentative mode of speaking. In extract 1 (lines 24–26), the process of thinking aloud involves the therapist's awareness of his limited understanding in the course of the session: *I understood this only in terms of his sensory faculties but not*—at this point the interviewee aborted his statement in a grammatical sense. It was, however, further continued by shifting into an observation *It is visible here that she is,* and after this unfinished sentence he added the interpretation, *she can be reached but he is frozen.*

In the second example, the practice of thinking aloud was particularly visible in lines 07–13; it starts again from the therapist's indicating his perception marked by

---

[11]In the first research design (see extract 1), the interviewer was more active, commenting the investigated segment herself/himself. In the second one (see extract 2), the role of the interviewer was more standardized asking questions about the cognitions and emotions during the session.

an interjection[12] *well, there I noticed.* Further on, the interviewee goes back and forth between the session and the interview situation, trying to give meaning to what he experienced and what he saw in the video *I thought it was very interesting how he behaved just there—it cannot be a coincidence > shakes his head from one side to the other < but can also be such a thing, well I need a distance i-it was not said in the therapy, the man did not say that there to um (4) it is a little bit that I have a feeling.* From a systemic perspective, we can observe the development of hypotheses by the therapist. In this case, the hypothesis is focusing on the husband, even giving him a direct voice, but not necessarily looking at the couple as a system.

To sum up, the analyses presented here indicate that thinking aloud can be treated as the particular IPR related storytelling practice which predominantly involves the narrator's insertions of subjective comments (Labov, 1972, 1982; Labov & Waletzky, 1967) and constant shifting in the narration between the time frame of the past and of the present.

Limitations, Methodological Reflections and Conclusions

As we brought two research projects together, both of them using IPR/SRI in couple therapy, we would like to conclude this chapter with some reflections on limitations, methodological similarities and differences we became aware of while doing the analyses.

First, we want to point out the challenge connected with the way of interpreting and presenting our data, which are translations from two different languages into a third one, of which none of us is a native speaker. We tried to solve this difficulty by starting the interpretation in the respective original language, discussing the interpretation with the translator and re-checking the translation in each language.[13]

With regard to similarities and differences in our projects, using IPR method-ology, we would like to indicate: in project 1, therapists (interviewees) as well as interviewers have the control to stop the video at the sequence they want to comment on. In extract 1 we can see in the conversation of therapist and interviewer (I: *I wanted to ask you exactly about his moment*) that both persons found this moment mean-ingful. In project 2, the clips shown are selected by a research-practitioner (in our case also the interviewer) according to the above-mentioned criteria. This means that the therapist of extract 2 has actually no choice but to comment on this segment (and we do not know to what extent this would have been an important sequence for him).

---

[12]Expresses spontaneous feeling or reaction, here used as a hesitation marker.

[13]The main concerns in presenting translations in scientific publications usually involve the level of transcription detail and the way the translations are physically present in the text (Nikander, 2008). We decided not to present the original transcripts due to the space in the chapter related to its double focus: presenting the IPR/SRI as a tool as well as presenting results. In order to make the translation transparent to the reader, we have needed to insert three lines: original talk, word-by-word translation in the next line (to give the reader information about structural details of the speech), and idiomatic English translation in the third line.

We see that this second context creates much more searching and probing of different positions in the talk of the therapist and fosters the thinking aloud process, while the therapist in extract 1 might have his story already at hand (although he might also be affected by watching the video and by the interviewer's questions, instigating new insights). Both methodological options are viable and should be chosen to suit one's own research purposes.

From our point of view, traditional versions of both—Interpersonal Process Recall and Stimulated Recall Interviews—are clearly biased with regard to recall and do not fully grasp the complexity of what is happening during the interview situation itself. The more descriptive "Self-Confrontation Interview" (Breuer, 1995) might be more adequate in researching the (re-) constructive processes, which happen while observing oneself being part of a therapeutic interaction.

The dialogical approach to research systemic psychotherapy proved to be a helpful methodological framework, especially with regard to the distinction between personal and professional selves. Although in both extracts the therapists were able to recall their professional voices, which were identified by them as emerging in the course of the therapeutic session, in the end it is not possible to establish the influence of the therapists' inner dialogue on their external conversation during the session (Rober, 2005). This might be easier if the psychotherapy under investigation was highly manualized and the therapist knew in advance (and hence also afterwards) what he/she is doing in the therapy session and with what intention. In non-manualized therapies, however (and that means, in most systemic approaches), the specific therapeutic session has to be understood as a process under (co-)construction. This particular process embeds a multitude of social identities and professional practices. From this perspective, the IPR/SR interview can be understood as one specific way of re-constructing ex post the construction of the therapeutic session, whereas this re-construction is happening in a new social interaction, influencing it.

Multi-actor psychotherapy, like couple and family therapy, involves a higher level of complexity in terms of interaction than individual therapy performed as a dyad: this should not be understood as a limitation for the IPR/SRI methodology in this therapy context but rather as a creative challenge. That is surely a part of its fascination.

References

Andersen, T. (1991). *The reflecting team: Dialogues and dialogues about the dialogues*. New York, NY: W W. Norton & Co.

Bakhtin, M. (1984). *Problems of Dostoevsky's Poetics*. Edited and trans. by Caryl Emerson. Minneapolis: University of Minnesota Press.

Bakhtin, M. (1986). *Speech genres and other late essays*. Austin, TX: University of Texas Press.

Bamberg, M. (1997). Positioning between structure and performance. *Journal of Narrative and Life History, 7*, 335–342.

Bamberg, M., & Georgakopoulou, A. (2008). Small stories as a new perspective in narrative and identity analysis. *Text and Talk, 28*(3), 377–396.

Bamberg, M., & Zielke, B. (2007). From dialogical practices to polyphonic thought? Developmental inquiry and where to look for it. *International Journal for Dialogical Science, 2*(1), 223–242.

Bloom, B. S. (1954). The thought process of students in discussion. In S. J. French (Ed.), *Accent on teaching: Experiments in general education* (pp. 23–46). New York: Harper & Brothers.

Borcsa, M., & Rober, P. (Eds.). (2016). *Research Perspectives in Couple Therapy. Discursive Qualitative Methods.* Cham, CH: Springer International. https://doi.org/10.1007/978-3-319-233 06-2.

Borchers, P., Seikkula, J., & Lehtinen, K. (2013). Psychiatrists' inner dialogues concerning workmates during need adapted treatment of psychosis. *Psychosis, 5*(1), 60–70.

Breuer, F. (1991). *Analyse beraterisch-therapeutischer Tätigkeit. Methoden zur Untersuchung individueller Handlungssysteme klinisch-psychologischer Praktiker* (Arbeiten zur sozialwissenschaftlichen Psychologie 22). Münster: Aschendorff Verlag.

Breuer, F. (1995). Das Selbstkonfrontations-Interview als Forschungsmethode. In E. König & P. Zedler (Eds.), *Bilanz qualitativer Forschung.* Bd. II: Methoden (pp. 159–180). Weinheim: Deutscher Studien Verlag.

Brown, J. M. (2010). The Milan principles of hypothesising, circularity and neutrality in dialogical family therapy: Extinction, evolution, eviction ... or emergence. *Australian & New Zealand Journal of Family Therapy, 31*(3), 248–265.

Bryniarska, A., Tomasiewicz, A. K., Janusz, B., & Józefik, B. (2019). Personal therapist's voices in the systemic first consultations. *Psychoterapia, 4*(191), 17–28. https://doi.org/10.12740/PT/115041.

Cegala, D. J., McNeilis, K. S., & Socha McGee, D. (1995). A study of doctor's and patients' perceptions of information processing and communication competence during the medical interview. *Health Communication, 7,* 179–203. https://doi.org/10.1207/s15327027hc0703_1.

Consuegra, E., Engels, N., & Willegems, V. (2016). Using video-stimulated recall to investigate teacher awareness of explicit and implicit gendered thoughts on classroom interactions. *Teachers and Teaching, 22*(6), 683–699.

Coupland, N. (2007). *Style.* Cambridge: Cambridge University Press.

Davies, B., & Harré, R. (1990). Positioning: The discursive production of selves. *Journal for the Theory of Social Behaviour, 20*(1), 43–63.

Deppermann, A. (2015). Positioning. In A. De Fina & A. Georgakopoulou (Eds.), *The handbook of narrative analysis* (pp. 369–387). Hoboken, NJ: Wiley.

Elliott, R. (1984). A discovery-oriented approach to significant events in psychotherapy: Interpersonal Process Recall and comprehensive process analysis. In L. Rice & L. Greenberg (Eds.), *Patterns of change* (pp. 249–286). New York: Guilford Press.

Elliott, R. (1986). Interpersonal Process Recall (IPR) as a psychotherapy process research method. In L. S. Greenberg & W. M. Pinsof (Eds.), *The psychotherapeutic process: A research handbook* (pp. 503–527). New York, NY: Guilford Press.

Elliott, R., & Shapiro, D. A. (1988). Brief structured recall: A more efficient method for studying significant therapy events. *British Journal of Medical Psychology, 61*(2), 141–153. https://doi.org/10.1111/j.2044-8341.1988.tb02773.x.

Elliott, R., & Shapiro, D. A. (1992). Client and therapist as analysts of significant events. In S. G. Toukmanian & D. L. Rennie (Eds.), *Sage focus editions, Vol. 143. Psychotherapy process research: Paradigmatic and narrative approaches* (pp. 163–186). London: Sage.

Freshwater D., & Rolfe, G. (2001). Critical reflexivity: A politically and ethically engaged research method for nursing. *NT Research, 6*(1), 526–537. https://doi.org/10.1177/136140960100600109.

Gale, J. (1992). *When research interviews are more therapeutic than therapy interviews.* The Qualitative Report, Volume 1, Number 4, Fall, 1992 (http://www.nova.edu/ssss/QR/QR1-4/gale.html).

Gale, J., Odell, M., & Nagireddy, C. S. (1995). Marital therapy and self-reflexive research: Research and/as intervention. In G. H. Morris & R. J. Chenail (Eds.), *The talk of the clinic: Explorations in the analysis of medical and therapeutic discourse* (pp. 105–129). Hillsdale, NJ: Erlbaum.

Gass, S. M., & Mackey, A. (2000). *Stimulated recall methodology in second language research.* Mahwah, NJ: Lawrence Erlbaum Associates.

Gergen, K. (2009). *Relational being: Beyond self and community.* New York: Oxford University Press.

Goodwin, C. (1986). Between and within: Alternative sequential treatments of continuers and assessments. *Human Studies, 9*(2–3), 205–217. https://doi.org/10.1007/BF00148127.

Goodwin, M. H. (1997). Byplay: Negotiating evaluation in storytelling. In G. R. Guy, C. Feagin, D. Schiffrin, & J. Baugh (Eds.), *Towards a social science of language* (Vol. 2, pp. 77–102). John Benjamins Publishing. https://doi.org/10.1075/cilt.128.08goo.

Harré, R., Moghaddam, F. M., Cairnie, T. P., Rothbart, D., & Sabat, S. R. (2009). Recent advances in positioning theory. *Theory & Psychology, 19*(1), 5–31.

Henretty, J., Levitt, H., & Mathews, S. (2008). Clients' experiences of moments of sadness in psychotherapy: A grounded theory analysis. *Psychotherapy Research, 18,* 243–255. https://doi.org/10.1080/10503300701765831.

Hermans, H. J. M. (2001). The dialogical self: Toward a theory of personal and cultural positioning. *Culture & Psychology, 7,* 243–281.

Hermans, H. J. M. (2006). The self as a theater of voices: Disorganization and reorganization of a position repertoire. *Journal of Constructivist Psychology, 19,* 147–169.

Hermans, H. J. M., & Dimaggio, G. (2007). Self, identity, and globalization in times of uncertainty: A dialogical analysis. *Review of General Psychology, 11*(1), 31–61; 1983, p. 22.

Janusz, B., Jozefik, B., & Peräkylä, A. (2018). Gender-related issues in couple therapists' internal voices and interactional practices. *Australian and New Zealand Journal of Family Therapy (ANZJFT), 39*(4), 436–449. https://doi.org/10.1002/anzf.1331.

Janusz, B., Matusiak, F., & Peräkylä, A. (2021). How couple therapists manage asymmetries of interaction in first consultations. *Psychotherapy.* Advance online publication. https://doi.org/10.1037/pst0000348.

Kagan, N. I. (1980). Influencing human interaction: Eighteen years with IPR. In A. K. Hess (Ed.), *Psychotherapy supervision: Theory research and practice* (pp. 262–283). New York: Wiley.

Kagan, N. I., Krathwohl, D. R., & Farquhar, W. W. (1965). *IPR–interpersonal process recall: Stimulated recall by videotape in exploratory studies of counseling and teaching-learning.* East Lansing: Michigan State University.

Karvonen, A., Kykyri, V.-L., Kaartinen, J., Penttonen, M., & Seikkula, J. (2016). Sympathetic nervous system synchrony in couple therapy. *Journal of Marital and Family Therapy, 42*(3), 383–395.

Labov, W. (1972). *Sociolinguistic Patterns.* Philadelphia: University of Pennsylvania Press.

Labov, W. (1982). Speech actions and reactions in personal narrative. In D. Tannen (Ed.), *Analyzing discourse: Text and talk* (pp. 219–247). Washington, DC: Georgetown University Press.

Labov, W., & Waletzky, J. (1967). Narrative analysis: Oral versions of personal experiences. In J. Helm (Ed.), *Essays on the verbal and visual arts* (pp. 12–44). Seattle, WA: University of Washington Press.

Laitila, A., & Oranen, M. (2013). Focused dialogues in training contexts: A model for enhancing reflection in therapist's professional practice. *Contemporary Family Therapy, 35*(3), 599–612.

Larsen, D., Flesaker, K., & Stege, R. (2008). Qualitative interviewing using Interpersonal Process Recall: Investigating internal experiences during professional-client conversations. *International Journal of Qualitative Methods, 7*(1), 18. https://doi.org/10.1177/160940690800700102.

Lucius-Hoene, G., & Deppermann, A. (2000). Narrative identity empiricized: A dialogical and positioning approach to autobiographical research interviews. *Narrative Inquiry, 10*(1), 199–222.

Lucius-Hoene, G., & Deppermann. A. (2004a). Narrative Identität und Positionierung. *Gesprächsforschung, 5,* 166–183.

Lucius-Hoene, G., & Deppermann. A. (2004b). *Rekonstruktion narrativer Identität: Ein Arbeitsbuch zur Analyse Narrativer Interviews.* Wiesbaden: VS.

Lyle, J. (2003). Stimulated recall: A report on its use in naturalistic research. *British Educational Research Journal, 29*(6), 861–878.

Macaskie, J., Lees, J., & Freshwater, D. (2015). Talking about talking: Interpersonal process recall as an intersubjective approach to research. *Psychodynamic Practice, 21,* 226–240. https://doi.org/10.1080/14753634.2015.

Nikander, P. (2008). Working with transcripts and translated data. *Qualitative Research in Psychology, 5*(3), 225–231. https://doi.org/10.1080/14780880802314346.

Nyman-Salonen, P., Vall, B., Laitila, A., Borcsa, M., Karvonen, A., Kykyri, V-L., ... Seikkula, J. (2020). Significant moments in a couple therapy session: Towards the integration of different modalities of analysis. In M. Ochs, M. Borcsa, & J. Schweitzer (Eds.), *Systemic research in individual, couple, and family therapy and counseling* (pp. 55–73). Cham, CH: Springer International.

Päivinen, H., Holma, J., Karvonen, A., Kykyri, V.-L., Tsatsishvili, V., Kaartinen, J., ... Seikkula, J. (2016). Affective arousal during blaming in couple therapy: Combining analyses of verbal discourse and physiological responses in two case studies. *Contemporary Family Therapy, 38*(4), 373–384.

Rober, P. (2002). Constructive hypothesizing, dialogic understanding and the therapist's inner conversation: Some ideas about knowing and not knowing in the family therapy session. *Journal of Marital and Family Therapy, 28*(4), 467–478.

Rober, P. (2005). Family therapy as a dialogue of living persons: A perspective inspired by Bakhtin, Voloshinov, and Shotter. *Journal of Marital and Family Therapy, 31,* 385–397.

Rober, P. (2014). The therapist's inner conversations in family therapy practice. *Person-centered and Experiential Psychotherapies, 7*(4), 37–41.

Rober, P., Elliott, R., Buysse, A., Loots, G., & De Corte, K. (2008). What's on the therapist's mind? A grounded theory analysis of family therapist reflections during individual therapy sessions. *Psychotherapy Research, 18*(1), 48–57.

Rober, P., Seikkula, J., & Latila, A. (2010). Dialogical analysis of storytelling in the family therapeutic encounter. *Human Systems: The Journal of Therapy, Consultation and Training, 21,* 27–49.

Rubin, H. J., & Rubin, I. S. (2005). *Qualitative interviewing: The art of hearing data.* Thousand Oaks, CA: Sage.

Sacks, H. (1992). *Lectures on conversation* (2 Vols). Oxford: Blackwell.

Schegloff, E. A. (1997). Whose text? Whose context? *Discourse and Society, 8,* 165–187.

Seikkula, J., Alakare, B., & Aaltonen J. (2011). The comprehensive open-dialogue approach in Western Lapland: II. Long-term stability of acute psychosis outcomes in advanced community care. *Psychosis, 3*(3), 192–204. https://doi.org/10.1080/17522439.2011.595819.

Seikkula, J., Karvonen, A., Kykyri, V. L., Kaartinen, J., & Penttonen, M. (2015). The embodied attunement of therapists and a couple within dialogical psychotherapy: An introduction to the Relational Mind research project. *Family Process, 54,* 703–715. https://doi.org/10.1111/famp.12152.

Selvini-Palazzoli, M., Boscolo, L., Cecchin, G., & Prata, G. (1980). Hypothesizing, circularity, neutrality: Three guidelines for the conductor of the session. *Family Process, 19,* 3–12.

Stivers, T. (2008). Stance, alignment, and affiliation during storytelling: When nodding is a token of affiliation. *Research on language and social interaction, 41*(1), 31–57. https://doi.org/10.1080/08351810701691123.

Tomm, K. M. (1984). One perspective on the Milan approach: Part I. Overview of development, theory and practice. *Journal of Marital and Family Therapy, 10,* 113–125.

Vall, B., Laitila, A., Borcsa, M., Kykyri, V. L., Karvonen, A., Kaartinen, J., ... Seikkula, J. (2018). Stimulated Recall Interviews: How can the research interview contribute to new therapeutic practices? *Revista Argentina de Clinica Psicologica, XXVII*(2), 284–293. https://doi.org/10.24205/03276716.2018.1068.

Voloshinov, V. N. (1976). Discourse in life and discourse in art (concerning sociological poetics). In V. N. Voloshinov (Ed.), *Freudianism: a marxist critique* (pp. 93–116). New York, NY: Academic Press.

West, W., & Clark, V. (2004). Learnings from a qualitative study into counselling supervision: Listening to supervisor and supervisee. *Counselling and Psychotherapy Research, 4*(2), 20–26.

Chapter 9
Bringing Mental Health Back into the Dynamics of Social Coexistence: Emotional Textual Analysis

Fiorella Bucci, Rosa Maria Paniccia, Felice Bisogni, Stefano Pirrotta, Francesca Romana Dolcetti, Giulia Marchetti, and Katia Romelli

Abstract Emotional Textual Analysis (ETA) is a psychoanalytically informed method of text and discourse analysis that was developed in the 1980s as a tool for psychological research and intervention with social groups, institutions, and organizations. ETA hypothesizes that emotions expressed in language are a fundamental organizer of relationships. By detecting clusters of emotionally dense words within a text (through a procedure that combines quantitative—software supported—and qualitative data analysis), this method enables the exploration of the unconscious emotional dynamics underpinning processes of sense-making within social groups and organizations. This chapter aims to discuss the contribution that the ETA methodology can offer today to mental health studies. We will present two case studies. (a) In the first one, ETA served to shed light on a new issue that has arisen in the mental health field: an unprecedented increase over the last few decades in psychiatric diagnosis related to children's difficulties at school. (b) In the second one, ETA was used

F. Bucci (✉)
Department of Psychoanalysis and Clinical Consulting, Ghent University, Ghent, Belgium
e-mail: fiorella.bucci@ugent.be

R. M. Paniccia
Department of Dynamic and Clinical Psychology, Sapienza University of Rome, Rome, Italy
e-mail: rosamaria.paniccia@uniroma1.it

F. Bisogni · S. Pirrotta · G. Marchetti
GAP, Rome, Italy
e-mail: felice.bisogni@gmail.com

S. Pirrotta
e-mail: stefanopirrotta@gmail.com

G. Marchetti
e-mail: giulia.ebasta@gmail.com

F. R. Dolcetti
Studio RisorseObiettiviStrumenti, Rome, Italy
e-mail: francescadolcetti@studio-ros.it

K. Romelli
Department of Maternal and Infant Health, ASST Valle Olona Hospital, Busto Arsizio, Italy
e-mail: katia.romelli@gmail.com

© Springer Nature Switzerland AG 2021   193
M. Borcsa and C. Willig (eds.), *Qualitative Research Methods in Mental Health*,
https://doi.org/10.1007/978-3-030-65331-6_9

within the framework of a 3-year intervention-research with a healthcare organization providing services for adult disability. The organization was stuck in a growing conflict with the family members of the service users. Our results corroborate the hypothesis that contemporary mental health risks—as well as demands and developmental trajectories—cannot be understood by looking solely at the individual; it is crucial to bring them back into the current dynamics of social coexistence, by means of methodologies that allow us to study the relationship between individuals and changing social contexts.

Keywords Textual analysis · Psychoanalytic theory · Psychosocial research · Institutional cultures · Inclusion · Diagnosis · Special educational needs · Client-staff relationship · Family-teacher relationship · Emotional symbolization

Introduction

Events on a global scale—such as the 2008 financial-economic crisis as well as the new migrations in Europe—have affected our social systems, in recent years, impacting so deeply on the experience of coexisting that, when dealing with "mental health," one cannot fail to take into account the social contexts in which the multiple issues we refer to with this term are situated. Thus, when it is said that mental health is rising to a global challenge, this means in our view that it is becoming all the more important in the present not to split mental health and mental illness issues from a more global understanding of the issue of social coexistence, in its affective and historical dynamics.

This would require a paradigm shift from the still dominant biomedical model toward psychosocially oriented models of analysis and intervention.

On the one hand, we could say that what sociology called individualization of problems and experiences (e.g., Beck, 1992; Giddens, 1991) has gained further momentum in the last few decades, along with an increasing effort to diversify and individualize patterns of health and social care (Needham, 2011). The case of education is a perfect example of this, with a worldwide surge in children diagnosed with learning disabilities (see, for example, Paniccia, 2012a, 2012b). On the other hand, from a different perspective, it becomes evident that the experience of being at risk of becoming socially marginalized, due to the impossibility of finding a place within the social system, affects more and more people, and this happens especially in countries where trust in legitimate institutions, and hence in the meaning and purpose of living together, is undergoing a deep crisis (Carli, 2017).

From this point of view, we believe that contemporary mental health risks—as well as demands and developmental trajectories—cannot be understood by looking solely at the individual; it is crucial to bring them back into the current dynamics of social coexistence, and in order to do that we need research methodologies that allow us to study the relationship between individuals and changing social contexts.

In this chapter, we shall examine a psychoanalytically informed method of text and discourse analysis, i.e., Emotional Textual Analysis (ETA), that was developed in the 1980s by Renzo Carli and Rosa Maria Paniccia to enable psychological research and intervention with social groups, institutions, and organizations (Carli, 2018; Carli & Paniccia, 2002; Carli, Paniccia, Giovagnoli, Carbone, & Bucci, 2016).

A significant development took place in psychoanalytic theory, especially in the 1970s, based on several international contributions leading to a new formulation of the unconscious as a symbolic meaning-making process unfolding within and through social relations (i.e., beyond the intrapsychic domain). The development of psychoanalytically informed methods of text analysis was in multiple ways connected to this theoretical shift, which inspired new active tools of social research and intervention. In the first section of the chapter, we describe some methodological features of ETA and the theory of mind and of social relationship inspiring it. We will also provide elements concerning the history of this tool, which is significant not just in terms of scientific innovation but also of the cultural context from which the method stemmed: a context of widespread interest in the functioning of social groups and organizations, as well as in the link between subjectivity and culture. It is important to bear this background in mind in order to grasp the difference between this methodological perspective and the present scientific and cultural context—epitomized by the radical shift to an individualistic paradigm in psychological sciences (Plamper, 2018)—and thus define the contribution that the ETA approach can make today to mental health studies.

In the following sections, we present two case studies, where ETA was used for different aims and levels of inquiry. In the first study, ETA served to shed light on a new demand that has arisen in the mental health field: that is, an unprecedented increase over the last few decades in psychiatric diagnosis related to children's difficulties at school. The meaning of this phenomenon remains still very unclear in the literature; we will propose a hypothesis based on our findings. In the second case, ETA was used within the framework of a 3-year intervention-research with a healthcare organization providing services for adult disability. The organization was stuck in a growing conflict with the family members of the service users, whose requests were perceived by the staff as apparently unlimited, pressing and intractable.

Incidentally, the two studies are closely interconnected: our results suggest that the rise of a diagnostic culture in school is undermining the precious socializing function that education had historically served in Italy. In a previous study carried out with the same methodology (Paniccia, Giovagnoli, Bucci, & Caputo, 2014), we found that families in central Italy perceived the school system as the only service attending a socializing aim for their children with disability. Reading together the results of the studies that we discuss here and the study from 2014, we can hypothesize that the spread of a diagnostic culture in school is also contributing to greater isolation for families with members with disability, particularly mental disabilities, whose requests toward the healthcare services become more and more pressing, demanding, and hopeless.

Emotional Textual Analysis

Theoretical Framework

Emotional Textual Analysis hypothesizes that emotions expressed in language are a fundamental organizer of relationships.

From a theoretical-epistemological viewpoint, ETA rests on a specific theory of emotion as a form of knowledge linked to the unconscious, which participates in the psychological construction of reality, according to rules that psychoanalytic theory has sought to explain. Specifically, the work of Matte Blanco and Fornari was central to the development of ETA. Both these authors started from a rediscovery and reinterpretation of Freud's first writings on the unconscious.

Matte Blanco (1975) considered all the spatial and structural models used in psychoanalysis until that time as inadequate in describing mental phenomena: in particular, the conceptualization of the unconscious as the region of repressed contents, which, being morally unacceptable or too distressing, are banished from consciousness. By introducing a radically different interpretation, Matte Blanco described conscious and unconscious in terms of *bi-logic*, that is, of two different modes of sense-making constantly interacting with each other: namely, while conscious thought follows the rules of cognition informed by the non-contradiction principle, the unconscious being is informed by the principles of symmetry and generalization, which found our emotional way of experiencing reality. This *bi-logic* implies that those aspects of reality that we perceive as endowed with a univocal sense in terms of cognition are, at the same time, polysemic—that is, they evoke multiple implicating experiences and associations—in terms of unconscious meaning (Bucci & Vanheule, 2020).

According to the Italian psychoanalyst Fornari (1976), this double level of meaning is reflected in language and can be inferred by studying language. The work of Fornari shed further light on the affective implications of unconscious semiosis, thereby contributing to a shift in psychoanalytic theory from a drive model to a semi-otic model of the mind. By *semiotic* we mean a model of the mind as an ongoing process of meaning-making that mediates our relation to the world and takes places by means of semiotic devices (such as language), the effectiveness of which depends on social exchange (Salvatore & Freda, 2011). Fornari maintained that unconscious symbolization transforms objects of reality into objects charged with affective value; that is objects that engage us in an affectively meaningful relationship[1]: i.e., friend or enemy, benevolent or threatening, vital or destructive instances. Without such a primal signification, Fornari says, sensory data coming from experience would be to us only raw data, quite irrelevant for the purposes of survival. At the same time, given the very way in which an *affective symbol* functions—i.e., given its symmetrical, arbi-trary, and polysemic nature—it intrinsically implies a confusion between the self and

---

[1]Fornari's theory of affective codes (1976) builds on Melanie Klein's object relations theory, in which we find for the first time a distinction between internal and external objects.

the other, between the inner and outer world, as well as between good and evil. This creates the basis for the incessant need in human beings to verify and negotiate the meaning of things intersubjectively—which happens through language—so as to establish socially effective cultural codes. Affective symbolization needs a cultural code to become effective in terms of reality (Fornari, 1981).

Renzo Carli and Rosa Maria Paniccia—founder members of Italian psychosociology—pushed this theoretical pathway forward by translating it into a theory of the technique of psychological intervention, not just with individuals but also with social groups, institutions, and organizations (see Carli & Paniccia, 1981, 2003). Their notion of *emotional collusion* (Carli, 2006a; Carli & Paniccia, 2003) gives form to a social model of the unconscious. The basic assumption is that every aspect of social experience, from the point of view of the unconscious knowledge, is polysemic in the sense outlined by Matte Blanco, that is endowed of multiple, potentially infinite emotional connotations. Within the social relationship, such a polysemy progressively reduces itself giving rise to a common symbolic process between the participants in a context. This process of sharing the emotional sense of reality between social actors is what Carli and Paniccia call *collusion* (from Latin *cum ludere*, literally, playing together) and it works as a sort of implicit premise that primes subsequent interpretative activity and interactions within a context: i.e., ways of interpreting events, evaluating, and decision-making (Salvatore & Freda, 2011).

Think for instance of a class in a primary school, whose progress evidently depends not just on the students' cognitive skills or the teachers' technical competences, but also on the relationship between students and teachers, underpinned by the way they reciprocally emotionally symbolize the process of learning, in its various components: e.g., the experience of making mistakes, of exploration and creativity, of competition and cooperation, of achieving goals, of being evaluated, and so on.

Carli and Paniccia's work within a broad, varied research and clinical field shed a new light on the functioning of social groups and organizations, by mapping emotional meaning-making activity inside them. They developed ETA with the goal of establishing a standardized tool for studying the emotional collusive dynamics underlying social relationships in social and organizational contexts, based on the analysis of texts produced by participants in the context. The outcome of these analyses could be used within the framework of psychosocial interventions in order to foster local relational and organizational competencies.

Operational Procedure

When using ETA, the process of inquiry most often starts from focus groups or individual interviews based on one initial open-ended question aimed to let the interviewees freely narrate their experience with regard to the research topic.[2]

The interviews are recorded, transcribed verbatim and put together in a single textual corpus, for the analysis of which ETA uses a specific procedure that integrates multivariate quantitative analysis and qualitative analysis. This procedure aims at breaking up the narrative order of the text, with the scope of allowing us to grasp a different order within it, which we assume to be an emotional order, based on the symmetrical logic of the unconscious.

One of the endeavors of ETA's authors was to exploit new chances for exploratory multivariate analysis of contingency data sets emerging in linguistics (in the wake of the work of Jean–Paul Benzécri [1973], for example), to pursue the new lines of inquiry that had opened in psychoanalysis with the hypothesis of a polysemic unconscious.

The quantitative analysis "starts by isolating in the textual corpus what we call *dense words:* that is, words whose emotional meaning (emotionally charged with polysemic values) is immediately evident even when we take the word out of its discursive context. *Dense* stands here for emotionally dense. For example, words such as 'to go away,' 'hatred,' 'failure,' or 'ambition' are characterized by a maximum of emotional density. By contrast, words like 'to go,' 'to think,' 'to do,' like modal, auxiliary and widely used verbs, or many adverbs, have a low emotional profile and do not indicate emotions except, at times, within a sentence (Carli et al., 2016)" (Bucci & Vanheule, 2020, p. 280). These are considered non-dense.[3] This is made possible by using software for text analysis, such as Alceste (Reinert, 1983, 1990) or T-Lab (Lancia, 2004), which generate a dictionary of all the words contained in the text, with related roots and frequencies, thereby allowing the research team to select only the dense words among them. Then, by means of multidimensional statistical analysis—i.e., factorial correspondence and cluster analysis—the software enables us to study how the dense words co-occur within the text forming stable and significant repertoires, which are then projected onto a factorial space so as to make their reciprocal relationships clear.[4] Finally, the meaning of the clusters inside the

---

[2]All the interviewees' associations, references, and the new connections they establish starting from the proposed question are significant for the detection of the emotional sense organizing their discourse, while the narrative coherence of their speech is deemed irrelevant in this kind of analysis.

[3]Depending on the context, a word may acquire particular emotional relevance. Thus, the dense words' selection is guided by knowledge of the local research context.

[4]To be precise, these programs cut the text into segments of similar length (sentences or fragments of sentences called Elementary Context Units, ECUs), which are automatically delimited by punctuation. Thus, once the dense words have been isolated and the context units delimited, the software constructs a matrix crossing ECUs and dense words. On this matrix the program conducts a cluster analysis (based on a factorial correspondence analysis) designed to classify the context units according to the similarity or dissimilarity of the words occurring in them so as to map the most significant lexical repertoires in the text. For each cluster we have a list of the dense words that

factorial space is interpreted through qualitative analysis. The interpretation is carried out by researchers specifically trained in the psychoanalytic models informing the ETA method (see Carli & Giovagnoli, 2011) and proceeds as follows: beginning with the dense words with the larger $\chi 2$ in each cluster, we first study the word's *etymology*, as a way to explore its *emotional polysemy*. This refers to the ability of a word—according to the symmetrical logic of the unconscious (Matte Blanco, 1988)—to evoke an intense multiplicity of meanings, that often only become clear if their historical roots in people's speech are addressed (Carli & Paniccia, 2002; Salvatore & Freda, 2011). Then, we study the associations between the words within a cluster, in descending order of $\chi 2$ (thus moving from the central word of the cluster toward those less significant), and subsequently the relationships between clusters within the factorial space. Through these various passages we are able to gradually grasp in a more precise and articulated way what meaning the problem we are dealing with acquires for the people that we interviewed from the point of view of their emotional implication.

The interpretative work is guided by a pool of analytic models elaborated by Carli and Paniccia (2002), building on the abovementioned psychoanalytic theoretical references.[5] Basically, these models distinguish different areas of emotional symbolization that all play a role in the adaptation process between the individual and its relational/social contexts. We can think of this process as of a continuum, starting with the primary emotional distinctions good/bad; friend/enemy, then passing through symbolizations linked to the experience of the body—e.g., the dichotomies inside/outside, bottom/top, or front/back. Then, we reach more elaborate, specific areas of emotional symbolization, connected with the experience of the other, that is of the relation to something external/extraneous to the self,[6] until we arrive to models regarding the social relation in its organizational, historically situated contexts.[7]

In the interpretation process, one goes constantly back and forth between the details of words, words' co-occurrences within the clusters, clusters' relationships within the factorial space, and the significance of these associations in terms of the analytic models. We will see an example of this interpretative work through the case studies to be discussed in the next sections.

---

characterize it, ordered by chi−square value ($\chi 2$). The larger this value, the more significant the occurrence of the word within the ECUs belonging to that cluster. This means that the words with larger $\chi 2$ in each cluster are those that most significantly distinguish one cluster from the other. We know also how the different clusters are in relation to the so−called *illustrative variables*, that is socio−demographic and other structural variables characterizing the interviews or the interviewees in a study (for greater detail on the ETA procedure see Carli & Paniccia, 2002; Carli et al., 2016).

[5] A comprehensive description of ETA's analytic models can be found in Carli and Paniccia (2002).

[6] The models included in this area describe a range of emotional dynamics whose common thread is to put barriers against the experience of foreignness which is inevitably implied in any social experience, such as the dynamics of provoking, controlling, reclaiming, possessing, mistrusting, complaining, feeling obligated.

[7] Models in this area include for example the emotional difference between compliance and commitment in organizational life or the difference between the organization experienced as a given entity or as a constructed entity.

It is important to notice that not the clusters alone but their factorial relationships too are central in ETA to the interpretation of the data. Factors delimit the space within which the clusters of dense words are defined and find a position, thereby allowing us to study how the clusters are related to each other as well as the meaning of such relationships (see Figs. 9.1, 9.2, and 9.3; and Tables 9.1, 9.2, and 9.3). Statistically, this is based on the fact that the cluster analysis from which the clusters of dense words are obtained is performed on a previous factorial correspondence analysis[8] (see above in Footnote 3). At the same time, at the level of the qualitative interpretation of the data, factorial relationships are essential because the goal of ETA is not to infer different themes or positions prevailing in a text (as it happens in other qualitative approaches, like thematic for example analysis), but instead to grasp the symbolic process that we assume emotionally organizes the relationship between the research participants and the specific object of inquiry. Namely, we aim to understand this emotional process in its articulation, that is in its dynamically interrelated multiple components.

While interpreting the clusters, in the qualitative part of ETA, we also study the link between the clusters and the interview content, as well as with relevant literature on the topic of study and with background knowledge of the research context and of the local culture. This is in order to understand how the emotional symbolizations that we have been examining give rise to specific social dynamics or are the outcome of specific historical and cultural processes.

The qualitative analysis is usually performed by a team of researchers, who operate in order to guarantee reliability of the interpretative procedure. Furthermore, final meetings devoted to discussing the results with the research participants allow the team of researchers to verify and further develop their conclusions. Such meetings are an important part of the ETA method, especially when this is used for psychological interventions with organizations, which most often start from a request from the organization itself to undertake a research action aimed at addressing a problem that they are facing. But also when ETA is used for research purposes, final meetings with the research participants are still essential to validate the researchers' interpretative hypotheses and at the same time prompt new thoughts and discussion on the problems examined.

A History of Integration Between Research and Intervention

ETA was developed in the early 1980s in Italy from many intervention experiences within manufacturing and service organizations carried out by a person with profound experimental and psychoanalytic knowledge: Renzo Carli. From a theoretical and methodological viewpoint, the integrated coexistence of three domains,

---

[8]Factorial correspondence analysis is a multivariate statistical technique developed by Benzécri and his research team, starting from the 1960s, particularly in order to study linguistic and textual data. More exactly, ETA uses multiple correspondence analysis, which enables the detection of underlying structures in a data set, by representing data as points in a multidimensional Euclidean space.

that is experimental research, psychoanalytic training, and organizational intervention, was not common at that time. There was an implicit rule that clinicians did not do research and researchers did not do clinical work. The division between clinical work and organizational intervention was less marked. It was strengthened later on, in a profound historical change, when from attention to cultures, relations, and subjective experiences we moved toward a growing individualism and an increasing focus on "facts," excluding, normalizing, and pathologizing subjectivity. To better understand the birth of ETA, we need to go back to the 1960s in Italy characterized by economic and cultural development. In that period a new emphasis was placed on companies and their responsibilities. What emerged from this was the concept of human resources to be developed instead of employees to control through rewards and punishments. It was a fervid cultural moment, which progressed further in the 1970s when French psychosociology, aimed at understanding social dynamics from a multidisciplinary perspective and informed by psychoanalytic expertise, encountered its Italian counterpart which was full of initiatives in that field.

In 1981, "Psychosociology of organizations and institutions" (Carli & Paniccia, 1981) was published. The book proposed to integrate the notion of organizational rationality, coming from economics, with psychosocial and psychoanalytic models. Carli and Paniccia worked within an intervention designed to change the culture of a leading Italian company: the hiring of a broad group of graduates was intended to revitalize the management, which had been unchanged for years. Carli and Paniccia felt it was necessary to know the culture of the company to be able to include and train the new entrants. In this way, the two authors wanted to avoid pursuing ideal purposes, at the risk of failure, and they looked for existing resources in the local context to accompany its development. They had experience in working with groups within organizations, aimed at reflecting on the participants' fantasies regarding the aims of the organization itself. They had formalized a pool of analytic models designed to translate the polysemy of the fantasies related to the organization they encountered into psychosocial and psychoanalytic categories that allowed new hypotheses on the meaning of the organizational experience. These were the premises of ETA where the two authors felt the need for a research method coherent with the theory of emotional collusion, to explore the culture of the company in question. Various resources were merged: the already mentioned pool of models, along with the new multivariate statistical techniques emerging at that time which allowed previously unimaginable amounts of data to be processed and exploratory research to be carried out in order to produce new hypotheses on certain themes, impossible without those data. The two authors thought they could investigate collusive emotional symbolizations with which members of an organization, institution, or social group requesting an intervention connoted their context of belonging even if the client could not afford long, expensive interventions. To this end, the authors designed two methods, both based on correspondence and cluster analysis. The first one was ETA, a discourse analysis, suited to the purpose of exploring the collusive fantasies of groups of people who could be reached with interviews and focus groups. The second one, called ISO (acronym for *Indicatori di Sviluppo Organizzativo*, Organizational Development

Indicators), was designed to analyze the data obtained through a specific question-naire developed ad hoc on different research themes and suitable for application to samples of large populations. The two methods could be adopted in sequence: once the collusive specificities of a population had been identified through ETA, these could be sampled through ISO, leveraging on the knowledge gained with ETA. Here we focus on ETA, but we have mentioned the whole procedure to clarify how such a research methodology unfolds.

The findings of the research that Carli and Paniccia conducted in the 1980s, mentioned above, were used in a ten-year intervention that led to the recruitment of about one thousand graduates. Later the two authors directed several other studies, often using both ETA and ISO. For example, for a public administration company providing information technology services, we measured the customer satisfaction linking it to cultural clusters that made it possible to understand the grounds for the different degrees of satisfaction detected; for a communication company, we investigated the local collusive dynamics over five years, inspiring changes that the top management planned based on our survey. We were able to map how the organizational culture was changing, after our intervention.

From the 1960s up to the early 1990s, Italian companies and institutions invested a great deal in organizational competences, linking them to the knowledge of organiza-tional cultures, which our research methods contributed to discern by shedding light on the emotional collusive dynamics underlying such cultures. Then, we registered an important shift, which was evident also in our research findings. The experience of an anomic country, controlled by elites that attacked instead of promoting competences, became predominant in those years. Meanwhile, as the financial sector, internation-ally, came to prevail over the "real economy," the interest in organizational cultures and in developing human resources dropped dramatically. In Italy, new demands for psychosocial research and intervention emerged: with rising crises inside social coexistence, young and older people in particular, as well as women, people with a psychiatric diagnosis, the unemployed and patients with chronic diseases, experi-enced new and increasing social risks. The case studies discussed here fall into this framework.

ETA to Inquire into the Meaning of Psychiatric Diagnosis in School

In 2015, the Italian school students diagnosed numbered 235,000, almost 2.7% of the whole student population. Compared to 10 years before, this group had increased by about 40% (MIUR, 2015). In 2017, the percentage rose further (Istat, 2018). Based on the review of the literature and from the observation of several cases, we thought that this phenomenon could not stem only from the refining of diagnostic criteria, or from a growth in pathologies, but was instead a sign of the emergence of a diagnostic culture in school. Diagnosis, we suggest, is not only a technical action performed by physicians; it is more broadly a cultural process that concerns the relationship between children and teachers, between teachers and families, between the children and their parents, and so on. In such a culture, disabilities, learning difficulties, and cultural differences tend to blur and overlap, all of them becoming deficits: namely, deficits with respect to a presumed unifying norm. At the same time, the descriptive taxonomy of pathologies (i.e., the ICD, International Classification of Diseases) seems to be expanding endlessly. What our study focused on was diagnosis as a culture, which implies shared emotional symbolizations. A full description of this work can be found in Paniccia, Giovagnoli, Bucci, Donatiello, and Cappelli (2019); here, we dwell more specifically on the kind and level of analysis that ETA can provide to understand the context from which new mental health demands currently arise.

The study's goal was to understand current school problems from the teachers' perspective and, in particular, explore how they experience the growing number of school children diagnosed.

We interviewed 82 teachers, divided in terms of the different stages of compulsory education in Italy: 22 worked in kindergarten, 34 in primary and in lower secondary school, 26 in high school.[9] The interviewees' age was classified as follows: up to 30 years (5 interviewees), from 31 to 50 years (52 interviewees), over 50 (25 interviewees). Only 9 teachers were male.[10] All interviewees worked in the province of Rome. The recruitment was based on snow-balling: starting from a small group of teachers, we asked them if they had colleagues that might be interested in taking part in the study.

We carried out individual interviews based on an initial open-ended question. We introduced ourselves as an academic research team interested in education and in listening to the interviewee's opinion about the important issues of school today as well as to his/her experience in his/her own school. We then listened without asking further questions. We asked permission to record the interview and declared our intention to discuss the research findings with any participants interested in doing so. We anticipated that the duration of the interview would be about 30 min. At the end, if they had not mentioned it, we asked the interviewees what they thought of the increase in diagnosis in school.

All interviews were transcribed verbatim and put together in a single textual corpus that was analyzed by Emotional Textual Analysis. The data analysis produced 5 clusters of dense words within a factorial space of four factorial axes. Figure 9.1 and Table 9.1 illustrate the factorial space and the statistical relationships between clusters and factors.

On the first factor, Clusters 2 and 4 (negative pole) are opposed to C 1 (positive pole). On the second factor, C 2 (positive pole) is opposed to C 3 and 4 (negative pole). C 5 is opposed, respectively, to C 1, on the third factor, and to C 3 on the fourth

---

[9]Education in Italy is compulsory from 6 to 16 years of age.

[10]Some contextual data: in Italy, 57% of primary and secondary school teachers are over 50 years of age, while on average in Europe only 36% belong to this age group (Eurydice, 2018). In European countries, most of the teachers are women. Italy is no exception (INDIRE, 2014).

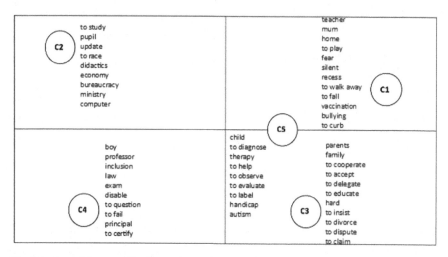

Fig. 9.1 Factorial space (The figure shows the key dense words in each cluster. *Note* The figure represents only the first and the second factorial axis: the first factor is represented by the horizontal axis, the second factor by the vertical axis. One should imagine the third and fourth factors as two other axes that cross the plane in the central point, thus generating a Euclidean 4-dimensional space. The central point represents the point of origin that cuts each factor into two semi-axes culminating in two opposite poles: a positive pole, on one side, and a negative pole, on the other [see Table 9.1])

Table 9.1 Relationship between clusters and factors (centroid coordinates)

	Factor 1	Factor 2	Factor 3	Factor 4
Cluster 1	**0.7588**	0.3788	**0.6465**	−0.0052
Cluster 2	**−0.6425**	**0.7296**	−0.2203	0.2852
Cluster 3	0.3946	**−0.4247**	−0.3321	**0.5810**
Cluster 4	**−0.5658**	−0.4199	0.3351	−0.1652
Cluster 5	0.3202	0.0417	**−0.5394**	**−0.6844**

Note The table shows the centroid coordinates of each cluster which indicate the cluster's position in relation to the factors; the higher this value (centroid coordinate), the more statistically significant the relation between cluster and factor. The most significant relationships are shown in bold

factor. As far as the illustrative variables are concerned, C 2 and C 4 are related to "high school," while C 1, C 5, and C 3 are related to "kindergarten."[11]

---

[11] As stated above, we call socio−demographic and other structural variables characterizing the interviews and the groups interviewed in a study *illustrative variables*: in this study, we took the different levels of education as an illustrative variable. Unlike dense words, these variables do not enter *actively* in the formation of the clusters. Nonetheless, the software that we use to support the quantitative part of ETA estimates the extent to which the different clusters of dense words are connected to the illustrative variables (this relation is also expressed in terms of chi−square value), which indicates, in our case, that certain associations between words occur more frequently in the speech of teachers who work in the primary school, for example, or in the secondary school, and

We comment first on C 2 and C 4, both positioned on the left side of the factorial space and in relation to the variable "high school."

C 2 is characterized by the words *to study, pupils, update, to race, didactics, bureaucracy, economy, ministry, computer.* It is useful to recall here what we mean with dense words, how the decision about which words are dense and which not is reached and what happens afterward, once we arrive at the clusters' interpretation. As stated above, we call dense words, those words in a text that more than others are endowed with emotional polysemy and with a low level of ambiguity; that is, words that are capable in themselves (even when taken out of the sentence) to evoke a full and intense multiplicity of meanings, in terms of emotionally significant experiences and associations. Actually, every word we use expresses polysemic connotations. However, in a text we find words, like articles, adverbs, pronouns, conjunctions, that have grammatical meaning rather than lexical meaning: i.e., their function is to establish relations between the full words; as well as we find ambiguous words, which make sense only when in relation to other words, like for example modal and auxiliary verbs. Of course, not all the dense words, chosen as such within a study, are equally capable to bring knowledge about the emotional symbolization process shared among the research participants; the degree of emotional density of a words depends, indeed, on the specific research context and research questions. For example, the most significant word in C 2 (the word with larger $\chi2$) is "to study." We chose it as a dense word because it evidently bares a full sense, charged with interesting polysemic connotations, as we will discuss in a moment. Nonetheless, this is such a widely used term in the discourse about school that, potentially, it could prove less informative than other words regarding the specific object of our inquiry: i.e., what issues teachers experience nowadays in their work, and particularly how they make sense of the growing use of diagnosis in schools. Probably, there are words, in this factorial space, that were more able than others to capture elements of the emotional-symbolic process that was in play in the interviews: for example, the word "to divorce" that we find in C 3. The teachers used this term in the interviews referring to the children's families, which in some cases are "divorced" families. Thus, on the level of communication, this word served to define a certain referent in the external reality; at the same time, on another level, that of emotional signification (on which ETA tries to shed light by pulling the word out of the grammatical bonds of the sentence), this term gives shape to a salient emotion that the teachers today experience in the relationship with the families. In this sense, we could say that "divorce" proved to be a particularly emotionally *dense* word in this analysis. We will return to the interpretation of C 3 below.

Going back to the analysis of C 2, thus we begin with studying the words' polysemy by retrieving their etymologies (where one finds clues on layers of shared meanings in the history of people's speech). Then, we go on studying the associations between the words in the cluster. Here we have an example of how the real

---

so on. If there are no statistically significant relationships with the illustrative variables, this means the cluster concerned has a wider relevance.

focus of the interpretative work in the AET is not the single words but the associ-ations between the words within the cluster. In fact, only studying the relationship between the words, the emotional polysemy brought out by each of them can be gradually reduced and we gain understanding of the emotional process expressed by the cluster as a whole. Finally, we will analyze how the clusters are related to each other based on their position on the factorial axes.

To study means dedicating oneself to learning, striving to achieve a goal. *Pupil, alunno* in Italian, comes from the Latin *al-dare,* that is, to nourish; the one who is raised and educated by someone other than their parents. The first words evoke the two main aims of the school: i.e., pursuing goals and competences, on the one hand, and educating, raising on the other. Now, school life, with these different training and educational aims which are often not easy to reconcile, is experienced by the teachers as a *race.* They have to update their skills to keep abreast of contemporary progress which seems to escape from their grasp, and, at the same time, they feel caught up in a routine of obligations that they have to fulfill (bureaucracy, recording expenses, complying with the ministerial programs). One cannot stop to think of what has been done: this seems to be the experience expressed in this cluster.

C 2 is opposed to C 4 on the second factorial axis. The latter depicts the school's problems from a different angle. The key dense words are: *boy, professor, inclusion, law, exam, disable, to question, to fail, principal, to certify.* In its etymology, "inclu-sion" means to close inside. In Italy, the verb "to include" (in line with a widespread use of the word "inclusion" in the international discourse on education) has almost replaced the term "to integrate," which previously played an important role in the Italian reflection on the participation of children with disability in school. Based on previous research and interventions within schools,[12] we could say that "inclusion" and "integration" describe deeply different emotional models of social interaction: while including, the prevailing fantasy is to assimilate something alien into a system by homologating it, that is by making it as normal as possible or, in other words, in line with the expectations regarding the main characteristics defining the norm in a given system. While with integrating, one recognizes that all the different elements that make a whole already belong to that system and help to define it (see, Paniccia, 2012a). In C 2, we find that the *inclusion* of students with disability seems all the more difficult to achieve within a school culture in which this is perceived as a duty, prescribed by *law,* and in which *examination* and *evaluation* (with the impending danger of the negative outcome: *to fail*) seem to emotionally saturate the sense of the experience.

We comment now on C 1, C 3, and C 5. These are all related to the variable "kindergarten."

C 1 is opposed to C 2 and C 4 on the first factorial axis. The first dense words in the cluster—*teacher, mum, home, to play*—tell us about the expectation that characterizes

---

[12]We have devoted several works over the years to investigating the education systems' problems (Carli, Dolcetti, Giovagnoli, Gurrieri, & Paniccia, 2015; Giovagnoli, Caputo, & Paniccia, 2015; Paniccia, 2012a, 2012b, 2013; Paniccia, Giovagnoli, Bucci, & Caputo, 2014: Paniccia, Giovagnoli, Di Ruzza, & Giuliano, 2014).

this initial stage of the school journey, more than any other, as a continuity between school and family. However, with the following words—*fear, silent, recess, to walk away, to fall, vaccination, bullying, to curb*—what seems to prevail in the experience of the teachers are emotions of fear and loss of control: toward the new little pupils with their unpredictable behaviors; but also toward the parents, with whom subjects of conflict can come up. The word *vaccination* evokes the harsh fight of the last few years in Italy, between school and the anti-vaccination movement among parents.

C 3 brings the conflict between school and family more evidently to the fore (*parents, family, to cooperate, to accept, to delegate, to educate, hard, to insist, to divorce, to dispute, to claim, mothering*). Teachers seem to think that families are not able to cooperate and educate because they are broken, not in step with the norm. But the divorce mentioned here refers also, in our interpretation, to the separation currently perceived between school and family, after the past union. The question at stake seems to be how school and family have to deal with the child.

C 5, lastly, is the cluster on diagnosis, which, when reading the words (*child, to diagnose, therapy, to help, to observe, to evaluate, to label, handicap, autism*), seems to proceed along a separate path, guided by its own logic, language, and techniques. C 5 is opposed to the conflicting C 1 and C 3, respectively, on the third and the fourth factor. In this cluster, we find no trace of conflict: conflict seems to be neutralized by the presence of the diagnosis. Here in particular, we see how factorial relationships are important in the interpretation of the data. We have not one but two clusters that are opposed to C 5 on two different factors. In both cases, on the one hand, we find traces of relationships with the children and the families, which the teachers experience with intense implication, albeit with distress (see the words *fear, to walk away, to fall,* and *bullying* in C 1) and conflict (see the words *hard, to divorce, to dispute, to claim*); on the other hand, in C 5, every word seems consistent with a diagnostic code, which in turn seems to create a world apart centered on the single child (word with the highest significance in the cluster) where no mention can be found of the aforementioned tensions.

In summary, we could say that the first factor tells us about a school that seems to be experienced by the teachers, in emotional terms, as a path of progressive assimilation of the students into the school routine and an inward-looking functioning: with an entry stage connoted by fear and danger (C 1) and a final stage where in many respects the feeling of obligation and the pressure to comply with the norm seem to prevail (C 4 and C 2). We find no mention in the clusters of a future that the school can help to envision, for and with the students; we will come back to this point in the conclusions of the chapter. A certain tendency toward looking inward is not a novelty in school.[13] We had found the same attitude also in the past (see, e.g., Carli, 2006b), but in a very different context, where school certification had a clear role in

---

[13] We use "inward-looking" to describe the tendency of an organization to function as a closed system, that is a system tending to assimilate any variability connected to the relationship with the external reality (including the relationship with the users/clients) in terms of an internal operative model designed to pursue given organizational patterns (Bucci & Vanheule, 2018; Thompson, 1967).

allowing social mobility,[14] and a greater cultural continuity tied families and school together. Nowadays, the fact that school is inward-looking appears rather as a form of defense, within which the diagnosis seems to aim at neutralizing the new knowledge potentially coming from criticalities (see the open, intense conflict with families) and restore the fantasy of routine. The diagnosis, we suggest, "sedates" the conflict, taking on the function of a new conformity, an alternative to the lost one. The "old" conformity, which was guaranteed by the cultural continuity between nursery school and families, seems to be replaced now by diagnosis as a surrogate conformity. This however changes the focus from the school's functioning to the individuals who diverge from the norm; a norm that ultimately remains unquestioned.

ETA as an Intervention-Research Tool for the Development of Healthcare Organizations

The second case study that we wish to discuss regards an organization that provides services for adult disability.

It is important to say that disability is a category developed in the medical field in the 1980s with the stated purpose of enlarging the potential range of action of the healthcare system beyond the limit of organic illness. WHO defines disability as a restriction or a lack, caused by an impairment, in carrying out an activity in a way or within a range considered normal for a human being, and it thereby re-defines illness as everything interfering with the individual capacity to fulfill the functions or obligations expected in a context (World Health Organization, 1980).[15] In this theoretical framework, disability is interpreted as an individual deficit, compared to what is considered normal in the context, that legitimates an intervention seeking to correct the deficit. This specific definition of disability establishes the possibility of classifying social behaviors as normal or pathological, regardless of the identification of etiopathogenic factors and through a classification process with unspecified reference parameters. This means that the classification process is determined mainly by the historically and culturally situated point of view of the operators conducting it. These staff members, to quote Canguilhem (1966/1975), may systematically confuse normality with what is considered socially desirable within their culture of belonging,

---

[14]Numerous studies highlight the crisis of the Italian school system as a driving force for social mobility (Almalaurea, 2018; Censis, 2018; OECD, 2018).

[15]*Disability* is part of a tripartite system that includes also *impairment* and *handicap*. Impairment is defined as "any loss or lack of any physiological, anatomical, psychological structure or function"; handicap is instead defined as "a disadvantage, for an individual, caused by an impairment or a disability, that limits or prevents the assumption of a role considered normal (in regards to age, sex, social and cultural factors) for that individual" (World Health Organization, 1980, p. 183). As in the case of the psychiatric syndromes of the DSM V (which includes intellectual disability), this is a categorial system that tends to be inward-looking since there is no external validator of the classification system itself (Di Ninni, 2004).

no matter what may be the subjective motivation bringing the clients to access the healthcare system.

Connected to this, Carli and Paniccia (2011) argued that the healthcare context tends to deem subjectivity as irrelevant for medical praxis, which does not consider the emotional relationship that the client establishes with the organization providing care and services to him/her. This can produce criticalities in the relationship between clients of the healthcare system and its staff.

In 2016, some of us, members of an association of psychologists that provides organizational consultancy services,[16] started a 3-year intervention-research project commissioned by an organization that is part of the Italian National Health System (for a full description, see Bisogni & Pirrotta, 2018; Pirrotta & Bisogni, 2018). Here, we specifically discuss how the use of ETA in this project enabled reflection on the emotional dynamics of the relationship between the organization and its clients—people with disability and their family members—and how this was helpful for the organization at a time when it was facing significant changes.

The Research Context and Design

The organization that commissioned the project was a Complex Operative Unit (COU) of a Local Health Authority in central Italy, composed of four Simple Operative Units (SOUs), each situated in a different territorial district. Work in the SOUs was carried out by multidisciplinary teams. The COU's tasks entail admission, assessment, and delivery of health and social care services to adults with physical and intellectual disability, between 18 and 64 years of age, at their home or in semi-residential and residential centers. Services also include professional training and work integration. At the time when we met the management of the organization, the COU was facing a growth in requests—increasing by 30% in the last few years—regarding especially young people with intellectual disability and autism spectrum disorders.

The staff complained about having to deal with requests by the clients to which it was difficult to give an answer. They perceived these requests as never-ending and often "inappropriate," not in line with the organization's aims. Both the management and the operators reported a climate of conflict with the clients and their family members.

We suggested that this conflict could be interpreted as the sign that there probably was a gap between the professionals' and the clients' expectations of the service. This is also in line with a healthcare culture that tends to intervene without dealing with the subjectivity of the clients, that is with their emotional involvement in the relationship with healthcare services, or with the emotional experiences of the healthcare professionals themselves. What the operators perceived as erroneous or inappropriate requests could suggest, in our view, the need to explore both their own and the clients'

---

[16]GAP was founded by Felice Bisogni and Stefano Pirrotta and provides organizational consultancy services for public bodies and third sector organizations (www.apsgap.it).

expectations of the service, and the relationships with each other. Starting from this hypothesis, we agreed with the management to carry out an intervention-research project, which ran in two phases.

Two Studies Using ETA to Explore the Culture of Staff and Clients

We conducted a preliminary study that involved 26 COU staff members and was aimed at exploring what they thought of the organizational functioning and of the relationship with the clients. Afterward, in a second study, which involved 90 clients—16 adults with intellectual disability and 74 family members (mostly parents, and 4 sisters)—we explored their expectations of the organization and of the problem that made them contact it. The families interviewed had been using the services of the COU for 7 years on average. The study involved mainly family members of people with intellectual disability; this choice was due to the staff's interest in understanding specifically the challenge this kind of user posed to the organization.

All participants were involved in individual open-ended interviews that were audio-recorded and transcribed. The interview transcripts were put together to form two textual corpora (one for the staff/one for the clients) which were processed through two separate Emotional Textual Analyses.

The Staff Culture

Regarding the staff culture, ETA produced 4 clusters of dense words within a factorial space made up of three factorial axes, which show how the clusters are related to each other (Fig. 9.2 and Table 9.2).

As far as the first factor is concerned, C 1 and C 3 (positive pole) are opposed to C 4 and C 2 (negative pole). On the second factor, C 4 is opposed to C 2. Clusters 1 and 3, which are associated with the first factor, are also opposed to each other on the third factor. We will now look at the meaning of these various oppositions and associations.

On the first factor, on one side (negative pole) we find two cultures (C 2 and C 4), which, in different ways, both seem to be based on evading the exploration of the clients' demand. The words in C 2 (*organization, team, to manage, operators, meeting, to decide*) describe the organizational dynamic as self-centered with no apparent connection with the clients' demand. The words in C 4 (*boy, parents, children, to live, patient, severe*) on the other hand highlight the tendency to infantilize the diagnosed adults and medicalize the relationship with them, thereby avoiding the exploration of the clients' own experience and expectations.

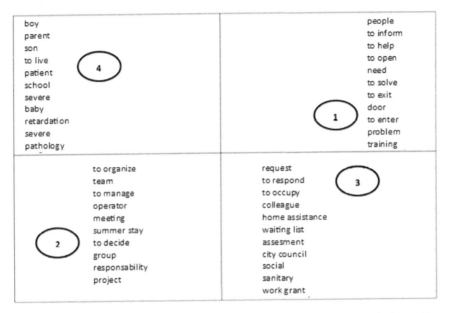

Fig. 9.2 Factorial space (operators) (The figure shows the key dense words in each cluster. *Note* The figure represents only the first and the second factorial axis: the first factor is represented by the horizontal axis, the second factor by the vertical axis. One should imagine the third factor as two other axes that cross the plane in the central point, thus generating a Euclidean 4-dimensional space. The central point represents the point of origin that cuts each factor into two semi-axes culminating in two opposite poles: a positive pole, on one side, and a negative pole, on the other [see Table 9.2])

Table 9.2 Relationship between clusters and factors (centroid coordinates)

	Factor 1	Factor 2	Factor 3
CL 1	**0.5018**	0.0972	**0.5717**
CL 2	**−0.5661**	**−0.7719**	0.1343
CL 3	**0.5087**	−0.1684	**−0.5972**
CL 4	**−0.4677**	**0.5769**	−0.1039

Note The table shows the centroid coordinates of each cluster that indicate the cluster's position in relation to the factors; the higher this value (centroid coordinate), the more statistically significant the relation between cluster and factor. The most significant relationships are shown in bold

In contrast, at the opposite pole of the first factor, we find two cultures (C 1 and C 3) in which the staff feel submerged by the clients' requests and somehow threatened. In C 3 (see the first words *request, to answer, to occupy, colleague, home assistance, waiting list*), the clients' requests are experienced as never-ending demands and, nevertheless, the organization is obliged to respond to them all, in an omnipotent way, because it operates as a public facility on behalf of the state. The words of C 1 (*people, information, to open, to help, need, to solve, to exit, door, to enter*) instead express a culture in which the relationship with the clients seems based on the values of openness, of giving help and hospitality to people in need.

C 1 and C 3 are also opposed to each other on the third factor, because in different ways both declare a difficulty in the relationship with the clients, due the impossibility of dealing effectively with their requests unless one adopts criteria to define discrete problems that one can treat. By contrast, both the sense of obligation and the reference to philanthropic values tended to create relationships based on a fantasy of omnipotence as a response to limitless need. At the same time, there was also the wish to reflect on problems and to be trained (C 1).

Based on these results, the management of the COU commissioned a second study in order to explore also the clients' point of view.

The Clients' Culture

In this second study, the ETA produced 5 clusters of dense words in a factorial space of four factorial axes, as showed in Fig. 9.3 and Table 9.3.

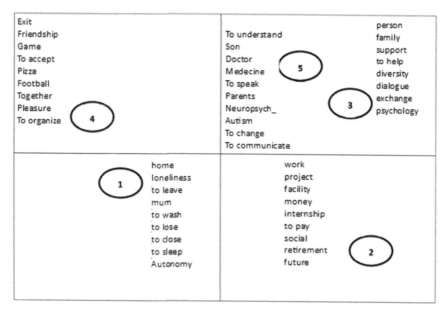

Fig. 9.3 Factorial space (clients) (The figure shows the key dense words in each cluster. *Note* The figure represents only the first and the second factorial axis: the first factor is represented by the horizontal axis, the second factor by the vertical axis. One should imagine the third and fourth factors as two other axes that cross the plane in the central point, thus generating a Euclidean 4-dimensional space. The central point represents the point of origin that cuts each factor into two semi-axes culminating in two opposite poles: a positive pole, on one side, and a negative pole, on the other [see Table 9.3])

Table 9.3 Relationship between clusters and factors (centroid coordinates)

	Factor 1	Factor 2	Factor 3	Factor 4
CL 01	−0.3879	−0.2657	**0.5346**	−0.0280
CL 02	**0.4272**	**−0.5395**	−0.3362	−0.0948
CL 03	**0.4534**	0.3119	0.1203	**0.7319**
CL 04	**−0.6648**	0.2625	**−0.4964**	0.0312
CL 05	**0.4468**	**0.5974**	0.1604	**−0.4902**

Note The table shows the centroid coordinates of each cluster that indicate the cluster's position in relation to the factors; the higher this value (centroid coordinate), the more statistically significant the relation between cluster and factor. The most significant relationships are shown in bold

We will not comment here on the analysis of the whole factorial space (on this, see Pirrotta & Bisogni, 2018). We focus on how discussing the clusters which emerged from the interviews with the users with intellectual disability and their families helped the staff discern the clients' demand in its various main emotional components. In this way, it was possible to disconfirm the representation of the clients as carriers of unlimited and all-encompassing requests, thereby defusing the persecutory emotion that was connected to such a representation. In particular, the study on the clients' culture allowed the clients' demand to be connected to a crisis in the cohabitation system within the family rather than to deficits regarding only the person diagnosed. This crisis concerned family relationships based on dynamics of unproductive dependency and reciprocal control that isolate the family (see in particular C 1) as opposed to the wish to construct an enjoyable, vital sociality (see in particular C 4) but also the difficulty in doing so. This appeared to be, in emotional terms, the core issue that motivated families of individuals with intellectual disability to request services: namely, the difficulty in building relationships based on the sharing of interests and wishes. We are talking about a problem that we can assume is linked with the failure of the parents' expectation of their children becoming progressively independent from them when adults, as well as to difficulties in the social and occupational integration of adults with disability.

By comparing the cultures which emerged from the two studies, we could see that both medical and social models of intervention, when failing to explore the clients' subjective motivation in contacting the healthcare organization and to define the problem on which to intervene in light of this motivation, risk hindering both the development of effective services and the mobilization of the clients' resources. It seems that the clients' problems cannot be taken for granted either as medical problems (illness to be cured) or as social problems (lack of job or social exclusion to be corrected, with respect to an expected norm). C 3 (in the second study) revealed the wish of the people with disability that we interviewed and that of the family members to have a dialogue with each other and with the professionals about the difficulties they experience in family life as well as in other social contexts. They also seemed interested in giving the organization their feedback so as to make it work more effectively. In order to support the possibility of such a dialogue, the two studies were followed by training activities with the staff and the family members involved, based on using the group as a tool for discussion and exchange.

In other studies using ETA in order to explore the emotional collusive dynamics underpinning organizational relationships and cultures (see, for example, Bucci & Vanheule, 2020; Paniccia, Dolcetti, Cappelli, Donatiello, & Di Noja, 2018), interviews with the different members of the organization (e.g., young new hires and their corporate mentors; staff members and guests in a migrant reception service) were merged in a single textual corpus, which was subsequently analyzed (the difference between the groups was traced as an illustrative variable).

In the case study that we have just discussed, on the contrary, we conducted two separate ETAs on two different data sets (one collecting the interviews with the staff and the other collecting the interviews with the clients) and then we compared the outcomes of the two analyses. This was primarily because the management of the COU commissioned a second study in order to explore the clients' point of view only at a later time, in light of the results of the first study which had involved the staff. In the two studies, we used slightly different trigger questions and thus we decided not to merge the data sets. At the same time, for such characteristics, this is probably an all the more interesting example of empirical study of the notion of collusion, as theorized by Renzo Carli. In fact, when comparing the two factorial spaces, one can clearly see how reciprocal expectations within a relationship are emotionally oriented in terms of a collusive process, whereby components of the feeling of one party find their mirror or complementary counterpart in the feeling of the other party. Nevertheless, elements of divergence, in the sense that they escape the collusive interplay, come also to the fore and the possibility to reflect upon and discuss about these dynamics gives awareness of the shared process in which one participates, as well as can lead to new perspectives.

Conclusions

The main application of ETA has historically been in two fields: psychological intervention within organizations, with the goal of promoting developments in the relationship between the organization and its clients, on the one hand; research on processes of cultural change impacting on the dynamics of living together, on the other. In this chapter, we wanted to provide insights on both these traditions by focusing specifically on contemporary mental health issues and demands.

The study on school is particularly significant, we believe, in revealing that splitting the individual from the context is inadequate in helping us understand mental health demands, particularly at the present time because the very notion of context is currently in crisis. In this chapter, when we use the notions of individual and context, we mean by the latter the historical experience of social systems endowed with more or less stable—symbolic—boundaries; that is, systems whose existence and role would be taken for granted, unless a crisis occurred. Nowadays, not just school, but more generally organizational, national, and family boundaries seem to be in question, in the sense that such systems are perceived as structurally in crisis, unless one takes care to retrieve and rethink their meaning.

Our findings suggest that the increase in diagnoses along with the spread of a diagnostic culture in school emerges as an attempt to restore a lost conformity, which was grounded on a cultural continuity between school and family (that has long been mediated by the Catholic Church in Italy). The diagnosis introduces a surrogate conformity which fails because, being built on an individualistic basis, it does not help the reconstruction of viable, shared purposes.

The conflict between schools and families, at the beginning of schooling, can be an important aspect of the development of the culture that we explored through our study. The conflict appears now not as a difference of positions, but as a mutual aggression. However, if the current confrontation with the families *becomes* a conflict, where the parties recognize the interest in sharing goals even if from different positions, this is the place where we can once again find a shared purpose for school.

Another aspect of development is the teachers' potential demand to reduce the gap they feel with the contemporary reality (e.g., present day languages, like the digital one, which would require or inspire innovations in teaching). The factorial space of the school does not tell us about the future, or of the function that school may serve in designing it. Nevertheless, in the individual interviews with teachers, there was no shortage of comments on the future and on other relevant issues, such as the loss of trust in education's power to provide important and useful skills. How should the absence of these themes in the factorial space be interpreted? There is no co-occurrence of dense words to evoke them: teachers do not share emotional codes and categories on these issues. Research studies like the one we have presented here intends to respond to this vacuum.

Olivetti Manoukian (2016) links the current crisis in health and social care organizations to a difficulty in defining and interpreting the problems motivating citizens' access to health and social care. The debate on disability, both scholarly and public, has historically been a place of strong divisions concerning the definition of disability (see, e.g., Bucci & Vanheule, 2018; Shakespeare, 2006; Söder, 2009). Carli and Paniccia have highlighted in several works (e.g., 2003, 2005, 2011) the difficulties related to the application of the medical paradigm, based on etiopathogenetic diagnosis and therapeutic prescription, beyond the limited field of organic illness. The medical paradigm, as we have seen, can prove to be ineffective in the mental health and disability fields. The ETA-based intervention-research that we have discussed in this chapter brings attention to the difficulty of healthcare organizations in considering the client's emotional relationship with the healthcare system itself and, at the same time, shows that ignoring this aspect can produce dissatisfaction and conflicts with the clients. We underline that dissatisfaction and conflicts emerge when the medicalization of problems is practiced and taken for granted. By contrast, we believe that the use of ETA allowed the operators to acknowledge the clients' dissatisfaction but also their interest in reflecting on the reasons for it. In this sense, ETA was a tool for organizational development, because it enabled the retrieval of emotional polysemy underpinning the participation in the shared organizational context by its different components, professionals, and clients, and thus of their subjective and mutual engagement.

References

Almalaurea. (2018). *XX Indagine Condizione occupazionale dei Laureati 2017. Sintesi del Rapporto 2018* [Analysis of the graduates' 2017 employment survey. Summary of the report 2018]. Retrieved from https://www.almalaurea.it/universita/profilo/profilo2017.

Beck, U. (1992). *Risk society: Towards a new modernity*. London: Sage.

Benzécri, J.-P. (1973). *L'Analyse des Données (tome 1 et 2)* [Data analysis (T.1 and T.2)]. Paris: DUNOD.

Bisogni, F., & Pirrotta, S. (2018). Research-intervention for the development of organizational competence in a sociosanitary service for adults with disability and their family members. *Rivista di Psicologia Clinica, 1*, 32–65.

Bucci, F., & Vanheule, S. (2018). Families of adult people with disability: Their experience in the use of services run by social cooperatives in Italy. *International Journal of Social Welfare, 27*(2), 157–167.

Bucci, F., & Vanheule, S. (2020). Investigating changing work and economic cultures through the lens of youth employment: A case study from a psychosocial perspective in Italy. *YOUNG, 28*(3), 275–293. https://doi.org/10.1177/1103308819857412.

Canguilhem, G. (1975). *Il normale e il patologico* [On the normal and the pathological]. Firenze: Guaraldi (Original work published 1966).

Carli, R. (2006a). Collusion and its experimental basis. *Rivista di Psicologia Clinica, 2*(3), 1–11.

Carli, R. (Ed.). (2006b). *La scuola e i suoi studenti, un rapporto non scontato. L'école et ses élèves, des rapports à ne pas tenir pour acquis. La escuela y sus estudiantes, una relaciòn que non se da por descontado* [School and its students, a relationship that cannot be taken for granted]. Milano: FrancoAngeli.

Carli, R. (2017). Il Ripiego: Una fantasia incombente [The fallback: An impending fantasy]. *Rivista di Psicologia Clinica, 2*, 5–24.

Carli, R. (2018). Inconscio, culture locali e linguaggio: Linee guida per l'Analisi Emozionale del Testo (AET) [Unconscious, local cultures and language: Guidelines for the Emotional Textual Analysis (AET)]. *Rivista di Psicologia Clinica, 2*, 7–33.

Carli, R., Dolcetti, F., Giovagnoli, F., Gurrieri, R., & Paniccia, R. M. (2015). La cultura locale del Servizio di assistenza specialistica nelle scuole della Provincia di Roma [The local culture of the special assistance service in schools of the Province of Rome]. *Quaderni della Rivista di Psicologia Clinica, 2*, 16–32.

Carli, R., & Giovagnoli, F. (2011). A cultural approach to clinical psychology: Psychoanalysis and analysis of the demand. In S. Salvatore & T. Zittoun (Eds.), *Cultural psychology and psychoanalysis: Pathways to synthesis* (pp. 117–150). Charlotte, NC: IAP-Information Age Publishing.

Carli, R., & Paniccia, R. M. (1981). *Psicosociologia delle organizzazioni e delle istituzioni* [Psychosociology of the organisation and of the institution]. Bologna: Il Mulino.

Carli, R., & Paniccia, R. M. (2002). *L'analisi emozionale del testo: Uno strumento psicologico per leggere testi e discorsi* [Emotional textual analysis. A psychological tool for reading texts and discourses]. Milano: Franco Angeli.

Carli, R., & Paniccia, R. M. (2003). *Analisi della domanda* [Analysis of the demand]. Bologna: Il Mulino.

Carli, R., & Paniccia, R. M. (2005). *Casi clinici: Il resoconto in psicologia clinica* [Clinical cases: The reporting in clinical psychology]. Bologna: Il mulino.

Carli, R., & Paniccia R. M. (2011). *La cultura dei servizi di salute mentale in Italia. Dai malati psichiatrici alla nuova utenza: L'evoluzione della domanda d'aiuto e delle dinamiche di rapporto* [The culture of the mental health services in Italy. From the psychiatric patient to the new users: The evolution of the demand for help and of relational dynamics]. Roma: Franco Angeli.

Carli, R., Paniccia, R. M., Giovagnoli, F., Carbone, A., & Bucci, F. (2016). Emotional Textual Analysis. In L. A. Jason & D. S. Glenwick (Eds.), *Handbook of methodological approaches to community-based research: Qualitative, quantitative, and mixed methods* (pp. 111–117). New York, NY: Oxford University Press.

Census. (2018). *52° Rapporto sulla situazione sociale del Paese* [52nd Report on the social situation of the country]. Retrieved from http://www.censis.it/rapporto-annuale/52%C2%B0-rapporto-sulla-situazione-sociale-del-paese2018-0.

Di Ninni, A. (2004). *L'intervento per la salute mentale dalle lezioni del corso di epidemiologia psichiatrica per psicologi* [The intervention for mental health from the leschildren of the course of psychiatric epidemiology for psychologists]. Roma: Kappa.

Eurydice. (2018). *La carriera degli insegnanti in Europa: accesso, progressione e sostegno* [Teachers' career in Europe: Entry, progress and support]. I Quaderni di Eurydice Italia, Ediguida S.r.l. Retrieved from http://www.eurydice.indire.it.

Fornari, F. (1976). *Simbolo e codice: Dal processo psicoanalitico all'analisi istituzionale* [Symbol and code: From psychoanalytic process to institutional analysis]. Milano: Feltrinelli.

Fornari, F. (1981). *I fondamenti di una teoria psicoanalitica del linguaggio* [Foundations for a psychoanalytic theory of language]. Torino: Bollati Boringhieri.

Giddens, A. (1991). *Modernity and self identity: Self and society in the late Modern Age*. Oxford: Polity.

Giovagnoli, F., Caputo, A., & Paniccia, R. M. (2015). L'integrazione della disabilità nella scuola primaria e secondaria di primo grado italiana: Una ricerca presso un gruppo di assistenti all'autonomia e alla comunicazione [Integration of disability at primary and lower secondary schools in Italy: A research study on assistants for autonomy and communication]. *Rivista di Psicologia Clinica, 1*, 167–200.

INDIRE. (2014). *Gli insegnanti in Europa e in Italia: contesto demografico, formazione e stipendi* [Teachers in Europe and in Italy: Demographic context, training and salaries]. Retrieved from http://www.indire.it.

Istat. (2018). *L'integrazione degli alunni con disabilità nelle scuole primarie e secondarie di primo grado* [The integration of pupils with disability in primary and secondary school]. Retrieved from https://www.istat.it/it/files//2018/03/alunni-con-disabilit%C3%A0-as2016-2017.pdf.

Lancia, F. (2004). *Strumenti per l'analisi dei testi* [Tools for text analysis]. Rome: Franco Angeli.

Matte Blanco, I. (1975). *The unconscious as infinite sets: An essay in bi-logic*. London: Gerald Duckworth.

Matte Blanco, I. (1988). *Thinking, feeling and being*. London: Routledge.

Miur. (2015). *L'integrazione scolastica degli alunni con disabilità a.s. 2014/2015*. Camera dei deputati, Servizio Studi, XVIII Legislatura. Retrieved from http://www.camera.it.

Needham, C. (2011). *Personalising public services: Understanding the personalisation narrative*. Bristol: The Policy Press.

OECD. (2018). *A broken social elevator? How to promote social mobility*. Retrieved from http://www.oecd.org/social/broken-elevator-how-to-promote-social-mobility-9789264301085-en.htm.

Olivetti Manoukian, F. (2016). *Oltre la crisi: Cambiamenti possibili nei servizi sociosanitari* [Beyond the crisis: Possible changes in the sociosanitary services]. Milano: Guerini e Associati.

Paniccia, R. M. (2012a). Psicologia Clinica e disabilità: La competenza a integrare differenze [Clinical psychology and disability: The competence in integrating differences]. *Rivista di Psicologia Clinica, 1*, 91–110.

Paniccia, R. M. (2012b). Gli assistenti all'autonomia e all'integrazione per la disabilità a scuola: Da ruoli confusi a funzioni chiare [Disability assistants for autonomy and social integration at school: From confused roles to clear functions]. *Rivista di Psicologia Clinica, 2*, 165–183.

Paniccia, R. M. (2013). Disabilità. La domanda rivolta alla psicologia attraverso i resoconti di esperienze di giovani psicologi. *Quaderni della Rivista di Psicologia Clinica, 1*, 80–87.

Paniccia, R. M., Dolcetti, F., Cappelli, T., Donatiello, G., & Di Noja, G. (2018). The culture of migrant reception services in Italy: An exploratory research. *Rivista di Psicologia Clinica, 2*, 93–120.

Paniccia, R. M., Giovagnoli, F., Bucci, F., & Caputo, A. (2014). Families with a child with a disability: The expectations toward services and psychology. *Rivista di Psicologia Clinica, 2*, 84–107.

Paniccia, R. M., Giovagnoli, F., Bucci, F., Donatiello, G., & Cappelli, T. (2019). The increase in diagnosis in the school: A study amongst a group of Italian teachers. *Rivista di Psicologia Clinica, 1*, 61–94.

Paniccia, R. M., Giovagnoli, F., Di Ruzza, F., & Giuliano, S. (2014). La disabilità nelle scuole superiori: L'assistenza specialistica come funzione integrativa [Disability in higher middle schools: The specialist assistance as integrative function]. *Quaderni della Rivista di Psicologia Clinica, 2*, 64–73.

Pirrotta, S., & Bisogni, F. (2018). The demand of the clients of a sociosanitary service for adults with disability and their family members: A research-intervention with the Emotional Text Analysis. *Rivista di Psicologia Clinica, 2*, 121–147.

Plamper, J. (2018). *The history of emotions: An introduction.* Oxford: Oxford University Press.

Reinert, M. (1983). Une méthode de classification descendante hiérarchique: application à l'analyse lexicale par contexte. *Les cahiers de l'analyse des données, 8*(2), 187–198.

Reinert, M. (1990). ALCESTE: Une méthodologie d'analyse des données textuelles et une application: Aurélia de Gérard de Nerval. *Bulletin de méthodologie sociologique, 26*, 24–54.

Salvatore, S., & Freda, M. F. (2011). Affect, unconscious and sense making: A psychodynamic, semiotic and dialogic model. *New Ideas in Psychology, 29*, 119–135.

Shakespeare, T. (2006). *Disability: Rights and wrongs.* London, UK: Routledge.

Söder, M. (2009). Tensions, perspectives and themes in disability studies. *Scandinavian Journal of Disability Research, 11*(2), 67–81.

Thompson, J. D. (1967). *Organizations in action.* New York: MacGraw-Hill.

World Health Organization. (1980). *International classification of impairments, disabilities, and handicaps: A manual of classification relating to the consequences of disease, published in accordance with resolution WHA29.* 35 of the Twenty-ninth World Health Assembly, May 1976. World Health Organization.

Chapter 10
Engraved in the Body: Ways of Reading Finnish People's Memories of Mental Hospitals

Saara Jäntti⊙, Kirsi Heimonen⊙, Sari Kuuva⊙, Karoliina Maanmieli⊙, and Anu Rissanen⊙

Abstract Finnish psychiatric practice has been heavily based on institutionalization. Mental hospitals have thus been part of Finns' lives in many ways. Our multidisciplinary research group has investigated how experiences in these institutions are remembered today by analysing writings by patients, relatives, personnel and their children, collected in 2014–2015 with the Finnish Literature Society. The memories cover phases of psychiatric care from the 1930s to the mid-2010s. This article presents multiple ways in which experiences that are often difficult verbalize can be interpreted, e.g. by drawing on perspectives from creative, artistic and cultural studies. Collecting and archiving the memories emphasizes their importance as part of national memory. Historical contextualization shows consistencies and inconsistencies in the treatment and organization of psychiatric care in Finland. The analysis of figurative language as a means of conveying traumatic experiences reveals narrative strategies employed to express abusive memories. Artistic research that includes somatic movement practice exemplifies possibilities of researching the memories through corporeality. The examination of the memories of the children of the staff in psychiatric hospitals provides new insights into historical psychiatric hospitals as emotional communities. The different ways of engaging—thematically, corporeally,

We wish to express our gratitude to Professor Vilma Hänninen for commenting both this chapter and the presentation in the QRMH7 conference in Berlin which this chapter is based on.

S. Jäntti (✉)
Department of Language and Communication Studies,
University of Jyväskylä, Jyväskylä, Finland
e-mail: saara.j.jantti@jyu.fi

K. Heimonen
University of the Arts Helsinki, Helsinki, Finland

S. Kuuva · K. Maanmieli
Department of Music, Art and Culture Studies,
University of Jyväskylä, Jyväskylä, Finland

A. Rissanen
Department of History and Ethnology,
University of Jyväskylä, Jyväskylä, Finland

conceptually, theoretically—with the texts complement each other, reveal the multi-layeredness of the memories and help create a richer understanding of the social, cultural and economic significance of the hospitals. Attention to the body, affects and emotions can help generate both new practices, new research questions and new ways of engaging the public with the results of academic research.

Keywords Mental hospital · Mental illness · History of psychiatry · Finland · Archives · Artistic research · Figurative language · Memory · Affect · Emotion · Corporeality · Multidisciplinary research

Introduction

As Finnish psychiatric practice has been heavily based on institutionalization, psychiatric hospitals and mental asylums have been part of the lives of Finnish people in many ways, and mental hospitals have played an important role in the everyday culture and history of Finland. Tens of thousands of people have been treated in them[1] and many more have visited their friends and family members there. The hospitals have also provided work and accommodation for the staff and their families. However, there has been little research on lay people's memories of their experiences of mental hospitals. The aim of this research was to collect and make known their memories.

The research is based on pieces of writing by patients, relatives, staff and their children that were collected and archived in the Finnish Literature Society in 2014–2015. The memories cover phases of psychiatric care from the 1930s to the 2010s, during which time the organization of psychiatric care underwent significant changes, which are reflected in the memories. The 92 pieces of writing that we obtained contain both painful and positive memories, and draw a rich, yet sketchy, landscape of the ways in which experiences related to the spaces of psychiatric institutions linger in Finnish people's memories. At a time when the Finnish healthcare system is about to undergo a major reform, it is crucial to make these experiences visible and heard, as, we argue, by making visible and tangible people's experiences, we can gain a better understanding of the social and cultural forces that shape attitudes to and ideas about psychiatric care, mental health problems and service users today.

Public discourse in the Finnish media nowadays often focuses on the lack of sick beds in psychiatric wards, and public action has been taken to protect some of the old institutions, such as the first mental asylum in Finland, Lapinlahti. Little attention has

---

[1]From the documents and statistics available, it is not possible to establish the exact number of patients as, especially in the past, the periods spent in the hospitals could last for years, and today, while patients often stay shorter times in hospital, the number of admissions per year has increased. For example, in 1972, when the number of hospital beds in Finland reached its peak, there were about 42000 patients in psychiatric hospitals. In 2000, however, the number of admissions was about 48000. It thus seems that while the number of beds has been reduced, the number of admissions has increased. It stood at around 34000 in 2017 (Source: Suomen virallinen tilasto: Terveys.1924-1981. Lääkintöhallituksen vuosikirjat, 1982-2017 Suomen tilastollinen vuosikirja).

been paid to the actual memories of people who have lived, worked or encountered various forms of treatment in psychiatric hospitals. The history of psychiatry has mostly been written from the point of view of doctors and other members of staff (Achté & Alanen, 1991; Parpola, 2013). The various histories written on the hospitals that are now being closed seldom include the experiences of patients and/or their family members. While new social histories around medicine, illness and psychiatry are emerging, there are still dominant discourses related to psychiatry. On the one hand, practitioners write a positive narrative of improved practices, treatment and care, and the development of medical treatments. On the other hand, public discourse and the media focus on the lack of treatment, and the unavailability of sufficient resources to help, treat and contain psychiatric suffering. The voices of service users often remain marginal and—as also our data shows—actual experiences in mental hospitals are permeated by stigma and shame.

This was the background against which the idea of establishing an archive of people's experiences emerged. Our multidisciplinary research group is now working on this historically and culturally contingent material, and we are focusing on the bodily, spatial, affective and multisensory aspects of the memories. By drawing on our backgrounds in history and art, and visual, cultural and literary studies, we seek to find novel ways of reading and interpreting the memories and new perspectives on the cultural meaning of mental hospitals. We do not strive for a shared truth about the memories, but rather seek to point out the multiplicity of interpretations. This chapter consists of a description of the collection of the written materials and a historical overview of the organization of psychiatric care in Finland. It presents three different analytic foci and ways of approaching the data, each of which sheds light on different aspects of the memories: (1) the use of figurative language, (2) patients' descriptions of space and (3) the memories of children who grew up on the hospital premises. Our aim was twofold: on the one hand, to point to the cultural significance of psychiatric hospitals in Finland and, on the other, to highlight ways of reading that value the writers' experiences and intentions.

Saara Jäntti: Organizing the Writing Collection

The memories were collected by the Network of Cultural Studies in Mental Health in collaboration with the Finnish Literature Society (SKS)[2] in 2014–2015. The idea was to obtain the recollections of as many different groups of people as possible in order to gain understanding of the various ways mental hospitals have affected people's lives, and of how their experiences are remembered and perhaps still affect the writers' attitudes towards life, psychiatry, mental health problems and their treatment, and family and other relations. By inviting people to write about their memories we also

---

[2] These archives document the written and oral cultural heritage of Finland. Their collections contain material on literature and cultural history, authors and literary figures as well as on traditional and contemporary culture (https://www.finlit.fi/en/archive#.XL7lTegzaUk).

wanted to convey the message that these memories matter, and that the writers' experiences deserve to be archived and become part of the national body of remembrance. I therefore took up the practical tasks of coordination, planning and collaboration with the Finnish Literature Society.

In October 2014, the society put out a call that was published in various places including the newspapers and magazines of organizations set up for users of mental health services and their families. These organizations were also contacted in the planning phases of the call and they contributed to the design of the request. Respondents were asked to write freely and describe, for example, their experiences of care, meaningful encounters and relationships that they remembered, how they now feel about their experiences and their effect on their lives, as well as the hospital building and its surroundings (see Appendix 1).

The writing began to appear slowly. Not everyone was willing to share memories: one day, the archivist at the Finnish Literature Society received a phone call from a former patient who was upset and furious with researchers for asking about something as painful as her experiences at the hospital. Most of those who wrote, however, were happy that they could share their memories, although some of them also mentioned that remembering was so painful that they had to leave some things unsaid. We were also approached by individuals and groups, for example from the former hospital of Lapinlahti, who wanted to conduct writing workshops to produce memories, and in the summer of 2015 Karoliina Maanmieli conducted a writing workshop in a rehabilitation community for thirty-one residents where she used to work. Apart from being shorter, the responses produced in these workshops did not differ significantly from the other responses, e.g. in content or style. Three pieces of writing were accompanied by drawings.[3]

It is worth mentioning that while the data collection was initially planned to end in June 2015, this was in fact the time when the responses really started coming in. It was therefore decided to extend the period until the end of September 2015. As a result, the number of responses doubled. The reason for this could be that awareness of the writing collection spread slowly, but it also points to the fact that painful and marginalized memories take time to form and develop. They may not be narratives people are used to sharing or share with ease, and they therefore take time to emerge. And of course, not everyone is used to writing at all.

All in all, our data now comprises around 500 pages from 92 people and covers different phases of psychiatric care from the 1930s to the 2010s. Half of the writers (45) had been patients.[4] The memories are related to a number of different hospitals in Finland. Many writers share their experiences from different hospitals, and many

---

[3]The workshops were advertised on the community's notice board and weekly meetings. Seven residents attended the workshop where Karoliina first handed them the call for writing and told them that they could share their memories in their own style, even by drawing or writing a poem, and that anything they would like to share would be valued. She did mention that she was especially interested in memories of coercion, but only one participant addressed this issue. The session lasted for an hour. Some participants wanted to continue writing on their own and gave Karoliina their work afterwards. Two participants dictated their memories to Karoliina.

[4]One piece of writing was sent after the collection period had ended.

have experienced the hospitals in different roles: as patients, family members and staff, for example. In some cases, the hospital experience is only a small part of the story, and the writers weave this experience into their life history, philosophy of life or their relatives' mental problems. Some of the memories describe everyday life as a mental patient in great detail. The length of the writing varies from a few sentences to extensive biographies. Some writers include poems, aphorisms, photos and pictures. Some writers discuss mental health, madness and their general understanding of it, rather than share their own actual impressions of hospital events.

Multidisciplinary Approach to the Memories: Description of Methodology and Methods

Handling the diversity of material with which we were presented was challenging. There was a wide variety of writers with different backgrounds and experiences related to different hospitals at different times in history, and the wide range of writing styles in which they wrote made interpretation difficult. Furthermore, experiences related to psychiatric care are often traumatic and affected by a social stigma, which calls for careful ethical and methodological consideration. One of the central questions in our multidisciplinary research enterprise is how to approach memories that are often hard to share—due to both the social stigma and the trauma related to them. While writers who participate in similar writing collections often seek to write coherent life stories, i.e. stories in which incidental events are combined into a single plot (Pöysä, 2015), painful memories are often characterized by gaps in content and difficulty in verbalizing them, and it can be difficult to weave them into the life continuum (see Fuchs, 2013; Holma, 1999). Also, in our data, many of the texts are anecdotal and fragmented, which—rather than disqualifying them from further analysis—reveals something important about the issue in question: in an increasingly text-based society, for example, where many services are moved online, these pieces of writing point to the enormous variation in people's ability to access written language and their own experiences through writing.

Our specific interests are related to the possibility of and ways of narrating embodied, affective and spatial experiences related to hospitals. Our respondents, rather than discussing for example the effects of legislative changes, convey subjective, bodily experiences and focus on the forms and impact of care—or on coercion, its related emotions and social relations. Thus, while our data is too limited to make generalized statements about the history of psychiatry, it does also provide evidence about and insights into the direct and indirect ways in which psychiatric practice affects families and communities.

In the following pages, three of our research team offer a reading of our multi-faceted material. As psychiatric patients' experiences are often painful and can be chaotic, unstructured and difficult to remember, verbalize and share (Jäntti, 2012; Stone 2004), poetry therapist Karoliina Maanmieli analyses the use of figurative language in the patients' writing and draws attention to the ways in which the patients seek to make their experiences understandable and, often, to convey the pain related to their physical experiences and the social hierarchies in the treatment. Artist-researcher Kirsi Heimonen explores the possibilities of relating to the bodily and spatial aspects of the memories through the artist-researcher's corporeality, developed by long-term engagement in a dance technique called the Skinner Releasing Technique. She examines how this way of relating to the memories can be employed in engaging with and sharing the memories with the public. Sari Kuuva engages with the memories of adults whose childhood was passed in psychiatric hospitals because their parents worked there. She explores the hospitals as emotional communities from the children's perspective.

All three approaches are based on close reading of the responses and careful selection of the data presented, and each researcher will explain and demonstrate her approach to the memories in their own section. To highlight the ways in which the researchers' backgrounds, methodological, conceptual and theoretical framework and choices affect their interpretations, the knowledge produced, and the ways in which these are conveyed, we chose to structure this chapter so that each researcher writes her own section in her own style and voice.

First, however, as legislation and organizational changes form the framework for medical and institutional practices within which the ideas and identities of the psychiatric patients and their families are shaped, Anu Rissanen provides a historical background to the memories. While few writers discuss them directly, legislation and treatments shape and produce historically and culturally contingent psychiatric cultures that affect patients', staff members' and family members' lives and ideas about what it means to be a patient and how patients can and should be treated. Some longer memories also reflect changes in the organization of care, such as the deinstitutionalization of the 1980s—and a number of them regret the closing of the hospitals, expressing concern for the patients' welfare. While many writers end on a positive note, they do also lament the difficulty of being admitted and being heard while in treatment, and criticize the standards of care.

Anu Rissanen: History of Mental Health Care in Finland in the Twentieth Century

The Development of Mental Hospitals in Finland

In Finland, it was not until the early 1900s that mental hospitals and confinement therein were introduced.[5] One reason for this was the country's late, gradual industrialization towards the end of the nineteenth century. As people began to participate in paid work on a larger scale, the changing society no longer had room for the mentally ill, lunatics and handicapped who were unable to provide for themselves, and they therefore became a burden on the community. A decree in 1889 on mental illness enabled the establishment of mental wards in poorhouses and communal mental hospitals. The idea behind the foundation of communal district hospitals was that they would care for docile, incurable patients. Soon after, larger cities and regional groupings founded district mental hospitals, and responsibility for organizing services shifted partly to the municipalities, which gradually took on the care of the mentally ill. Altogether fourteen district mental hospitals with a total of 5000 beds were built before 1939 (Hyvönen, 2008; Pietikäinen, 2013; Törrönen, 1978).

In our data, one memory dates from this time.[6] It likens the mental hospital to the communal poorhouse (SKS/MKM 088-089, patient, mid-1930s). The cities' poor relief administrations and their referrals show that in the early twentieth century some patients were sent to mental institutions on account of their poverty rather than illness. As elsewhere, so too in Finland, psychiatry and mental institutions were regarded and used as a tool for social control. Nevertheless, they also provided shelter for those whose socio-economic status was poor and who had no family connections (Pietikäinen, 2015; Rissanen, 2018a).

The Mental Illness Act of 1952 profoundly altered mental health care in Finland. It marked the beginning of the local administration of psychiatric care. Local authorities were made responsible for organizing mental health services while the state remained responsible for the funding and long-term planning of psychiatry and forensic psychiatry and the care of dangerous mentally ill patients. Finland was divided into Mental Health Districts. The former district mental hospitals became their central hospitals, also known as A-hospitals. Their task was to treat acute patients and chronic patients who were considered too difficult to treat in other hospitals. The 1952 law also obliged Mental Health Districts to establish a Psychiatric Outpatient Centre, the

---

[5]In Finland, as elsewhere, the mentally ill and disabled were traditionally looked after by their family and their village. The system of psychiatric treatment was established on the basis of old leper colonies, and the first decree that regulated mental health was promulgated in 1840. The first mental institution, Lapinlahti asylum in Helsinki, with 70 sick beds, was founded in 1841. The 1840 decree made the state responsible for organizing care for the mentally ill, but the lack of funds and the ensuing shortage of sickbeds affected how their care developed.

[6]This hundred-page manuscript was sent in by members of the writer's family. It had originally been written as a memoir or testimony of the writer's experiences in mental hospitals, and it describes life in hospital in detail.

number of which rose slowly from the beginning of the 1970s (Hyvönen, 2008; Salo, 1992).

Ironically, the same law that legislated outpatient care also led to a rapid increase in the number of psychiatric hospital beds. Contrary to the general opinion of psychiatrists themselves, the law continued the tradition of dividing psychiatric treatment into acute and long-term care. Between 1952 and 1970 over 40 small, local, mental hospitals were founded for non-violent chronically ill patients as the state financially supported this development. At the same time, then, as the rest of Western psychiatry was turning to dehospitalization and care in the community, following the introduction in the 1950s of new pharmaceuticals and the rise of social psychiatry and psychotherapy, the number of sickbeds in Finland increased rapidly due to the establishment of these so-called B-hospitals. In 1970, Ireland and Finland had more hospital beds per capita than any other countries in Europe. The difference was that Ireland was reducing their number as rapidly as Finland was increasing theirs.[7] Although the move towards psychiatric dehospitalization developed in the 1960s, it was only in the late 1970s that policy moved in the same direction with the enactment of the partly revised Mental Illness Act. It strengthened outpatient treatment, set up new housing arrangements and emphasized the importance of rehabilitation for both psychotic and non-psychotic patients in hospital and outpatient treatment. It also introduced new day hospitals that provided outpatient services, which at least some patients felt was a relief (Alanko, 2017; Hyvönen, 2008; Pietikäinen, 2013; Salo, 1996).

The 1980s was an era of economic growth and optimism in Finland. This also meant stable funding for public health care. In psychiatry, the National Board of Health transferred resources from institutional care to outpatient care and the number of hospital beds was reduced by 40%. Several projects were launched to examine psychiatric disorders and their treatment, and to find resources and tools to prevent suicide and reduce the number of new long-term schizophrenic patients. New legislation for special health care brought psychiatry and somatic health care under the same administrative agency, which was managed at the regional level (Alanko, 2017; Hyvönen, 2008; Kärkkäinen, 2004).

This positive development culminated in the new Mental Health Act, which came into force in 1991. For the first time, mental well-being was recognized as important, and mental health care was perceived as a tool to improve psychological well-being and prevent mental disorders. One way to improve mental health was to improve citizens' living conditions. Unfortunately, the era of optimism was interrupted by an economic depression in the early 1990s. Public financing was seriously curtailed and tax revenues contracted considerably. Local authorities reduced their funding for many things, including staffing and outsourced services, and this affected especially counselling services in alcohol and substance abuse, and care of the disabled and mental health care. A large number of people were hastily dehospitalized, and in

---

[7] The importance of institutional care is shown in these numbers: in 1900 there were 1300 patients (0.5/1000), in 1940 almost 8400 patients (2.27/1000) and in 1970 almost 20000 patients (4.2/1000).

outpatient care, many therapeutic services were either reduced or closed. Psychiatrists view the 1990s and the beginning of the new century as an era of turbulence; it certainly was a period of chaos for psychiatric patients (Hélen, Hämäläinen, & Metteri, 2011; Hyvönen, 2008; Kärkkäinen, 2004; Korkeila, 1998; Salokangas, Saarinen, & Honkola, 1997).

The problems that transpired in the 1990s persist today in Finnish psychiatry. The number of out-patients has risen steadily at the same time as the number of hospital beds fell to less than 4000 in 2015. This comes out in the testimonies as difficulty in being admitted to hospital. There is a severe shortage of therapy services due especially to the lack of therapists and funds. Therapy services are geographically unequally distributed, and such services have become concentrated in Southern, Western and Central Finland (Hélen et al., 2011; Hyvönen, 2008; Mikkola, Rintanen, Nuorteva, Kovasin, & Erhola, 2015).

Treatment in Mental Hospitals

In the first decades of the twentieth century, treatments included bed rest therapy, deep sleep therapy, hydrotherapy, wet pack therapy, malaria fever therapy and sedatives. Work therapy, namely Simon's Active Therapy, reached Finland at the end of the 1920s and was taken up by every hospital. Most of these treatments are mentioned in the writing recalling the 1930s. Shock treatments (cardiazol and insulin coma therapy) were introduced in the 1930s. Their arrival in hospitals' treatment policies was met with high expectations and great enthusiasm. At first, the nursing staff's enthusiasm for insulin coma treatment, for example, had a therapeutic impact on patients, but as it proved to relieve only some of the symptoms of manic-depressive disorder instead of schizophrenia and other psychosis diseases, the enthusiasm tended to fall and with that also the therapeutic effects. Electroshock therapy was introduced in the 1940s and, after some modifications, has remained in use until today (De Young, 2015; Pietikäinen, 2013, 2015; Rissanen, 2018b).

In the 1950s, new pharmaceuticals revolutionized psychiatry. Together with coercion and isolation, these are the forms of treatment most discussed in our data. New drugs like chlorpromazine (Largactil®), thioridazine (Melleril®) and melperone (Bunil®) became "the magic bullets of psychiatry", as many historians (e.g. Pietikäinen, 2013, 2015) call them. As a result, the wards became quieter and more peaceful, which is reflected especially in the memories of those who grew up in and around the hospitals. Many patients seemed to calm down and improve their social functioning. Drugs helped many, but the side effects, such as drooling, dizziness, motoric restlessness and tremors, were often quite severe—and still today seem to constitute the most difficult aspects for many of our writing patients. Atypical antipsychotic Clozapine was used for a time at the beginning of the 1970s and again after 1990. The use of psychotropic drugs increased strongly in the 1990s, when SSRI antidepressants such as sertraline and citalopram came onto the market (Huttunen & Javanainen, 2004; Shorter 2009).

Ways of Reading the Memories

Karoliina Maanmieli (Former Kähmi)—Figurative Language and Memories of Abuse

My approach to these writings is influenced by my background as a practical nurse and poetry therapist. I have worked with people diagnosed with schizophrenia for fifteen years, using poetry therapy as a method of rehabilitation. This makes me particularly interested in the writers' use of figurative language, its meaning and its function in the memories. I am also interested in the therapeutic value of this type of writing, which I studied in my doctoral dissertation (Kähmi, 2015). This study with a poetry therapy group for people diagnosed with psychosis showed that figurative language is a powerful tool to express what is painful, as it provides the necessary distance and safety. When one is in a state of psychosis or crisis, words may provoke unusual, conflicting images and an emotional content that can be understood in the context of poetry therapy.

My present research focuses on memories of violence and coercion in hospitals. This choice was originally grounded in my professional background and awareness that service users experience mental hospitals as a source of trauma. Nevertheless, I was surprised by the number of negative hospital memories in our research material especially as they were not explicitly asked for in the call. Patients from the 1930s and 2000s alike reported a lack of supportive relations and unnecessary, violent policing, for example, in the form of punishments such as dispossession and seclusion. The prevalence of such coercive practices is, unfortunately, confirmed by other research (e.g. Keski-Valkama, 2010; Koivisto et al., 2004; Kontio et al., 2012; Kuosmanen, 2009), despite the fact that research (e.g. Vuorela & Aalto, 2011) also shows that they have no positive impact on recovery.[8] In the following, I explore the patients' use of figurative language that conveys painful emotions in psychiatric treatment. They are predominantly but not exclusively linked to coercion.

Figurative Language as a Means of Conveying Traumatic Experiences

My main methodological focus is the relation of metaphor to the intelligibility of texts. While Pöysä (2015) maintains that writers responding to the type of invitation we sent out often seek to write a coherent life story, in which incidental events are combined into a single plot, with the sort of sudden, traumatic events that surround a mental hospital (Holma, 1999, p. 213), this is a difficult task. In these cases, narrative coherence may be found in the metaphors.

---

[8]Recent efforts, such as the Mieli [Mind] project in 2009–2015, have sought to improve patients' status, and to reduce seclusion and other restrictions.

Savolainen (2015) considers the use of metaphors to be a way of distancing oneself from the painful story one is trying to tell by making it fictional. Metaphors help to find new dimensions in a manageable form, and to transmit an effective message from a safe distance (Moon, 2007). In poetry therapy, what may commonly be viewed as a mad way of writing can be discussed and interpreted as poetry and thus a legitimate way of expressing one's experiences and emotions (Kähmi, 2015). Some of the texts in our data display artistic freedom. They are written in an aphoristic or poetic style, with pictures and drawings on the side. In the light of theories on the therapeutic effects of art, writing may also have benefited the writers therapeutically. Indeed, according to Mertanen (2009), poetry helps writers to release and structure their own life stories, as well as to process their emotions.

My approach to the interpretation of metaphors is informed by Lakoff and Johnson's cognitive metaphor theory. According to cognitive metaphor theory, metaphors are an intrinsic part of all our thinking, not just a linguistic phenomenon (Lakoff & Johnson, 1980). Metaphors work in our everyday life by linking ideas and helping us understand. All this suggests a continuum between conventional metaphors, which are not commonly noticed, and so-called fresh metaphors. In consequence, also the seemingly common metaphors are worth exploring and should be viewed as meaningful and important attempts to communicate suffering. According to therapeutic writing researchers such as Bolton and Latham (2004), this is often the only way to illustrate experiences that are hard to verbalize.

Among the wealth of metaphors and similes in the material, I chose to focus on those referring to force and coercion, because I noticed that the most common metaphors used refer to totalitarian institutions such as a prison, army or concentration camp. Other widely used categories were animals and inanimate things.

Heaven and Hell

The same person tended to produce dramatically different accounts of different hospitals: one hospital could be described as heaven and another as hell. This juxtaposition sometimes seemed to work as a rhetorical means to create a humorous effect, and raises questions about the author's situation prior to the hospitalization:

> My main experience of being in hospital I call heaven and hell. […] First X.[9] In 1999. It was like from a horror movie, only much more scary. […] That hospital was the most agonizing place I have known thus far […] Years passed. Then one day I cracked up. […] Funnily enough, this time the hospital appeared as a perfect nest of happiness. The nurses were nice and fair, doctors downright geniuses, and there was rehabilitation available during my stay and afterwards. […] My mind and memory are filled with gratitude and relief. (SKS/MKM 385–386, patient, 1970s)

---

[9] As our data in regard to each hospital is too limited to make general statements about any particular hospital and our main purpose is to discuss phenomena related to psychiatric hospitals rather than particular hospitals, we have anonymized them here.

The Oppressive Institution: Prison, Concentration Camp or a Rubbish Dump

Many writers regard the mental health care system as a means to implement social control and stigmatization, rather than to provide individual care and rehabilitation. From their point of view, the function of the treatment culture and diagnoses in hospitals is to control the behaviour of the patients in the wards. Välimäki, Taipale, and Kaltiala-Heino (2001) and Kuosmanen, Hätönen, Malkavaara, Kylmä, and Välimäki (2007) have used the concept "deprivation of liberty" to describe methods that are used to control patients in psychiatric wards. The aim of these measures is to reduce risks, but they are also routinely used as part of the treatment. These methods include restrictions on leaving the ward and on communication, the confiscation of property, and various other coercive measures. Losing one's liberty can be understood as losing one's autonomy and self-ownership.

In some memories, the hospital is compared to a totalitarian institution and is represented as a prison or a concentration camp, or simply as a rubbish dump (see also Maanmieli 2018). According to research, this kind of comparison is a typical way of describing feelings of shame (Kaufman, 1989; Malinen, 2010). My own observations both in relation to this data and in poetry therapy suggest that restrictions affect the patients' thoughts about themselves and strengthen their belief in their own worthlessness. Prisons are not only a place one is confined to, but also a place where one loses one's dignity and self-ownership:

> This imprisonment in the isolation room started when I demanded my wallet and keys and I was told that they are not here. (SKS/MKM 404–413, patient, 1980s)

Prison metaphors point both to locked doors and strict rules and to a psychological condition of being unable to process what is happening or to find a way out of the anxiety (Maanmieli, 2018). Psychotic symptoms may make one feel that one is behind locked doors. For example, in one memory the writer describes "being double locked" due both to the staff's requirement to socialize and a panic attack:

> Then, shockingly, you are supposed to socialize with others after this treatment. I go into a kind of double lock (panic) I got drugs for it. (SKS/MKM 414-415, patient, no indication of the time of hospitalization)

According to previous research, psychiatric medication may increase the feeling of being in a cage, since it may block brain activity and reduce one's ability to function (Tandon, 2011; Wingo, Wingo, Harvey, & Baldessarini, 2009). One writer particularly describes the difficulty of remembering:

> I would have liked to process my relationship with my father in the hospital, but it was not done. I only got this strong medication that made me forget. (SKS 0416, patient, 1990s)

Portraying the hospital as a concentration camp rather than a prison highlights the inevitability and existential quality of the situation: one is sent to prison for committing a crime, but is sent to a concentration camp for qualities such as race or mental disability:

> My perceptions of mental hospitals are filled with horror, like Nazi concentration camps as seen by the victims. (SKS/MKM 273–277, patient, 1993–2006)

The patient who wrote the oldest memory in our data, referring to the 1930s, even claims that rather than prolonging the suffering of patients who have no hope of getting better, poisoning should be adopted as a hospital policy. He refers to the hospital as a rubbish dump, which summarizes his opinion that hospitals were useless and did not provide any relief for mental health problems. According to this writer, the staff were mostly uneducated and unpleasant, and the rules arbitrary. Although standards of care have changed substantially since the 1930s, also some of the most recent memories also portray the staff as treating mental patients as worthless and inhuman (Maanmieli, 2018).

Animals and Inanimate Things

Patients referred to animals a lot to describe their lack of power, the attitude of nurses towards them, or the effects of medication. One newly arrived patient describes how she perceived the other patients as animals made sick by the side effects of medication. Another patient perceived co-patients as furry animals in their cages. Comparisons to inanimate things were used in the oldest and newest memories alike. According to another one, being hospitalized felt like being a canned pineapple. In the oldest memory, the writer calls patients *society's rubbish*, but also some of the newest memories present the status of patients very negatively. One writer describes a nurse's hurtful behaviour through the following image:

> Shivering, I raised my hand towards a nurse. I was hoping she would help me stand up. Her reaction was somewhat disgusted. She recoiled as if I was a filthy animal. (SKS/MKM 482–486, patient, 2010s)

Here the writer uses both institutional and animal images to send a message about human nature:

> Mental hospital was a prison to me. The Doctors there are kings, the nurses are citizens, and the patients only slaves and jesters. We are never on the same level. Never! And I feel like throwing up, I really do, for the misuse of power! I would cry if I had tears. I would scream if I had a voice […] We surrender because it is our position in the mental hospital setting. We, patients, are like puppies, helpless puppies incapable of doing anything independently other than gnawing bones in the corner. MAN IS A WOLF WHO, WITH THE TASTE OF BLOOD IN HIS MOUTH, ATTACKS OTHERS WHEN THEY ARE AT THEIR WEAKEST. (SKS/MKM 387–389, patient, 2010s)

This writer sees the mental hospital as a kingdom that imprisons patients and makes them only slaves or jesters of the system. Using figurative language, he tries to convey the extent to which he experiences powerlessness and a lack of basic humanity and care. The image of man as a wolf with a taste of blood in his mouth emphasizes the perceived cruelty. Horrifying feelings of emptiness and strangeness underlie these kinds of expressions. For patients with a traumatic background, the hospital may become somewhere where the nightmarish experiences of childhood are repeated (Maanmieli, 2018). In the worst cases, the gulf between oneself and others becomes a chronic condition and way of perceiving oneself (Stolorow, 2008).

In their writing, patients report the staff's failure to listen, empathize or respect, strict arbitrary rules, the unnecessary use of force, and compulsory or over-strong medication. Through metaphorical expressions, they convey emotions related to these experiences. Research can bring these traumatic experiences and the patients' voices to the surface and open up the meanings of the metaphors used.

Many writers say that writing was essential to their recovery, both during and after hospitalization. The initiative to collect mental hospital memories may thus also have worked therapeutically for some and inspired them to write about the time they spent in hospital. Some studies suggest that simply writing down stressful events can improve health and increase the quality of life (Pennebaker & Seagal, 1999; Smyth & Delwyn, 2002). According to Gillie Bolton (1999), metaphors are windows through which we can reach areas of life that we have chosen to forget or marginalize. This collection has enabled the sharing of painful memories which, according to Bolton, is also safe: we can trust the writing hand, because it will not write anything that we are not ready to face.

Kirsi Heimonen: Researching Through Corporeal Attunement

As an artist-researcher with a background in dance and somatic movement practices, I am interested in how corporeality and movement appear in the written memories. For me, approaching the written memories of mental hospitals has meant immersing myself in the material, attuning to it with a subtle corporeal attention, and offering a kind of interpretation through movement in order to create corporeal insights into the memories. This approach belongs to artistic research, which is singular, trans-disciplinary and multi-medial by nature. It operates both in the field of art and in the field of research (Kirkkopelto, 2012; Schwab & Borgdorff, 2014). In artistic research, research takes place through art-making, which involves material thinking and thinking by doing. Artistic knowledge is reflexive knowledge that is equal to but separate from other forms of knowledge (Mersch, 2015; Rouhiainen, 2017). Thus, for example, performances are considered forms of knowledge and research outputs. They comprise methods, and form the content and research results, along with research articles. They do not, however, translate themselves into writing, as writing and moving exist in different realities (Heimonen, 2009).

As is common in artistic research, I draw on various disciplines, including the phenomenological approach, in which the focus is on the lived experience, the attitude of wonder and the human's interconnectedness with and within the world (Heimonen

& Rouhiainen, 2019; Merleau-Ponty, 2005/1945). I also draw on new materialism (Bennett, 2010; Coole & Frost, 2010).[10]

Artistic research deals with non-verbal processes, so the challenge lies in trying to articulate and communicate forms of knowing that are non-linguistic. However, I hope that writing about it can evoke intersubjective, corporeal experiences and offer an alternative approach to mental health research. This approach does not make value judgements of the memories. They are appreciated as such. The question of ethicality, however, is embedded in the art-making, since I inhabit and treat the memories in a particular way in and through corporeality. Hopefully, respect for each writer of the memories comes through in the artistic deeds. Here, I invite the reader to follow some traces of this methodological path, which can hopefully cast light on insights that have emerged within it.

Corporeal Attunement and Embodied Hauntology

The notion of attuning in and through corporeality permeates the whole process of researching. The main phases are reading the written material, visiting mental hospitals and realizing selected memories through movement. These phases are interlinked and overlap, and each one in turn sheds fresh light on the phenomenon. A particular attunement to listening through porous corporeality happens that resembles the notion of listening put forward by Jean-Luc Nancy, who writes how listening forms one's perceptible singularity, "to be *at the same time* outside and inside, to be open *from* without and *from* within" (Nancy, 2007/2002, p. 14).

The first stage for me in this particular process, what first caught my attention when reading the written material and attuning to it through corporeality, was the way in which some patients and visitors describe their attachment to the premises of the mental hospital. This suggested that the materiality and immateriality of the premises of a mental hospital are intertwined in human perception and feelings about them, and pointed to the patients' sensitivity to, e.g., the size, texture, colour or light of their sites. This oriented my selection of material and its exploration in and through movement. One example of the excerpts I picked out is:

> I was mentally prepared for my mother to scream and cry and be upset, but she was frighteningly calm, and as expressionless and pale as the hospital building itself. (SKS/MKM 339, daughter of a patient, 2000s)

The second important stage in my research path has been attuning to the premises of mental hospitals when myself visiting various of them in Finland with the research team. Walking inside those institutions, pausing and breathing the layers of histories sedimented in those spaces offered particular atmospheres that invited me to linger.

---

[10]The various approaches in new materialism have common features: they abandon the terminology of matter as an inert substance, recognize the plural, complex, relatively open process of materialization, and the immersion of humans with the productive contingencies of materiality (Coole & Frost, 2010).

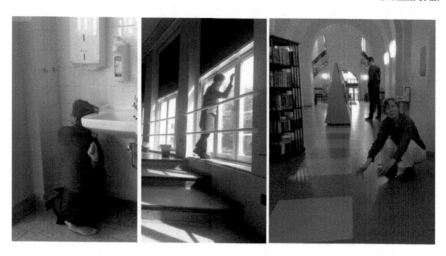

Fig. 10.1 Kirsi moving at the Material Cultures of Psychiatry conference in Hamburg (two images on the left by Sari Kuuva), and in an art event in a public library in Helsinki (by Karoliina Maanmieli)

So as the memory above suggests, I have lived the whiteness of the walls inside hospitals when walking along the corridors, and that has affected the way I have moved or written about the memories.

Thirdly, fleshing out some memories through movement in live dance events at conferences and art happenings has given me important opportunities to share the memories. On these occasions, my research colleagues have read aloud selected fragments of the memories as I have lived through them by moving (see Fig. 10.1). What has made those events unique has been the performance site, the participants, the time of day and corporeal conditions. Along with the movements, I have found myself speaking, repeating some words of the text and wondering about the place. A kind of continuation of the memories or an alternative path has emerged through moving and speaking, and my corporeality has been available for the moves and sentences to emerge.

This method of corporeal attuning ranges from reading the written memories to moving. This has led to my being haunted by the memories: some fragments of memories have overtaken me in everyday life—when walking, eating or sleeping— insisting that I pay attention to them. A slow, intense process keeps happening. This resonates with Lisa Blackman's (2015) notion of embodied hauntologies. According to Blackman, embodied hauntologies "work with traces, fragments, fleeting moments, gaps, absences, submerged narratives, and displaced actors and agencies" (Blackman, 2015, p. 26). Blackman also states that this kind of methodological orientation requires a mediated form of perception that exceeds conventional modes of perception. My commitment to a somatic method, the Skinner Releasing Technique (SRT), has intensified and cultivated the vulnerability of corporeality, and allowed memories to haunt me, and me to perceive things that are beyond conventional research methods.

Somatic Movement Practice as a Research Method

The porousness of corporeality, a particular kind of attunement and openness, a way of perceiving the world, is offered to me by the Skinner Releasing Technique, which has therefore affected how some memories haunt me. This somatic practice[11] has influenced everything I do: reading, writing, speaking, breathing and moving. The principles of the technique, such as letting go, multidirectional alignment, a watchful state, effortless effort and suppleness, have become embedded in corporeality, which has turned out to be an important way of approaching the writings (Dempster, 1996; Lepkoff, 1999). Letting go—the most important principle, with which all the others are interlocked—entails giving up one's habits and conventions, ranging from stiff muscles to ways of thinking, that prevent one from perceiving what is unfolding in each moment. It has brought an alertness that encourages one to question one's own actions.

The incorporation of the Skinner Releasing Technique has happened to me slowly over the years, and still it keeps unfolding, changing my corporeality, including my perspective on the world. Theatre practitioner and researcher Ben Spatz (2015) stresses how immersion in bodily practices brings insight, and argues for the embodied technique as knowledge. My orientation to the research material has emerged slowly—slowness is essential: listening, pausing and attuning to the written memories is about letting something emerge without pushing forward one's own agenda.

Affects Within Memories and Movement

Here are some excerpts from the memories that have haunted me, dwelled in this corporeality and that I have fleshed out through movement. In each performance, I "was caught up" (Blackman, 2012, p. 102) by them.

> In some wards, I paid attention to the wide corridors that gave rise to a feeling of space when walking there… and that brought imagination into play. (SKS/MKM 395, patient from the 1970s to the 2010s)

> During the three-month treatment period I couldn't sleep at all. I sat on the window sill in my room, I liked that, it was painted white, a broad concrete shelf. I watched the outside world till the early hours. Watching the falling snow brought a kind of beautiful fulfilment, it

---

[11] The Skinner Releasing Technique (SRT), a creative approach to movement training, was developed by Joan Skinner in the 1960s in the United States of America. Skinner is a former member of the Martha Graham and Merce Cunningham dance companies. SRT includes image-guided instructions to ease tension, promotes an effortless way of moving, and alignment with the whole self. It integrates technical and creative aspects in moving (Dempster, 1996; Eddy, 2016; Skura, 1990). In order to understand what this method is about, one needs to take part in lessons, to live it, since it is neither easy nor desirable to give a definition of a somatic practice (Reed & Whatley, 2009). Other somatic practices include Alexander, Klein and Feldenkreis techniques and Body Mind Centering. More information about SRT: http://www.skinnerreleasing.com/aboutsrt.html.

calmed down the accumulation of anxiety that was swirling around inside me. (SKS/MKM 483, patient, 2000s and 2010s)

These descriptions of corridors or snowfall can be taken as vital materiality that interweaves with the state of the writer; or we could say that those materialities and immaterialities create their state of being. Jane Bennett describes vital materiality as something that "captures an 'alien' quality of our flesh", and thus reminds humans of the "very *radical* character of the fractious kinship between the human and the nonhuman" (Bennett, 2010, p. 112).

These excerpts suggest a sensitive relationship between the experiencer and the environment. This kinship with the nonhuman may be intensified by the fact that the patients often report that nobody listens to them, or that they do not want to become acquainted with other patients. Because of their sensitive attachment to the physical environment, I have sensed the kinship between my corporeality and theirs. In my performances, each excerpt guided me to a particular spot or area on the site, like a corner, and that location offered its own architectural-material-atmospheric qualities, which have become part of the memory in question. The site, atmosphere and excerpts have all permeated the corporeality, and the contours of the corporeality have become blurred.

The corporeal attunement through memories and the physical locations in mental hospitals have created various atmospheres for exploration. The notion of atmosphere links together the relationship between human and nonhuman, as in the fragments above, and affects. Affects refer to the capacity of bodies to affect and be affected (Blackman, 2008); here, the bodies of patients, visitors, my body and the bodies of the spectators of these performances. Lisa Blackman's description of affect, which "is disclosed in atmospheres, fleeting fragments and traces, gut feelings and embodied reactions and in felt intensities and sensations" (Blackman, 2015, p. 25), resonates with this porous corporeality, since affect is transpersonal: it refers to processes of life and vitality that circulate and pass between bodies (Blackman, 2012). Affectivity is taken here as the ability of corporeality to mediate something of the atmosphere of mental hospitals through movement. The vagueness and yet the power of the notions of atmosphere and affect create space around the memories that transcends the individual experience, and makes it inseparable from the environment, including the treatment. Attuning to the fragments of memories means that the researcher is part of the research; there is no possibility of detachment. That concerns also embodied hauntologies and exploring affectivity (Blackman, 2015; Trivelli, 2015). However, the idea is not to take hold of the phenomenon and determine it, but to let oneself be taken up by it and live through it by moving.

Trusting corporeality gives no clear answers, since it is in constant flux. The knowledge that is produced through moving is partial, in a state of becoming, and unnamed (Heimonen, 2009). Hence, turning these written memories into physical movements and then writing about it entails paradoxes. First, shifting from writing to the realm of moving means moving beyond language while trying to share something of its qualities. Second, the attempt (here) to convey something of the dance by writing can be seen as betraying the reality of dancing since, as Lepecki (2006) puts it, wordlessness is not a defect of dance, but a way of being. Approaching writing by moving is neither translation nor representation. Instead, these paradoxes lead to a diverse group of non-representational methods and theory that seek ways to cope with more-than-human and more-than-textual, multisensory worlds. Rather than reporting and representing, "non-representational work aims to rupture, unsettle, animate and reverberate" (Vannini, 2015, p. 5). In my study, the notion of subjectivity here is not that of a fixed, self-contained subject but that of a becoming subject and human agency intertwined with materialities, as is argued, for example, in new materialism (Coole & Frost, 2010).

Performing Memories

One way to describe the sharing of memories through movement with audiences is the notion of corporeal empathy. Corporeal empathy shifts the focus from imagination, perception and rationality to recognizing feelings through corporeal experiences, valuing experiences and avoiding the dominance of rational knowledge (Aaltola, 2017). When I have moved excerpts from these written memories in public events, the reception has varied: sometimes the audience have been attentive and still, sometimes they have burst into laughter. Sometimes the atmosphere in the events has been somewhat hesitant, which has affected me, too. Often, spectators have approached me later. Researchers have been amazed how the moving of the memories brought out the corporeality and humanity of the writers. On one occasion, a spectator shared her own experiences in mental hospital and said that "everything you did was just like how people acted there". The corporeality has been open, allowing a range of reactions; some of the affects emerging from memories, movement or a site have triggered a response in spectators, and affects have moved through people and materials. Something is being presented through moving, since I am dealing "with forms of knowing that exceed rational, conscious experience" (Blackman, 2012, p. 24).

The method I have described here encourages researchers to approach their research material by pausing and listening to their corporeality, without preconceptions, letting the space and time create an atmosphere where questions, hunches and spontaneous reactions can all emerge.

Sari Kuuva: Psychiatric Hospitals as Emotional Communities—Fear, Topophilia and Topophobia in the Memories of the Children of the Staff

One unexpected part of our research data was the memories of people who had lived on hospital premises as children because their parents worked in the hospitals.

Particularly during the 1940s and the 1950s,[12] the staff in Finnish psychiatric hospitals frequently lived within the hospital grounds with their families, and this group of writers, the "hospital children" as I will call them, were mostly the offspring of nurses, but also of doctors and other groups. Most of the children had relatively similar living conditions, and they form a more homogeneous group than the other writers, patients, relatives and staff, who have more varied social and cultural backgrounds.

As I familiarized myself with the data, I noticed that those who had spent their childhood in the hospital observed their environment from perspectives that had not been so thoroughly investigated earlier as the experiences of patients or staff, and that there was little research literature on this issue (e.g. Arbaeus, 1993). The hospital children included descriptions of forbidden spaces in the hospital environments, and they were actually able to move around in their surroundings rather more freely than most adult members of their community. Therefore, the hospital children did not have fixed standpoints or attitudes to the otherwise hierarchically organized life, spaces and practices of psychiatric hospitals, but had got to know the hospital and the people living and working there through movement and play. What is interesting in the texts written by the hospital children are the connections between motion and emotion. As children frequently observe their environment from different perspectives from those of adults, their emotional experiences are different, too.

I have approached the hospital children's memories by focusing on their emotional content. My earlier studies have mainly focused on the cultural aspects of emotions (Kuuva, 2007, 2010, 2018). I assume that, compared to other children living in the countryside, or in residential areas like factories and military bases, as well as the other people who lived, worked and visited in mental hospitals, the children who lived in these hospitals formed their own special kind of emotional communities (cf. Rosenwein, 2006). To some extent, the emotional experiences of these children resemble the experiences of contemporary children living outside hospitals as well as the experiences of patients, staff and relatives in the context of hospitals, but there are also differences.

The key questions guiding my analysis are: (1) What kinds of emotions did the hospital children (who are now adults) experience when they moved in and around the hospitals? (2) What terms of emotion do the hospital children use explicitly when they describe their childhood experiences? (3) Which emotions are implicitly present in the texts, and how are these emotions constructed? (4) What kind of conceptual relationships are there between the most important emotions in the texts by the hospital children?

---

[12] Mental hospitals and their surroundings formed miniature hierarchical communities within society and the villages and municipalities they were placed in. Partly this was due to legislation, decrees and hospital rules, which, for example, until the 1950s, required that doctors and nurses live on the premises. After the Second World War, there was a severe shortage of mental nurses, and decent accommodation was an asset with which hospitals tried to attract medical staff. It was common for the staff to find their spouses among the hospital staff, and families with children lived in the hospital grounds from the 1940s to the early 1970s. Hospitals frequently had utilities like a bank, a shop, barbers' shops and day care on the premises (Nieminen, 2015; Tuovinen, 2009).

My method is conceptual analysis, and I focus especially on emotion concepts by analysing the ways in which emotions are present in the texts, either explicitly or implicitly. By studying the uses of emotion concepts I aim to clarify how emotional experiences are constructed in the texts (cf. e.g. Bal, 2002; Saariluoma, 2002; Wilson, 1963; Wittgenstein, 1953/2001). This approach is based on Wittgenstein's later philosophical investigations where it is argued that the meaning of concepts derives from their context whereby it is related to thematic and discourse analysis. For example, when studying the hospital children's experiences of fear or a sense of security, which are explicitly mentioned in their texts, I analyse the content associated with these concepts. In my analysis, fear and the sense of security are connected to the concepts of *topophilia* and *topophobia*, which are frequently used in cultural geography. Topophilia refers to a strong, positive emotional bond between a person and a place; topophobia refers to fear related to a certain place (Tuan, 1974/1990, 1977). Although these concepts are not explicitly used by the hospital children, both the fear and the sense of security described by them are repeatedly linked with mental hospitals as places. Therefore, it can be argued that notions relating to topophilia and topophobia are implicitly present in the hospital children's texts, and it is therefore reasonable to use these concepts in the analysis of these texts. The use of these concepts links the hospital children's memories to the perspectives of cultural geography. These concepts appear in the texts as emotional attitudes towards the childhood environment and the people and phenomena that were encountered there.

Fear, Topophilia and Topophobia

Fear is the most frequently used term of emotion in the texts of the children of the mental hospital staff, but its counter term, a sense of security, is also frequently mentioned. Typically, the hospital children say that they were not afraid to move around in the area of the hospital. This can be taken to contradict the assumption of people living outside hospitals that there was something frightening about the hospitals. As described by one writer in this group:

> We were relatively isolated in the grounds of the psychiatric hospital, where outsiders were not allowed. […] It seems that people living in town were almost so afraid of 'the fools' that they avoided us, too. (SKS/MKM 491, hospital child)

Living in hospital accommodation was stigmatizing. Emotions related to the stigma are processed in the writing, for example, by denying the fear and by emphasizing the feeling of security that derives from the communal life of the hospital.

Although fear is frequently denied, there are people and situations which are experienced as frightening. For example, the hospital children describe certain patients as aggressive, and it can be assumed that their aggressiveness aroused fear in the children. Also, the patients' screaming and certain psychiatric treatments, like electroshock therapy or lobotomy, made them afraid. Sometimes fear is implicitly present in the texts. For example, when the writers explain how the patients sometimes committed suicide, terms like fear or melancholy are not always explicitly used, but these emotions are present as descriptions of situations etched in the memory and in ideas about the heaviness of the atmosphere:

> At least twice someone drowned themselves in the pond in the summer... Once, during the celebration of Midsummer, we saw that one of the patients tried to jump into the bonfire. (SKS/MKM 535, hospital child)

> I remember the heaviness and sorrow that the parents experienced when a patient committed suicide or died. (SKS/MKM 345, hospital child)

In these citations, fear is not explicitly mentioned, but the context and the presence of death, which shocks and saddens the whole community, creates an atmosphere where fear is also continuously present. Suicides and death affect the staff and their children alike, and they undermine the children's sense of security both directly, when they witness suicide attempts, and indirectly, through the sadness of their parents which, according to the writers, often goes unexplained. In the mid-twentieth century, parents did not commonly discuss their emotions with their children or explain what had happened. The inexplicable emotional reactions of the adults thus sometimes frightened the children.

Fear is one of the strongest emotions, and it can alter the experience of place and change topophilia into topophobia (Koho, 2014; Tuan, 1974/1990, 1977). In the memories of the hospital children, this shift from topophilia to topophobia can be seen in the following lines:

> It felt quite safe to live there. Long after I had moved away from there, my mother called me and said that terrible things had happened near the hospital. A schoolchild had been killed at the very same bus stop where I used to wait for the bus, often alone. The person who did it was not found immediately, and the whole hospital was afraid. Then it turned out that the offender was a patient who had been regarded as harmless and had ground privileges. We knew many patients of this kind. (SKS/MKM 477, hospital child)

This shows how a place that was earlier felt to be safe suddenly becomes frightening when something unexpected happens.

While fear is a central emotion in the wider emotional community of a psychiatric hospital, what it consists of is different for different groups. For example, fears related to psychiatric treatments are different for patients, staff and their children. The fear of people living outside a psychiatric hospital is more abstract than the fear of people living within the hospital boundary: the outsiders' fear is not softened by positive emotions such as the sense of community and of security that the children experienced. It is therefore important to analyse what causes a particular emotional experience and how this experience is conceptually constructed.

Empathy

With reference to psychiatric hospitals and psychiatric care, an interesting feature is the children's ability to feel empathy. Through their observations, movement and play, they gain multiple perspectives and reflect situations from the perspective of their friends, parents and the patients, too. Although children do not know the details of different medical treatments, they observe the influence of these treatments on patients, and also on their own parents. For example, the hospital children noted how hard it sometimes was for their parents to witness the impact of lobotomies on their patients. The children also did not distinguish between patients and other people:

> All of us who spent our childhood and youth at the district hospital from the 1940s to the mid-1960s learnt to see the human mind as a subjective and experiential whole. We did not make much distinction between patients and non-patients. (SKS/MKM 217, hospital child)

The hospital children's texts show what complex emotional environments psychiatric hospitals were. They were not just places of psychiatric care but also places where people worked, lived and played. The childhoods of the children who lived there resemble the childhoods of agrarian children in general (cf. e.g. Gutman, 2013; Korkiakangas, 1996; Nieminen, 2015; Stearns, 2013; Toivola, 2005). Because of the emotional peculiarity of a psychiatric hospital, the children of the hospitals can offer new perspectives not only on the study of psychiatric care, but also on the study of emotions related to childhood.

Discussion

Our multidisciplinary approach, drawing on the history of psychiatry and various methods of cultural and artistic research, throws light on the numerous ways in which memories of mental hospitals can be interpreted, and how different approaches shape the knowledge that is gained from such memories. Our data offers a sketchy, yet important and unique window onto the ways in which mental and psychiatric hospitals are remembered today. In some cases, the memories also reveal how the writers' experiences still affect their lives, attitudes and their families and communities today. With our data collection method, the collection of written responses in collaboration with the Finnish Literature Society, we reached people beyond the usual reach of media representations and published autobiographies, for example. However, as severe mental health problems can limit people's access to language and as memories related to psychiatric disorders and treatments can be too hard or too painful to remember, the writing project only reached a limited number of people. With our research and the public events that we have organized to discuss our findings, however, we have sought to create spaces for the further remembering and sharing of memories.

Remembering breeds remembering, and the sharing of memories related to psychiatric hospitals can help heal wider cultural trauma related to institutionalization. The possibility of sharing memories through research and writing offers those who have experienced trauma the chance to voice experiences that cannot be discussed with families or in public, and also to express criticism without the fear that this might prevent the writer from getting proper treatment now or in the future. Psychiatric patients are especially vulnerable because they are so dependent on the health care system. Awareness of this is also evident in the fact that many writers emphasize that they are not bitter and do not wish to criticize anyone. Although a significant number wanted to remain anonymous, others positively wanted to have their memories filed in the archives under their own name.

It can be detected from the memories that many writers used the opportunity given by our call to both remember and to structure their memories in ways that could communicate their experiences to others. The memories reveal pain, anger, worry and remorse, but also gratitude, acceptance and hope. Many writers also commented on their writing: on the way they were (or were not) able to express their experiences and feelings, on the opportunity to write about the memories and on what they had written. This points to the fact that, as the historian Joan Scott (1991) has put it, experience is an interpretation of events that is itself in want of interpretation. Our aim in this article has been to provide insights into different ways of reading, relating to and producing knowledge about the heterogeneous body of memories of mental hospitals. This can create a space for sharing further memories, and it can encourage people to think about their own relation to an institution and also share painful, joyful and contradictory memories related to institutions that have brought people together in so many ways and in such different roles.

The different ways of engaging in dialogue with the memories offered in this chapter suggest that it is not only through language and discourse that memories work on the one who remembers and the one who reads and interprets those memories. The memories engage and can be interpreted affectively, and reading the memories can also affect the reader well beyond language: they are experienced—and their meaning can be interpreted and understood—through extra-lingual means such as dance. The different ways of engaging—thematically, corporeally, conceptually, theoretically— with the texts reveal the multilayeredness of the memories.

Karoliina Maanmieli's examination of the figurative expressions in patients' testimonies shows how metaphors and similes are used to convey the strong emotions related to negative and traumatic experiences. Sari Kuuva's approach brings to light a group of people whom we do not customarily associate with mental hospitals: children who grew up at the hospital provide interesting insights into the life of hospital communities. Their responses about childhood in the hospital also show that the emotional burden of the parents' workplace affected their homes. They are now yet another group of people who are affected by the ways in which psychiatric care is organized, and they deserve further study. Their emergence also points to the further and wider cultural effects of psychiatric care.

Kirsi Heimonen's approach takes us beyond discursive and representational ways of being in the world. Emphasizing the bodily, corporeal relation to the materiality of the world, her approach helps us to understand the richness of experience that lies beyond words and manifests itself in relation to the nonhuman. For those relying on language as the primary means of making sense of others and ourselves, the way she reads the writings with, in and through corporeality and dance provides a lens to the possible reality that lies beyond language and discourse. It reminds us that not all aspects of illness, experience and treatment are translatable into concepts and words.

The different methods complement each other, yet their co-presence also points to each one's limitations. The ways of reading the memories presented here seek to evoke understanding and empathy, in a way re-humanize people in mental hospitals, a goal that is in line with Dainius Puras' (2018) call for a change of paradigm to one that prioritizes human rights in the planning of health services. The experiences and viewpoints presented in our data point both to the failings in treatment from the point of view of staff and patients, and to the attitudes and emotions that support or prevent change. This type of research highlights embodied and corporeal experiences within psychiatry and sets psychiatry in its wider cultural context. It also points to the perhaps unforeseen effects on unforeseen groups of people, such as children brought up at the hospital, and may increase awareness of the range of experiences related to psychiatric care.

This has also been the purpose of the public events we have organized, where we have shared our research with the public, and the writing workshops that Karoliina has developed inspired by the first public event in 2017 where Kirsi danced some memories. In the discussion that followed, the audience reported that the dance made the memories more touching and accessible, and aroused feelings of empathy towards the patients. This inspired Karoliina to create a writing workshop based on traumatic memories. She selected parts of the patients' most painful memories, which the participants read and then wrote down their own imaginary, mental hospital memory. The texts were then used for reference in the discussion. The participants reported that the workshop helped them to relate to the patients' experiences and to recognize the need for kindness at times of crisis. This method could be implemented in professional education and guidance to help nurses understand their patients' experiences. The dance performance and creative writing workshop are only two examples of the numerous ways in which creative methods can be used to develop psychiatric care and raise awareness and empathy towards people who suffer from mental health problems and their treatment.

Conclusion

The study of psychiatric care is often guided by strong and established cultural metaphors, narratives and imageries. However, the goal of study should not just be to repeat and confirm what is already known (cf. Pietikäinen, 2013). New perspectives, such as those that open up from the testimonies of those who lived in psychiatric hospitals as children, can generate new research questions and help create a richer understanding of the social, cultural and economic significance of the hospitals. Historical study shows the consistencies and inconsistencies in the treatment and organization of psychiatric care. Approaches from the perspective of creative, artistic and cultural studies can reveal new aspects of experiences that are difficult to convey and verbalize. Attention to the body, affects and emotions can help generate both new practices, new research questions and new ways of engaging the public with the results of academic research.

Funding The research has been funded by the Kone Foundation in 2017–2021.

Appendix 1 Our Call for Memories

Memories and Experiences of the Mental Hospital
Collection of memories from Oct. 15, 2014 to May 31, 2015 (later extended to September 30, 2015)

In one way or another, mental hospitals have been part of many Finnish peoples' lives. Thousands have been treated in them. Many have worked in them, and many have visited their friends or family members in them. The patients and staff members of the hospitals may also have been part of many local peoples' lives.

We are now collecting memories related to mental hospitals. First experiences related to the hospital are often strong. For the patients and the staff mental hospitals, however, can be a site of everyday life. We are also interested in such descriptions as well as local people's memories and experiences of mental hospitals and their functions.

Write about your experiences! You may use the questions below:

- Have you been treated in a mental hospital? What kind of memories do you have of this period, treatments, staff, other patients or the locality? Tell us about your experiences.
- How did you fell about the ward you were in? What kind of treatment did you receive? What kind of rehabilitation was available? Were you heard? What was the most meaningful encounter for you in the hospital?
- What was the everyday life like in the hospital? What about celebrations? How did you keep in contact with your family, friends or relatives? Did you have visitors? How did it feel to receive them?
- Have you been a member of staff in a mental hospital or have you worked in one? Tell us about your experiences.
- Has your family member (e.g. your spouse, parent, child or sibling), relative, girl or boy friend, friend or acquaintance been treated or worked in a hospital? Tell us about your memories.
- How was it to live in or near a mental hospital? How has the hospital affected your own life or the environment or locality?
- How have your personal experiences of mental hospitals affected your earlier ideas about mental hospitals or their operation?
- Have you noticed changes in the operation of a mental hospital in the long run? How have you experienced these changes? Tell us about your observations and experiences.
- You can also describe the hospital as a physical environment. What was the building like? How did it look inside? What were the surroundings like? How did it feel to travel to the hospital or to visit one? How did it feel to leave the hospital?
- What did the hospital mean to you? Your experience is important.

The collection is organized by researcher Saara Jäntti and the Network of Cultural Studies in Mental Health at the University of Jyväskylä together with the Finnish Literature Society.

The writings will be archived in the Finnish Literature Society for researchers. You can also send us photos or recordings related to the mental hospital or life in them or use them to refresh your memory.

Guidelines
Write in your own language and style. You can also record your memories or interview a person who has stories, memories or experiences related to mental hospitals. Your reply must be accompanied by your own and your possible interviewee's consent to store the material you

send to the collection with your name or a pseudonym in the archives of the Finnish Literature Society.

Familiarize yourself with the guidelines for archiving in the Finnish Literature Society's archives www.finlit.fi/luovutus_ja_keruuohjeet.

Send us your writing by May 31, 2015

- by using the online form at www.finlit.fi/mielisairaalat or
- by post at Suomalaisen kirjallisuuden seura, kirjallisuusarkisto, PL 259, 00171 Helsinki, write "Mental hospitals" on the envelop or
- by email as an attachment to keruu@finlit.fi with the subject title "Mental Hospitals".

There will be a lottery of books for those who reply.

Further information: Finnish Literature Society, phone: 0201131240, keruu@finlit.fi

Saara Jäntti, saara.jantti@jyu.fi

References

Archived Material

SKS/MKM The Archives of the Finnish Literature Society, Literature and Cultural History Collections. Muistoja ja kokemuksia mielisairaalasta. Muistitiedon keruu 2014-2015.

Literature

Aaltola, E. (2017). Ruumiillinen empatia. In E. Aaltola & S. Keto (Eds.), *Empatia. Myötäelämisen tiede* (pp. 74–91). Helsinki: Into.

Achté, K., & Alanen, Y. O. (1991). *150 vuotta psykiatriaa: Lapinlahden sairaalan historia 1841-1991.* [Klaukkala]: Recallmed.

Alanko, A. (2017). *Improving mental health care: Finnish mental health policy rationale in the era of dehospitalisation.* Helsinki: University of Helsinki.

Arbaeus, K. (1993). Att berätta sin barndom. Teoksessa: Alf Arvidsson (red.), *Muntligt berättande. Verklighetskonstruktion och samhällsspegel* (pp. 47–60). Etnologiska institutionen: Umeå universität.

Bal, M. (2002). *Travelling concepts in the humanities. A rough guide.* Toronto: University of Toronto Press.

Bennett, J. (2010). *Vibrant matter: A political ecology of things.* Durham and London: Duke University Press.

Blackman, L. (2008). *The body: The key concepts.* Oxford, New York: Berg.

Blackman, L. (2012). *Immaterial bodies: Affect, embodiment, mediation.* London, California, New Delhi, Singapore: Sage.

Blackman, L. (2015). Researching affect and embodied hauntologies: Exploring an analytics of experimentation. In B. Timm Knudsen & C. Stage (Eds.), *Affective methodologies: Developing cultural research strategies for the study of affect* (pp. 25–44). Basingstoke, Hampshire and New York, NY: Palgrave Macmillan.

Bolton, G. (1999). "Every poem breaks a silence that had to be overcome": The therapeutic power of poetry writing. *Feminist Review, 62,* 118–133. https://doi.org/10.1080/014177899339225.

Bolton, G., & Latham, J. (2004). Every poem breaks a silence that had to be overcome: The therapeutic role of poetry writing. In G. Teoksessa Bolton, S. Howlett, C. Lago, & J. K. Wright (Eds.), *Writing cures: An introductory handbook of writing in counseling and therapy* (pp. 106–122). London: Routledge.

Coole, D., & Frost, S. (2010). *New materialisms: Ontology, agency, and politics.* Durham and London: Duke University Press.

Davies, K. (2001). "Silent and censured travellers"? Patient's narratives and patients' voices: Perspectives on the history of mental illness since 1948. *The Social History of Medicine, 14*(2), 267–292.

De Young, M. (2015). *Encyclopedia of asylum therapeutics, 1750-1950s.* Jefferson, NC: McFarland.

Dempster, E. (1996). The releasing aesthetic. An interview with Joan Skinner. *Writings on Dance, 14,* 16–26.

Eddy, M. (2016). *Mindful movement: The evolution of the somatic arts and conscious action.* Bristol and Chicago: Intellect.

Fuchs, T. (2013). Depression, intercorporeality and interaffectity. *The Journal of Conciousness Studies, 7*(8), 219–238.

Gutman, M. (2013). The physical spaces of childhood. In P. S. Fass (Ed.), *The Routledge history of childhood in the western world* (pp. 249–266). London and New York: Routledge.

Heimonen, K. (2009). *Sukellus liikkeeseen–liikeimprovisaatio tanssimisen ja kirjoittamisen lähteenä.* Helsinki: Theatre Academy.

Heimonen, K., & Rouhiainen, L. (2019). Notes on and examples of embodiment in artistic research of dance and performance. In V. L. Midgelow, J. Bacon, P. Kramer & R. Hilton (Eds.), *Researching (in/as) motion: A resource collection.* Helsinki: Theatre Academy of the University of the Arts Helsinki. https://nivel.teak.fi/adie/topics/somatics-embodiment-and-subjectivity/.

Hélen, I., Hämäläinen, P., & Metteri, A. (2011). Komplekseja ja katkoksia – psykiatrian hajaantuminen suomalaiseen sosiaalivaltioon. In I. Hélen (Ed.), *Reformin pirstaleet. Mielenterveyspolitiikka hyvinvointivaltion jälkeen* (pp. 11–69). Tampere: Vastapaino.

Hirvonen, H. (2014). *Suomalaisen psykiatriatieteen juuria etsimässä: Psykiatria tieteenä ja käytäntönä 1800-luvulta vuoteen 1930.* Joensuu: University of Eastern Finland.

Holma, J. M. (1999). Psykoosi narratiivina. In J. Haarakangas & J. Seikkula (Eds.), *Psykoosi – uuteen hoitokäytäntöön* (pp. 206–219). Tampere: Kirjayhtymä.

Holmes, D., et al. (2004). The mentally ill and social exclusion: A critical examination of the use of seclusion from the patient's perspective. *Issues in Mental Health Nursing, 25*(6), 559–578.

Huttunen, M., & Javanainen, M. (2004). *Lääkkeet mielen hoidossa.* Helsinki: Duodecim.

Hyvönen, J. (2008). *Suomen psykiatrinen hoitojärjestelmä 1990-luvulla historian jatkumon näkökulmasta.* Kuopio: Kuopion yliopisto.

Jäntti, S. (2012). *Bringing madness home. Janet Frame's Faces in the water, Bessie Head's A question of power and Lauren Slater's Prozac diary.* Doctoral dissertation, University of Jyväskylä, Jyväskylä.

Kähmi, K. (2015). Kirjoittaminen on tie minuun, minusta sinuun: ryhmämuotoinen kirjoittaminen ja metaforien merkitys psykoosia sairastavien kirjallisuusterapiassa. Väitöskirja, Jyväskylän yliopisto.

Kärkkäinen, J. (2004). *Onnistuiko psykiatrian yhdentyminen somaattiseen hoitojärjestelmään?.* Helsinki: Stakes.

Kaufman, G. (1989). *The psychology of shame. Theory and treatment of shamebased syndromes.* New York: Springer.

Keski-Valkama, A. (2010). *The use of seclusion and mechanical restraint in psychiatry. A persistent challenge over time.* PhD Thesis, University of Tampere.

Kirkkopelto, E. (2012). Inventiot ja instituutiot: Taiteellisen tutkimuksen kritiikistä [Inventions and institutions: On the critique on artistic research]. *Synteesi, 3*(2012), 89–96.

Kirmayer, L. (2001). Broken narratives: Clinical encounters and the poetics of illness experience. In C. Mattingly & L. Garro (Eds.), *Narrative and the cultural construction of illness and healing* (pp. 153–180). Berkeley: University of California Press.

Koho, S. (2014). Hyväksikäytetyn lapsen paikka ja maisema Maria Peuran romaanissa on rakkautes ääretön. In T. Saresma & S. Jäntti (Eds.), *Maisemassa*, Nykykulttuurin tutkimuskeskuksen julkaisuja 115 (pp. 159–190). Jyväskylä: Jyväskylän yliopisto.

Koivisto, K., Janhonen, S., & Väisänen, L. (2004). Patients' experiences of being helped in an inpatient setting. *Journal of Psychiatric and Mental Health Nursing, 11*(3), 268–275.

Kontio, R., Joffe, G., Putkonen, H., Kuosmanen, L., Hane, K., Holi, M. & Välimäki, M. (2012). Seclusion and restraint in psychiatry: Patients' Experiences and practical suggestions on how to improve practices and use alternatives. *Perspectives in Psychiatric Care, 48*(1), 16–24.

Korkeila, J. (1998). *Perspectives on the public psychiatric services in Finland: Evaluating the deinstitutionalisation process*. Helsinki: Stakes.

Korkiakangas, P. (1996). *Muistoista rakentuva lapsuus. Agraarinen perintö lapsuuden työnteon ja leikkien muistelussa*. Helsinki: Suomen Muinaismuistoyhdistys.

Kuosmanen, L. (2009). *Personal liberty in psychiatric care—Towards Service User Involvement*. University of Turku. http://urn.fi/URN:ISBN:978-951-29-3840-7.

Kuosmanen, L., Hätönen, H., Malkavaara, H., Kylmä, J., & Välimäki, M. (2007). Deprivation of liberty in psychiatric hospital care: The patient's perspective. *Nursing Ethics, 14*(5), 597–607.

Kuuva, S. (2007). *Content-based approach to experiencing visual art*. Doctoral dissertation, University of Jyväskylä, Jyväskylä.

Kuuva, S. (2010). *Symbol, Munch and creativity: Metabolism of visual symbols*. Doctoral dissertation, University of Jyväskylä, Jyväskylä.

Kuuva, S. (2018). Mielisairaalan varjoista. Nostalgia ja melankolia mielisairaala-alueella asuneiden lapsuusmuistoissa. *J@rgonia, 16*(31), 12–41.

Lakoff, G., & Johnson, M. (1980). *Metaphors we live by*. Chicago: The University of Chicago Press.

Lepecki, A. (2006). *Exhausting dance: Performance and the politics of movement*. New York: Routledge.

Lepkoff, D. (1999). What is release technique? *Movement Research Performance, 19*, 2–5.

Maanmieli, K. (2018). Suomalaiset käenpesät. Väkivallan metaforat ja traumakokemuksen kuvaus mielisairaalamuistoissa. *Psykoterapia, 37*(1), 37–48.

Malinen, B. (2010). *The nature, origins, and consequences of Finnish shame-proneness. A grounded theory study*. Doctoral Dissertation, University of Helsinki.

Merleau-Ponty, M. (2005/1945). *Phenomenology of perception*. London: Routledge.

Mersch, D. (2015). *Epistemologies of aesthetics* (L. Radosh, Trans.). Zurich-Berlin: Diaphanes.

Mertanen, H. (2009). Poeettinen ja metaforinen kieli hoitotyössä. In J. Ihanus (Ed.), *Sanat että hoitaisimme. Terapeuttinen kirjoittaminen* (pp. 233–254). Helsinki: Duodecim.

Mikkola, M., Rintanen, H., Nuorteva, L., Kovasin, M., & Erhola, M. (2015). *Valtakunnallinen sosiaali- ja terveydenhuollon laitospaikkaselvitys*. [Helsinki]: Terveyden ja hyvinvoinnin laitos.

Moon, B. L. (2007). *The role of metaphor in art therapy: Theory, method, and experience*. Springfield, IL: Charles C. Thomas Publisher.

Nancy, J.-L. (2007/2002). *Listening* (C. Mandell, Trans.). New York: Fordham University Press.

Nieminen, A. (Ed.). (2015). *Piirin lapset kertovat. Elämä Törnävän sairaalan yhteisössä 1930–1970-luvuilla*. Seinäjoki: Etelä-Pohjanmaan terveydenhuollon perinneyhdistys ry.

Parpola, A. (2013). *Toivo/Häpeä. Psykiatria modernissa Suomessa*. Keuruu: Otavan kirjapaino Oy.

Pennebaker, J. W., & Seagal, J. D. (1999). Forming a story: The health benefits of narrative. *Journal of Clinical Psychology, 55*(10), 1243–1254.

Pietikäinen, P. (2013). *Hulluuden historia*. Helsinki: Gaudeamus.

Pietikäinen, P. (2015). *Madness: A history*. London: Routledge.

Pöysä, J. (2015). *Lähiluvun tieto. Näkökulmia kirjoitetun muistelukerronnan tutkimukseen*. Helsinki: Suomen Kansantietouden tutkijain Seura.

Pūras, D. (2018, September 20). *Mental health and human rights: A need for the paradigm shift*. Presentation at the 7th Qualitative Research on Mental Health conference, Berlin.

Reed, S., & Whatley, S. (2009). The universities and somatic inquiry: The growth of somatic movement dance education in Britain. In M. Eddy (Ed.), *Mindful movement: The evolution of the somatic arts and conscious action* (pp. 149–163). Bristol and Chicago: Intellect.

Rissanen, A. (2018a). *Silmitön ja väkivaltainen: Erään mielisairaalapotilaan ura 1900-luvulla.* Historian ja etnologian laitoksen tutkijat ry, Jyväskylän yliopisto.

Rissanen, A. (2018b). Treatment and rehabilitation: Patients at work in Finnish mental institutions. In T. Laine-Frigren, J. Eilola, & M. Hokkanen (Eds.), *Encountering crises of the mind: Madness, culture and society, 1200s-1900s* (pp. 196–221). History of Science and Medicine Library, 57. Brill.

Rosenwein, B. H. (2006). *Emotional communities in the early middle ages.* New York: Cornell University Press.

Rouhiainen, L. (2017). On the singular and knowledge in artistic research. In J. Kaila, A. Seppä, & H. Slager (Eds.), *Futures of artistic research: At the intersection of Utopia, academia and power* (pp. 143–153). Helsinki: The Academy of Fine Arts, Uniarts Helsinki.

Saariluoma, P. (2002). Does classification explicate the contents of concepts? In I. Pyysiäinen & V. Anttonen (Eds.), *Current approaches in the cognitive science of religion* (pp. 229–259). London: Continuum.

Salo, M. (1992). *Luonnosta laitoksiin: Hulluuden muodonmuutokset ja mielisairaalalaitoksen vakiintuminen: tapaustutkimus julkisen mielisairaalahoidon synnystä ja vakiintumisesta Englannissa.* [Helsinki]: Sosiaali- ja terveyshallitus: VAPK-kustannus -distributor].

Salo, M. (1996). *Sietämisestä solidaarisuuteen: Mielisairaalareformit Italiassa ja Suomessa.* Tampere: Vastapaino.

Salokangas, R., Saarinen, S., & Honkonen, T. (1997). Psykiatristen sairaansijojen väheneminen ja skitsofreniapotilaiden selviytyminen. Kotiutettujen skitsofreniapotilaiden hoito. *Suomen Lääkärilehti, 52*(24), 2659–2667.

Savolainen, U. (2015). *Muisteltu ja kirjoitettu evakkomatka. Tutkimus evakkolapsuuden muistelukerronnan poetiikasta.* Vantaa: Multiprint.

Schwab, M., & Borgdorff, H. (2014). Introduction. In M. Schwab & H. Bogdorff (Eds.), *The exposition of artistic research: Publishing art in academia.* Leiden: Leiden University Press.

Scott, J. (1991). The evidence of experience. *Critical Inquiry, 17*(4), 773–797.

Shorter, E. (2009). *Before Prozac: The troubled history of mood disorders in psychiatry.* Oxford and New York: Oxford University Press.

Skura, S. (1990). Releasing dance: Interview with Joan Skinner. *Contact Quarterly, 15*(3), 11–18.

Smyth, J. M., & Delwyn, C. (2002). Translating research into practice: Potential of expressive writing in the field. In S. J. Lepore & J. M. Smyth (Eds.), *The writing cure: How expressive writing promotes health and emotional well-being* (pp. 257–278). Washington, DC: American Psychological Association.

Spatz, B. (2015). *What a body can do: Technique as knowledge, practice as research.* Abingdon: Routledge.

Stearns, P. (2013). Childhood emotions in western history. In P. S. Fass (Ed.), *The Routledge history of childhood in the western world* (pp. 158–173). London, New York: Routledge.

STM [Sosiaali- ja terveysministeriö]: Plan for mental health and substance abuse work. Proposals of the Mieli 2009 working group to develop mental health and substance abuse work until 2015. Reports of the Ministry of Social Affairs and Health, Finland 2009, 3.

Stolorow, R. D. (2008). The contextuality and existentiality of emotional trauma: Psychoanalytic dialogues. *The International Journal of Relational Perspectives, 18*(1), 113–123.

Stone, B. (2004). Towards a writing without power: Notes on the narration of madness. *Auto/Biography Studies, 12,* 16–32.

Tandon, R. (2011). Antipsychotics in the treatment of schizophrenia: An overview. *Journal of Clinical Psychiatry, 72,* 4–8.

Toivola, R. (2005). *Moision lapset: muistoja Moision sairaalan alueella 1900-luvun puolivälissä asuneiden lasten elämästä.* Helsinki: [Ritva Toivola].

Törrönen, S. (1978). *50 vuotta työtä mielenterveyden hyväksi.* [Papinsalmi]: Mielisairaanhuoltopirien liitto.

Trivelli, E. (2015). Exploring a 'remembering crises': 'Affective attuning' and assemblaged archive' as theoretical frameworks and research methodologies. In B. Timm Knudsen & C. Stage (Eds.),

Affective methodologies: Developing cultural research strategies for the study of affect (pp. 119–139). Basingstoke, Hampshire and New York, NY: Palgrave Macmillan.

Tuan, Y.-F. (1974/1990). *Topophilia: A study of environmental perception, attitudes, and values.* With a new preface by the author. New York: Columbia University Press.

Tuan, Y.-F. (1977). *Space and place: The perspective of experience.* Minneapolis: University of Minnesota Press.

Tuovinen, S. L. (2009). *Inhimillinen Nikkilä: Helsingin suuri mielisairaala Sipoossa 1914-1999.* [Helsinki]: Helsingin kaupungin terveyskeskus.

Välimäki, M., Taipale, J., & Kaltiala-Heino, R. (2001). Deprivation of Liberty in psychiatric treatment: A finnish perspective. *Nursing Ethics, 8*(6), 522–532. https://doi.org/10.1177/096973300 100800606.

Vannini, P. (2015). Non-representational research methodologies: An introduction. In P. Vannini (Ed.), *Non-representational methodologies: Re-envisioning research* (pp. 1–18). New York: Routledge.

Vuorela, M., & Aalto, I. (2011). Häpeäleima tekee elämästä raskaan. In J. Korkeila, K. Joutsenniemi, E. Sailas, & J. Oksanen (Eds.), *Irti häpeäleimasta* (pp. 32–37). Bookwell Oy: Porvoo.

Wilson, J. (1963). *Thinking with concepts.* Cambridge: Cambridge University Press.

Wingo, A. P., Wingo, T. S., Harvey, P. D., & Baldessarini, R. J. (2009). Effects of lithium on cognitive performance: A meta-analysis. *The Journal of Clinical Psychiatry, 70*(11), 1588–1597.

Wittgenstein, L. (1953/2001). *Philosophical investigations.* Oxford: Blackwell.

Skinner Releasing Technique. http://www.skinnerreleasing.com/aboutsrt.html.

Chapter 11
Conclusion: Qualitative Research in Mental Health: Reflections on Research Questions, Methods and Knowledge

Carla Willig and Maria Borcsa

Abstract This chapter reflects on the use of qualitative research methodology in the studies described in this volume. Although all studies were concerned with the ways in which meaning is negotiated, modified or reproduced when people engage with phenomena that are relevant to mental health, they deployed a wide range of research designs including textual analysis (including various types of discourse analysis; linguistic interactional analysis; emotional textual analysis), theme-focused types of analysis (including grounded theory; thematic analysis; metasynthesis), reflexive methods (including autoethnography; interpersonal process recall; corporeal attunement and hauntology) as well as phenomenological approaches. To help readers differentiate between these approaches and to clarify their purpose and rationale, we present a systematic reflection on the types of research question they address, the methods of data collection and analysis they utilise, the voice and style in which they present their findings, and the type of insights they can generate. We also pose the question of what makes qualitative research 'research' and argue that despite their differences, all studies were designed to increase our understanding of the social processes that underpin 'mental health' and to contribute to the literature in the field. The chapter concludes with a discussion of future directions and challenges for qualitative mental health research.

Keywords Qualitative mental health research · Research questions · Qualitative research design · Diversity in qualitative research · Textual analysis · Theme-focused analysis · Reflexive methods · Phenomenological approaches

The chapters included in this book share a commitment to increasing our understanding of the social processes that underpin 'mental health' through the use of

C. Willig (✉)
Department of Psychology, City, University of London, London, UK
e-mail: C.Willig@city.ac.uk

M. Borcsa
Institute of Social Medicine, Rehabilitation Sciences and Healthcare Research, University of Applied Sciences Nordhausen, Nordhausen, Germany
e-mail: borcsa@hs-nordhausen.de

© Springer Nature Switzerland AG 2021
M. Borcsa and C. Willig (eds.), *Qualitative Research Methods in Mental Health*,
https://doi.org/10.1007/978-3-030-65331-6_11

qualitative research methods. The studies presented are all, in one way or another, concerned with meaning-making and with the ways in which meaning is negotiated, modified or reproduced when people engage with phenomena that are relevant to mental health. Within that shared endeavour, different methodological approaches can be employed, and the chapters in this book showcase a wide range of qualitative research designs that can help shed light on the processes involved in shaping experiences relevant to mental health. These include varieties of textual analysis (including various types of discourse analysis; linguistic interactional analysis; emotional textual analysis), theme-focused types of analysis (including grounded theory; thematic analysis; metasynthesis), reflexive methods (including autoethnography; interpersonal process recall; corporeal attunement and hauntology) as well as phenomenological approaches. And although most of the studies used qualitative interviews to generate their data, there are also examples of alternative forms of data collection such as the use of written accounts, personal journals, published accounts, secondary data, and focus groups, as well as innovative forms of interviewing including the walking interview and interpersonal process recall in multi-actor therapies. We hope that our readers have been stimulated by the chapters included in this volume, and that the richness and diversity of the qualitative approaches showcased here have provided inspiration and motivation to those planning to conduct research in this field of study.

Four Types of Research Question

We do realise, however, that such diversity and multiplicity of approaches can feel like a lot to handle, and that being exposed to such variety may raise questions about how to choose between them. In what follows, we hope to clarify how the different approaches presented in the chapters relate to one another and how researchers may best differentiate between different types of methods so as to enable them to make meaningful choices.

One helpful way of grouping methodological approaches is on the basis of the types of research questions they are designed to address (see Table 11.1)[1]. For example, a common type of research question seeks information about the presence and content of theoretically derived constructs in the data. Such constructs can reference cognitive (e.g. beliefs, attitudes, perceptions) as well as more social, process-oriented (e.g. communication styles, interactive patterns) phenomena. For example, Sargent and Abela's (Chapter 2) research used thematic analysis to extract and represent psychiatrists' perceptions of schizophrenia from interview data, and Krivzov et al. (Chapter 3) used metasynthesis to identify different kinds of therapeutic processes evident in published psychotherapy case studies. This type of research question pre-supposes the relevance of the construct which informs the search for

---

[1] Please note that as some chapters discuss several studies, there may be reference to more than one type of research question in any one chapter.

Table 11.1 Types of research questions, examples from the chapters and methods

Types of research question	Examples	Methods
Type 1: *What is there? What is going on?*	What are psychiatrists' perceptions of schizophrenia and recovery from schizophrenia? What are the therapeutic processes that characterise treatment of medically unexplained symptoms?	Thematic analysis; metasynthesis
Type 2: *What is it like to experience X? What does this experience mean to the person?*	How do forensic psychiatric clients experience transitioning from hospital to living in the community? What is it like to be diagnosed with cancer? What does it mean to live with terminal cancer?	Autoethnography; phenomenological methods; grounded theory; metasynthesis
Type 3: *How is an experience constructed through language?*	How is the experience of living with cancer (or of childbirth, or unemployment, or mental health problems, or 'being at risk') constructed through language? What are the dominant discourses in circulation, and what are their implications for how people can experience these events?	Foucauldian discourse analysis; critical discourse analysis; linguistic interactional analysis
Type 4: *What lies behind that which presents itself?*	What drives the demand for certain types of mental health diagnoses? Which emotions are difficult to access and how may they be expressed through people's accounts of their experience of living in a mental hospital?	Emotional textual analysis; Dialogical analysis: figurative language focus and conceptual analysis with a focus on implicit emotional content; corporeal attunement and hauntology

relevant themes (in our examples, 'perceptions', and 'therapeutic process'), and it demonstrates a commitment to the idea that aspects of social reality can be captured through research. Such research draws upon existing knowledge of the phenomenon under investigation and builds upon existing research in the field to expand the knowledge base.

A second type of research question concerns itself with the nature and quality of particular experiences, seeking to capture their texture and meaning so that they can be better understood. For example, Kinney (Chapter 4) used walking interviews to obtain data that could shed light on participants' experiences of transitioning from a forensic psychiatric hospital to the community, and Willig (Chapter 5) used autoethnography as well as hermeneutic phenomenology to gain a deeper under-standing of the lived experience of cancer. This type of research question seeks to produce phenomenological knowledge to enable people who have not had that partic-ular experience to obtain some insight into its nature and quality. Phenomenological research questions are based upon the assumption that it is possible to capture and communicate the meaning and texture of experience in ways that makes it at least somewhat accessible to those who have not had the experience themselves.

A third type of research question focuses on the role of language in shaping human experience. Here, the focus is on how experience is talked about, and what this might tell us about its construction and possibilities. Methods used to address this type of research question involve fine-grained analysis of language and language usage. For example, Willig (Chapter 5) and Challenor et al. (Chapter 6) used forms of discourse analysis to identify dominant discourses and trace their implications for the production of subjectivities and experiential possibilities in relation to significant life events such as cancer (Willig) and mental health issues, childbirth and unemployment (Challenor et al.). In a similar vein, Lorke et al. (Chapter 7) conducted a linguistic interactional analysis (with a focus on lexical and semantic features) of interview data to shed light on the complex linguistic negotiation of participants' 'at risk' status and its implications for their experience of themselves as being 'at risk'.

Research questions that focus on the constructive dimension of language are based upon a social constructionist perspective, which is concerned with the social processes producing particular social and psychological realities. Language and language use are chief amongst the means by which the social construction of reality comes about, and most social constructionist research uses discourse analytic methods to analyse texts, although images (see Challenor et al., Chapter 6) can also be included.

A fourth type of research question is concerned with accessing latent meanings in the data that are understood to underpin the more overt, manifest content. Such latent meaning can take the form of unconscious dynamics, emotional tensions or conflicts, or taken-for-granted, unacknowledged social imperatives, and will be informed by the theoretical framework the researcher is working with. For example, Bucci et al. (Chapter 9) used emotional textual analysis to access what they conceptualise as the collective collusive fantasies of groups of people (here, school teachers, and healthcare staff and their clients) in order to better understand their choices and demands, and how these relate to the sociocultural and historical contexts within which they are being made. Jaentti et al. (Chapter 10) deployed a figurative language focus on metaphor use as well as conceptual analysis to reveal difficult emotional content as well as implicit emotional content in written memories of life in a mental hospital. This type of research is based on the assumption, informed by theory, that people's overt behaviour and their declared views and opinions as well as the stories they tell about themselves are driven by underlying motivations and desires, which are not immediately evident to either the researcher or the research participant. To access such latent meanings, the researcher needs to employ methodical procedures, which will allow them to bring to light what is normally hidden from view. Borcsa and Janusz (Chapter 8) used interpersonal process recall interviews, dialogical and story-telling analysis to examine the interplay between couple therapists' personal and professional voices as they reflect on their experience of a therapy session.

Closely related to this approach is research that uses data collection methods that can capture meaning not easily expressed in words. For example, Jaentti et al. (Chapter 10) used the researcher's bodily movement inspired by texts (patients' memories) and by space (the mental hospital) to access deeper, embodied meanings of the experience of living in a mental hospital. And Challenor et al. (Chapter 6) analysed images of childbirth posted on social media to access meanings that were excluded from textual accounts.

The methods presented in Table 11.1 are primarily methods of data analysis (rather than data collection). The reason for this is that methods of data analysis are designed to answer particular types of research question whilst methods of data collection can be deployed more flexibly and across a variety of qualitative research designs. For example, semi-structured interviews can be used to collect data, which can then be analysed in a variety of ways including thematic analysis, discourse analysis and phenomenological analysis. However, there are some methods of data collection, which are more specifically suited to a particular research design and a specific approach to analysis. For example, the walking interview and interpersonal process recall interviews are examples of data collection methods that have been designed to generate data that is suitable to provide answers to quite specific questions about research participants' experiences and motivations. Finally, there are approaches that are characterised by a combination of data collection and analysis procedures, which work in conjunction to produce specific insights and answer the research question. Such approaches include grounded theory, autoethnography and metasynthesis.

It is important to acknowledge that what has been presented here is only one way of grouping the studies, and that there are many other ways in which this could have been done (e.g. in terms of subject matter, epistemological orientation, use of the self/reflexive involvement of the researcher and many more). Types of research question were chosen as a focus here because the formulation of the research question is the first step a researcher takes when designing a new study. And as we hope to inspire researchers to embark upon qualitative research in the field of mental health, this is where we concentrated our attention. In addition, we recognise that there are many more research methods that can be used to address the four types of research question identified in Table 11.1, and that the methods referenced in the table only constitute a small selection of methods.

Diversity with a Purpose

The type of research question that underpins a study has implications for the epistemological orientation of the study, the methodological choices made and the way in which it is written up. This is why the chapters in this book vary quite significantly in the tone, style and manner in which they are presented. Type 2 research questions, for example, require the researcher to be more obviously present in the research and its reporting. As a result, we often see the researcher using the first-person voice to report phenomenological research. By contrast, research driven by Type 1 research questions normally use a more traditional third-person perspective in the write-ups, whilst social constructionist (Type 3) research reporting can incorporate the researcher's own voice in their reflections on how discourse structures social and psychological life. Studies based on Type 4 research questions necessitate that the researcher positions him/herself as someone capable of accessing deeper and perhaps hidden meanings and is, therefore, likely to speak with some degree of expert authority about the analysed material. Again, there is no law-like relationship between types of research questions and writing styles, but rather degrees of compatibility and researcher preferences. In the end, every qualitative researcher will need to decide for themselves what may be the most appropriate and effective way of reporting their research.

The chapters contained in this book demonstrate that qualitative research is characterised by a great diversity of approaches to the generation of knowledge and insight. As we have seen, important choices need to be made by the researcher, for example in relation to the formulation of the research question, the choice of methods for data collection and analysis, and the style in which the study is written up. A further range of options emerges from the fact that qualitative research is often interdisciplinary which means that qualitative researchers often have access to theories, perspectives and methods from more than one discipline. In particular, pluralistic qualitative research which is designed to look at a phenomenon from different angles tends to incorporate diverse vantage points and diverse ways of accessing understanding, and these are often drawn from different disciplines. An excellent example of such an approach is Jaentti et al.'s research (Chapter 10) in which a multidisciplinary research group came together to analyse pieces of writing about life in a mental hospital by patients, relatives, staff and their children. The researchers drew on their backgrounds in history, art, cultural, visual and literary studies to provide readings of the written accounts which paid attention to their bodily, spatial and affective aspects. Willig's research programme into the experience of living with a cancer diagnosis (Chapter 5) also demonstrates how multiple methods can be used to illuminate a phenomenon (in this case, cancer-related distress) from different angles and for different purposes, ranging from the fine-grained scrutiny of individual experiences to an examination of the sociocultural context in which those experiences take place. The field of 'mental health' is, of course, itself an interdisciplinary field of study, and mental health researchers come from diverse disciplines including sociology, history, psychiatry, nursing, various sub-disciplines of psychology (e.g. clinical psychology, counselling psychology, health psychology, social psychology) and others. Mental health research can focus on the experiences of people diagnosed with mental health issues, on experiences of emotional and/or psychological distress in the general population, on the history of mental health services, on representations of mental distress in literature and the media, on the experiences of mental health professionals and/or those supporting people who experience mental distress and many more. Mental health research is an extremely wide-ranging field of study in which a multitude of methodological approaches can be used to address a large variety of research questions. As such, it is difficult to clearly delineate mental health research as a distinct field of study. This means that alongside the richness and diversity in approaches taken to study social and psychological processes relevant to mental health, there is also the challenge of how to stay on top of such a heterogeneous field, and how to compare and evaluate the disparate body of work that constitutes it. Given that qualitative mental health research can take so many forms, be driven by very different types of research questions, and use radically different styles of reporting its findings, the question arises of what binds all this work together. And what makes it 'qualitative research' rather than something else such as journalism, philosophy or creative writing?

What Makes Qualitative Research 'Research'?

We propose that despite their differences in approach, qualitative researchers in mental health are engaged in a pursuit of knowledge, which is motivated by the desire to improve our understanding of social and psychological processes relevant to mental health. This means that descriptions of and reflections on experiences relevant to mental health can be part of qualitative research but they are not sufficient in and of themselves to render a piece of writing qualitative mental health research. Willig (2019) proposed three criteria for deciding whether a piece of work qualifies as qualitative research: (i) the presence of a specific research question, (ii) contribution to a body of knowledge and (iii) a clearly identified method of inquiry. We believe that the various studies presented in this book do meet these criteria. Ensuring that qualitative research is based on clear, coherent and rigorous methodological perspectives and procedures is especially important at a time when the very notion of qualitative research is being called into question by the emergence of 'post-qualitative research'.

Post-qualitative research is based on a critique of conventional qualitative research and argues that qualitative research ought to abandon its attempt to contribute to the production of knowledge about the human condition. Post-qualitative research is more concerned with the potentialities inherent in human and non-human practices and with what can be produced/created through them rather than with establishing 'what is'. From a post-qualitative perspective there is no reason why we should privilege data over other sources of information (such as theory or researcher reflexivity) as it is argued that the former does not provide us with privileged access to social or experiential realities as these do not actually exist as meaningful entities in their own right. Post-qualitative research positions the researcher as someone whose interactions, their 'intermingling' or 'entanglement' with other people's words and actions sparks 'wonder and creativity' (Brinkmann, 2017, p. 118) in them which can lead to the generation of ideas about how things could be or what could be(come). By contrast, we would argue that although different qualitative research methodologies produce different kinds of insights, qualitative researchers are still engaged in the pursuit of knowledge as their overarching objective (see Willig, 2016). All types of knowledge generated by qualitative research (even 'relativist' knowledge) make claims about how something happens or what form something takes, be that people's thoughts and feelings, their actions and practices, the way they make sense of the world, the discursive resources they deploy and how they deploy them, and so on. And these claims are based upon the application of systematic, transparent procedures that are designed to extract meaning from the data which can provide answers to specific research questions. As we have seen, research questions that inform qualitative mental health research vary widely, and they can be concerned with a broad range of aspects of human experience; however, there is always a specific research question that identifies a gap in our knowledge which the researcher seeks to answer, and it is the answer to the research question that makes a contribution to knowledge (ideally, by telling us something that we did not know before). So, despite their differences in approach to methodology, all forms of qualitative research seek to ground their knowledge claims in methodical, systematic and transparent analyses of data and can, therefore, be described as empirical. This is what differentiates knowledge claims based on research from insights produced by other means.

Of course, most qualitative researchers accept that there is no unproblematic, direct access to the phenomena they are interested in (be that people's thoughts and feelings, the meanings of their actions, or the processes by which social and psychological events unfold), and that qualitative data never speaks for itself but needs to be made sense of. The qualitative scientist is required to interpret (i.e. give meaning to) the data and this process inevitably means that a transformation of the data through the researcher necessarily takes place during the process of investigation (see Willig, 2012, for a discussion of the role of interpretation in qualitative psychology). Researcher reflexivity is required to ensure that the qualitative investigator keeps an eye on their own contribution to meaning-making during the research process and takes this into account in any conclusions they may draw from their findings. Qualitative scientists do recognise the complexity of the process of knowledge generation and they acknowledge the contribution of the investigator's choices and preferences to the form that the resultant knowledge will take. However, the purpose of qualitative research cannot be to simply create and share new meanings in order to engage and stimulate readers to think about something in new and different ways. If qualitative scientists were primarily concerned with inviting their audience to engage with new ideas and meanings, we would not be justified in describing this activity as research. If there is no claim as to what these ideas and meanings represent, and if the sole objective is to evoke a response that widens the audience's experiential field/repertoire, then perhaps we have moved from the realm of research into the realm of the arts.

Trends and Challenges

The richness, range and diversity associated with qualitative research in mental health presents both opportunities and limitations. On the plus side, there are now many different data collection and analysis methods to choose from, and innovation particularly in the use of visual methods (e.g. see Reavey, 2020) continues at pace. This means that researchers are able to select methods that are best suited to help them answer their research questions, rather than having to limit the scope and ambition of their questions due to a limited range of available methods. As a result, qualitative researchers in mental health can ask all manner of research questions including 'what' questions (e.g. 'What is it like to experience cancer-related distress?'; 'What do psychiatrists think about schizophrenia?'), 'how' questions (e.g. 'How do patients make sense of the transition from hospital to the community?'; 'How do patients negotiate their 'at risk' status?'), and 'why' questions (e.g. 'Why has there been an increase in psychiatric diagnoses for school children?'; 'Why is there so much conflict between staff and the family members of service users?').

We are still a long way from including service users sufficiently in mental health research but in this area, too, particularly over the last 10 years or so, progress has been made. Building on the work of pioneers in this emerging field (e.g. Faulkner & Layzell, 2000; Rose, Wykes, Leese, Bindman, & Fleischmann, 2003; Faulkner, 2004), Wallcraft, Schrank and Amering's (2009) 'Handbook of Service User Involvement in Mental Health' provided a broad overview of the field, its history, politics, rationale and practicalities, based on the experiences of researchers in several countries. Since then an increasing number of papers have been published which examine the processes and outcomes of such research collaborations, and which identify challenges and possibilities associated with them (e.g. Callard & Rose, 2010; Happell et al., 2019; Mugisha et al., 2019; Sangill, Buus, Hybholt, & Lauge Berring, 2019). There is an emerging consensus indicating that for collaborative research in mental health to be productive, meaningful and ethical, it needs to develop research practices which avoid the reproduction of power inequalities and which move beyond a tokenistic involvement of service users (Sangill et al., 2019). Qualitative research in mental health in general and the chapters included in this volume in particular share such a commitment to confront and challenge the inequalities and disempowerment that is so often both cause and consequence of people's struggles with their mental health.

Conclusion and Future Directions

As we write this chapter, we find ourselves in the middle of the initial phase of humanity's encounter with a novel coronavirus (COVID-19). The emergence of this new virus and the seriousness of the disease that it can give rise to constitute a major challenge to governments, health systems and populations across the world. It has become apparent very quickly that hardly any aspect of life has remained unaffected by the presence of the virus and the measures that are required to control it. Hospitals, care homes, schools, universities, public transport, food distribution, the travel and leisure industry, in fact, all human enterprises that involve face-to-face contact between people have had to be re-organised or suspended altogether.

The emergence of COVID-19 demonstrates very powerfully just how quickly and how easily our established and familiar ways of doing things can be disrupted by something unexpected. The challenge of COVID-19 has significant implications for affected populations' mental health, and we anticipate that this crisis will generate a body of work dedicated to exposing, understanding and ameliorating some of its negative effects on people's mental state, as has happened in response to similar threats (e.g. HIV-infection). The numerous ways in which COVID-19 can impact on people's mental health demonstrate yet again just how interdisciplinary and wide-ranging a field mental health research is, and indeed needs to be. The impacts of the suspension of face-to-face counselling and psychotherapy, of experiences of isolation due to lockdown measures and quarantine, of multiple bereavements, of the economic depression and job losses that will follow in the pandemic's wake, of the increased at-risk status of vulnerable sections of the population, of the reduction of physical contact between people, and of the significant increase in uncertainty about the future are just some examples of the kinds of topics that mental health researchers will be focusing on in the coming months and years.[2]

Such research will help us understand better how people are making sense of the extraordinary changes that their lives have undergone and how people's experiences of themselves in their everyday lives are taking shape in response to these changes. The great variety, versatility and inventiveness that characterises qualitative mental health research and which has been demonstrated in this book, will no doubt ensure that qualitative mental health researchers will make an important contribution to our developing understanding of the impact of a pandemic and its effects on people's mental health and well-being.

References

Callard, F., & Rose, D. (2010). *Mental health service user leadership in research*. https://www.euro.who.int/__data/assets/pdf_file/0008/124559/E94376.pdf.

Faulkner, A. (2004). *The ethics of survivor research: Guidelines for the ethical conduct of research carried out by mental health service users and survivors*. Bristol: Policy Press (printed for the Joseph Rowntree Foundation).

Faulkner, A., & Layzell, S. (2000). *Strategies for living: A report of user-led research into people's strategies for living with mental distress*. London: Mental Health Foundation.

---

[2]Indeed, there are already examples of qualitative research currently in progress which have come to our attention. Naomi Moller (Open University, UK) and Virginia Braun (The University of Auckland, New Zealand) are conducting an online COVID-19-related story completion study to explore responses to the COVID-19 lockdown in the UK and New Zealand in which participants are being asked to write two short stories about different scenarios featuring characters in COVID-19 lockdown. And Virginia Eatough (Birkbeck, University of London, UK) is collecting data in the form of written descriptions of ordinary experiences, which people encounter in new ways due to the context within which they are taking place (i.e. the COVID-19-related lockdown in the UK); the aim of the study is to shed light on experiences of what the researcher calls 'the precious ordinary' (after a phrase from the novel 'Benediction' by the Colorado novelist Kent Haruf).

Happell, B., Platania-Phung, C., Scholz, B., Bocking, J., Horgan, A., Manning, A., … Biering, P. (2019). Changing attitudes: The impact of expert by experience involvement in mental health nursing education: An international survey study. *International Journal of Mental Health Nursing, 28*(2), 480–491.

Mugisha, J., Hanlon, C., Knizek, B. L., Ssebunnya, J., Vancampfort, D., Kinyanda, E., & Kigozi, F. (2019). The experience of mental health service users in health system strengthening: Lessons from Uganda. *International Journal of Mental Health Systems, 13*(1). https://doi.org/10.1186/s13033-019-0316-5.

Reavey, P. (Ed.). (2020). *A handbook of visual methods in Psychology: Using and interpreting images in qualitative research.* Hove: Psychology Press.

Rose, D., Wykes, T., Leese, M., Bindman, J., & Fleischmann, P. (2003). Patients' perspectives on electroconvulsive therapy: Systematic review. *British Medical Journal, 326,* 1363–1366.

Sangill, C., Buus, N., Hybholt, L., & Lauge Berring, L. (2019). Service user's actual involvement in mental health research practices: A scoping review. *International Journal of Mental Health Nursing, 28*(4), 798–815.

Wallcraft, J., Schrank, B., & Amering, M. (2009). *Handbook of service user involvement in mental health.* Chichester: Wiley-Blackwell.

Willig, C. (2012). *Qualitative interpretation and analysis in Psychology.* New York, NY: Open University Press (McGraw-Hill Companies).

Willig, C. (2016). Constructivism and 'the real world': Can they co-exist? *QMiP Bulletin, 21*(Spring), 33–38.

Willig, C. (2019). What can qualitative research contribute to psychological knowledge? *Psychological Methods, 24*(6), 796–804.

Index

© Springer Nature Switzerland AG 2021

M. Borcsa and C. Willig (eds.), *Qualitative Research Methods in Mental Health*,

https://doi.org/10.1007/978-3-030-65331-6

Printed by Printforce, the Netherlands